THE DIABETIC DETECTIVES

THE SEARCH FOR THE CAUSE AND THE CURE OF TYPE2

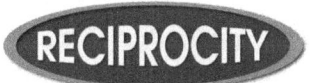

First Edition published by Reciprocity in 2021
All rights reserved.

WRITERS
Brian Bain and Gordon Ritchie

NUTRITIONAL ADVISOR
Gordon Ritchie

DESIGNER
David Joyce

Copyright © Brian Bain and Gordon Ritchie, London 2021

All Rights Reserved. No part of this publication may be reproduced, stored in a retrieval system, or transmitted, in any form, or by any means, electronic, mechanical, photocopying, recording or otherwise, without the prior permission of the publisher and copyright holder.

Disclaimer
The information in this book is provided on the basis that neither the authors nor the editors nor the publishers shall have any responsibility for any loss or damage that results or is claimed to have resulted from reading it. Some of the recipes contain nuts or nut milk. If you have a nut allergy please avoid those particular recipes.

CONTENTS

Preface 8

THE DIABETIC DETECTIVES
Brian and Gordon 9
Anti Gravity Levitation 10
The Life of Brian 13
The first tour of the West Indies in HMS Sirius (1972-1973) 15
The second tour of the West Indies in HMS Ariadne (1977) 16
Civilian Life 17
Homage to Steve McQueen and his Great Escape 20
1990-2010: Gyms, Health Clubs and House Boats 22
First Diagnosis 22
2014-2018 Lowestoft 22
The Thames with spaceships 1st stroke 23
Air France and my 2nd Stoke 23
Gordon Gets Religion 24
High Status Lies versus Negative Status Truths (conspiracy theories) 27
Diabetes 30
Life of Brian Part 2 36
The Big Break 38
How Type2 Works 44
The Cure 48
Conclusion 51
Final Advice and Tips 52

THE RECIPES
Introduction 54

BREAD & PIZZAS
Flax and Chia Seed Bread 58
Low Carb Buns 59
Low-Carb Tortillas 59
Garlic Bread 60
Low Carb Naan Bread 60
Low Carb Pizza 61
Pizza Toppings

CONTENTS

Margherita 62
Anchovies/Tuna with Capers 62
Barbecue Chicken 63
Barbecue Sauce 63
Beef and Basil 64

BREAKFASTS
Flax Porridge 66
Classic Full English Breakfast for Two
    Pork Chops or Roast Pork Slices 67
    Poached Eggs 67
    Scrambled Eggs 67
    Soft/Hard Boiled Eggs 68
    Fried Egg 68
    Bubble and Squeak 69
    Garlic Mushrooms 70
    Fried Tomatoes 70
    Spicy Baked Kidney Beans 71
    Low Carb Fried Bread 72
    Cauliflower or Turnip Hash Browns 72
Bubble and Squeak with an Egg 73
Huevos Rancheros with Minced Beef 74

SMOOTHIES
Asparagus Anthem 76
Tomato Twist 76
Green Breeze 76
Fruity Boost 77
Bok Choy and Broccoli Collection 77
Carrot and Chlorella Royale 77
Green Lagoon 78
Rocket loves Orange 78
Orange and Asparagus Refrain 78

SOUPS
Vegetable Stock 80
Vegetable Soup 80

CONTENTS

Broccoli & Stilton Soup with Crispy Croutons 81
Creamy Tomato Soup 82
Cream of Asparagus Soup 82
Bortsch Ukraine 83
Pennsylvania Chowder 84
Creamed Tomato Soup with Sage 84
Mushroom Bisque 85
French Onion Soup 86
Broccoli Egg Drop Soup 87
Cream of Pea Soup with Tarragon 88
Mulligatawny Soup 89

SAUCES

Savoury Brown Sauce 91
Classic Tomato Sauce 91
Red Wine and Tomato Sauce 92
Green or Red Pesto 93
Mayonnaise 94
Worcestershire Sauce 94
Horseradish Sauce 95

PASTRY DISHES

Low Carb Flaxseed Pastry 97
French Onion Tarts 97
Quiche Gruyère Chanterelle 98
Chicken and Mozzarella Pie 100
Spinach and Goat's Cheese Pie 101
Mushroom Flan 102
Winter Vegetable Pie 103

MISCELLANEOUS MAIN DISHES

Chilli Con Carne 105
Cheese Aubergine Bake 106
Stuffed Aubergines 106
Fried Chicken in the Hole 107
Turnip Topped Cumberland Pie 108
Classic Shepherd's Pie 109

CONTENTS

White Tuscan Pie 111
Spiced Turnip Mini Shepherd's Pies 112
Lancashire Hotpot 113
No Pasta Lasagne 113
Broccoli and Cauliflower Chicken Gratin 115
Burgers with Tomato Relish 115
Green Cabbage Casserole 117
        TexMex Seasoning 117
Garlic Chicken with Mash 118
Brussel Sprouts and Hamburger Gratin 118
Tortilla with Minced Beef and Salsa 119
        Salsa 119
        Mexican Seasoning 120
Aubergine and Mushroom Parmigiana 120
Spanish Cauliflower 121
Watercress Soufflé 122
Chinese-Style Vegetables 122

ROASTS

Roast Paprika Chicken 125
Roast Lamb with Garlic and Rosemary 126
        Mint Sauce 126
Roast Pork with Garlic and Rosemary 127
Roast Paprika Turnips or Swede 127
Yorkshire Pudding 128
Sage and Onion Stuffing 129
Macadamia and Mushroom Roast 130
Slow-Cooked Pot Roast with Creamy Gravy 131
Roast Beef with Roasted Vegetables 132
Layered Cheese and Tomato Nut Roast 133

FISH

Fish Pie 135
Dill Weed Salmon Pie 136
Fish Casserole with Mushrooms & Mustard 137
Salmon with Pesto and Spinach 138
Lemon Baked Salmon 138
Cheesy Tuna Casserole 139

CONTENTS

CURRIES
Garam Masala Chicken 141
        Garam Masala 141
Thai Fish Curry 142
Curry Chicken with Broccoli & Green Beans 143
Chicken Curry Pie 144
Chicken and Spinach Balti 145
Lamb Curry 146

EGGS
Spanish Turnip Omelette 148
Mediterranean Eggs 149
Curried Eggs 149
Piperade 150
Eggs Primavera 151
Eggs Florentine 151
Scotch Eggs 152

ACCOMPANYING VEGETABLES
Vegetable Preparation and Cooking Times 154
Ratatouille 156
Spiced Cider Carrots 156
Stuffed Courgettes 157
Turnip Paprika Goulash 158
Lemon Broccoli 158
White Turnip Rydan Celtic Mash 159
Spiced Shredded Green Cabbage 160
Spiced Cauliflower or Broccoli Rice 160
Swede or Turnip Paprika Chips 161
Salt and Vinegar Courgette Crisps 162
Creamed Green Cabbage 162
Mushroom Paté 163
Stuffed Artichoke Tomatoes 164
Onion Rings 165
Stuffed Peppers 165
Leek and Mushroom Gratin 167
Cauliflower Mash 167
The Ultimate Mash 168

CONTENTS

Pickled Onions *168*
Dill Pickled Gherkins *169*

SALADS & DRESSINGS

Mixed Green Salad *172*
Summer Salad *172*
Classic Tomato Salad *173*
Greek Salad With Feta Cheese *174*
Classic Coleslaw *174*
Tuna & Tomato Salad *175*
Chicken Caesar Salad *175*
Caesar Salad Dressing *176*
Vinaigrette Dressing *177*

DESSERTS

Strawberry Egg Custard *179*
Brandy Pancakes *179*
Chocolate Brownies *180*
Sponge Cakes *181*
      Strawberry Vanilla Cake Filling *181*
      Macadamia Vanilla Cake Filling *182*
      Lemon Cake Filling *182*
      Chocolate Cake Filling *182*
French Custard Strawberry Tart *183*
Vanilla Cheesecake *184*
Marbled Strawberry Cheesecake *185*
New York Cheesecake *186*
Carrot and Cinnamon Cake *186*

Trans Atlantic Food Name Differences *188*

Oven Temperatures *189*

Conversions (UK/US) *189*

Glossary of Cooking Terms *190*

Appendix I: The Demonic Origin of COVID19 .... *193*

PREFACE

Gordon had very bad type 2 diabetes, first diagnosed in November 2012. Brian had very damaging diabetes, first diagnosed in 2010. This is the story of how these two sugarholics risked everything to find the cause and the cure for this disease. It is not the story of how to reverse your sugar numbers for that is already known - not widely enough or prominently enough to the medical profession, but more to diabetics themselves and complimentary practitioners. A ketogenic (very low carb) diet combined with a cardio type exercise routine (long walks, comfortable pace spin bike sessions etc.) will do that. No, it is the story of the journey that these two gluconauts took to discover the cause of Type2 and then to formulate a cure. Gordon is now fully cured. He can, and does eat whatever he wants (from chocolate cake to roast potatoes and rice) and does almost no exercise (one 45 minute walk every 2 weeks), but maintains an HbA1c of 5.0%. Brian is lagging slightly behind and needs to do one exercise for 30 minutes each day to keep his sugar below 6.0 mmol/L (108 mg/dl).

The purpose of this book is to reveal the cause and the cure of type2 and at the least, to entertain the reader in the process, if not actually prevent him from getting or from suffering from this terrible disease any longer. Neither author is a medical doctor. But Gordon did do a year of Cell Biology at Cambridge.

The reason that the medical profession has not yet discovered the cause or the cure is that it falls into the great and sad divide between traditional pharmaceutical medicine and alternative or complimentary medicine.

This book gives mankind the chance to eradicate Type2 Diabetes. 1/7th of all NHS cases in the UK are Diabetes related and over 450 million people suffer from this lethal and debilitating disease as of 2021. It is the authors' sincere hope that people will start curing themselves with the protocol described in this book and that clinical trials will convince the medical profession to confirm and improve their findings.

In the meantime, in the spirit of Lorenzo's oil, they invite the reader to come along on the journey they took from the immovable rock of type2, to the unstoppable bulldozer of human ingenuity.

BRIAN AND GORDON

The Quintessential positive creative relationship of the 20th century must have been Sir Paul McCartney and John Lennon. The last time the two met was a tragedy. They had been on good terms for a while. And Paul turned up with his guitar, unannounced, at John's place, as he had done countless times before. But John turned him away. John described the situation as follows...

"That was a period when Paul just kept turning up at our door with a guitar. I would let him in, but finally I said to him, 'Please call before you come over. It's not 1956, and turning up at the door isn't the same anymore. You know, just give me a ring.' He was upset by that, but I didn't mean it badly. I just meant that I was taking care of a baby all day, and some guy turns up at the door." John Lennon, 1980

John was murdered later that year. The two never met again. I have always thought that John was a better song writer than Paul when they were apart. But Paul was a better song writer than John when they were together. And regardless of who is better than whom, the pair of them, when together, healed the emotions of a generation.

It has taken me a long time to understand the dynamics of relationships and their value. Indeed we all spend a lifetime learning about that subject. But creativity, which is perhaps the most powerful manifestation of individuality, appears to germinate, to grow best and to yield the most wonderful fruit, in the soil of a partnership.

That is why Sir Paul kept turning up at the Dakota with his guitar. John was the key to his creativity.

It is the same way with Brian and myself. I am creative in the absence of Brian. But his energy empowers me to be unstoppable. In the battle to find a cure for Type2 Diabetes, I had run most of the course by myself with the help of an enormous amount of work published on the internet. But I would never have jumped the final hurdle without the courage of Brian.

Having spent 15 years in the Navy Brian has a good understanding of people's characters and enjoys pushing them to the limit - whatever that limit may be. I remember on one occasion we went to the Water Margin Chinese restaurant in Kingston. The proprietor fancied himself as an Elvis impersonator. So Brian said to me: Watch this, it's gonna be free saki all round. He then produced a series of hilarious platitudes which dragged Elvis2 out of his shell and the King was reborn. From that point onwards, everyone spent the rest of the evening either performing, or in hysterics at the performance of others, whilst free saki was flowing everywhere.

This is Brian's gift. He sees what you are capable of before you show it to him and he brings out the best performance you have, a performance that you yourself may not have seen before. He should have been a film director. Actually he was peripherally associated with that industry whilst at Living Images in Hampton.

Whereas John Lennon brought out the best performances Paul had. I remember an interview where John said: I wish I had written All my loving, But I think I wrote a pretty mean rhythm guitar for it. But in my opinion he did co-write it, in the sense that Paul would not have written it without the energy of their partnership and without the presence of John both musically and emotionally. And that rhythm guitar was a key component to the astounding beauty of the song (although Paul always plays it too fast for my taste).

But that is the wonder of partnerships. Life is too short to learn all of its lessons in 100 years. But for every lesson you have failed to grasp, there is someone somewhere who has totally nailed it. That is the power of partnerships.

The tragedy is that even if your best supporting actor or actress forms a partnership with you for a sufficiently long period of time to bear fruit, nothing much is transferred unless there is love between the two parties. Love gives to each party the power of both parties. Whereas hate can take away each party's power.

At one point in the story of our cure for Diabetes, we both thought (not entirely erroneously) that I would either die or have a stroke or heart attack if I did not immediately drink 2 bottles of Fitou. Brian's response to this crisis was to bring me every bottle he had of the stuff - immediately - and leave them all with me in circumstances where he was not in much better shape that I was. And his partner was of the same mind as him.

So here is the story of the 35 year relationship between Brian and Gordon which resulted in a discovery that we hope will one day fix as many people's metabolisms as the Beatles fixed people's hearts.

ANTI GRAVITY LEVITATION

It was the start of the 80s. I was in my room at Cambridge designing what was to become the Quadrocopter. The student next door was designing a microcomputer. George Lucas had just had Yoda lift an X wing out of a swamp using the force. I was captivated. I came out of the Odeon Cinema at Marble Arch and tried to levitate a plant pot outside the Kebab shop. I was most disappointed to discover that the force was not with me.

But I am nothing if not tenacious and if George Lucas could do it then someday so would I.

The rationale behind my desire for anti gravity levitation was not merely its face value spectacularity, however. No, indeed. For I am at heart an engineer, and early 80s Sci-Fi was about personal transport in more than one dimension. The visionaries of the cinema had seen the beauty and perhaps even the necessity to escape from the traffic jams of our road systems. And I wanted to make that escape into a reality. I wanted to transfer it from the movie screen to the car showroom.

At the time helicopters were very, very mechanically complex and had rotor heads which could change the pitch of each helicopter blade both collectively and cyclically (during each revolution of the fan). This was necessary to stop the thing falling over in forward flight. I knew that they would never be safe for consumer transport with that level of mechanical complexity - there were just too many things that might go wrong. In fact I will not travel in a Helicopter today because the crash rate is around 40x greater than that for aeroplanes. There are just too many single points of failure. My favourite is the Jesus bolt on the top of the rotor head. If that comes off you have only one option!

So what was needed was 4 solid fans controlled by 4 electric motors, which had almost no mechanical complexity at all. The collective pitch control would be replaced by altering the power to each of the 4 motors and the cyclic pitch by having 2 fans rotating one way and two fans the other so that the tendency of a chopper to roll in forward flight due to the difference in lift between the advancing and retreating blades would be cancelled out by said contra rotation.

So I took my mother's old Hoover, bent a piece of aluminium into a rotor blade and put a light dimmer between the motor and the mains switch and spun the thing up. After a few attempts I got it to take off. It travelled into our neighbours Garden still attached to the mains lead, which very much upset our neighbours but delighted my mother.

The secret to inventing things is to get as fast as possible to the proof of concept stage. I had just proved the concept. Now it was time to spend some money. So I purchased 4 electric helicopters from the model shop and attached them to the 4 corners of an aluminium frame. This was the first electric quadrocopter. I thought of patenting it and probably should have done so. But there was already in existence the Benson Skymat, which had a whole mat of rotors on a frame which were petrol driven rather than electrical. Had I patented the electric version of the Skymat, drone technology might have been 20 years ahead of where it is now.

In the event I decided to do a PhD at Imperial College in London in Aerodynamics, mainly to investigate the Quadrocopter. But as has now been learned from the disaster of the UK government's lockdown response to Coronavirus, Imperial College is not in the same league as Cambridge (where I studied first natural sciences and then maths) or Oxford (which I briefly attended for part of a PhD in Pure Maths). Imperial would not fund my Quadrocopter. So, instead I spent my time there solving the equations of airflow to second order accuracy. Something that all the academics at Imperial said was impossible notwithstanding the fact that the Americans had already done it. I myself then did it and was awarded a two year SERC fellowship as a result.

But before I could start it, the Professor threw me out because I insisted on putting in my PhD thesis that he had told me that I would never be able to do what I eventually did and that fortunately I thrive just as much on discouragement as I do on encouragement.

I truth being half Scottish and one quarter Irish if you tell me I cannot do something I will spend the rest of my life trying to do it!

But I was not too upset at being thrown out and denied my PhD (actually the deal was that I would be given a PhD only if I signed over the money for my 2 years SERC fellowship to the Professor). That was a deal that I could and did refuse. So I am not Dr Ritchie. I am Gordon Ritchie MA Cantab, a degree from a true university, rather than what in my experience was a den of self interest.

My favourite day at Imperial (apart from when I got my finite difference alternate direction implicit Navier Stokes solver to work to second order) was sitting in a lecture and another professor said: The reason that we use the Hanning Window is that nobody knows what Fourier Transforms into a square box. And the Hanning window is a reasonable approximation in these circumstances. I then put my hand up and said: Well I know what Fourier transforms into a square box. The professor said: You do - what is it?

I said: It is the inverse Fourier Transform of a square box, which is a diffraction function, and that is where all your extra errors are coming from. That Professor was more of an academic. He saw what I said and did not try to discourage me or cancel me. I was secretly glad to leave aerodynamics research because my goal was still to defy gravity like George

Lucas had done in Star Wars and I had invented a magnetic levitator and wanted to market it as an executive toy.

So I taught myself electronics using the wonderful Horowitz and Hill text book and built a magnetic Levitator and patented it. The patent I got was any magnetic levitation device with a gap of more than 10 mm between the levitated and levitating components. This was in order to distinguish it from monorails and such like which were designed not for visual effect but for maximum performance and so had much smaller gaps.

This thing had an electromagnet and an infrared eye. It would levitate an object placed below the electromagnet so long as said object had a powerful neodymium permanent magnet inside it just under its top and so long as the top of the object had and reflective and matt surface for the infrared eye to see.

Due to Laplace's equation, a static magnetic field cannot be stable in all 3 dimensions at the same time (because all 3 second derivatives must add to zero so they cannot all 3 be positive which is required for stability. One derivative, representing one axis, one direction, one coordinate, is always going to be negative and therefore unstable). So you cannot just balance one magnet on top of another. You have to keep changing the field to achieve that.

The infrared eye would detect how far away the levitated object was by the amount of light reflected off the object back to the eye in the electromagnet. Then it would adjust the power of the electromagnet accordingly. That creates actually an unstable feedback loop. So then one needs to create an electronic shock absorber which is best done with phase advance.

Once you have mastered that, the levitator is beautiful. You could throw a ball or cigarette box or oil can or car into the device and it would catch it instantly and hold it a few inches below the electromagnet.

So I got the thing built and tried to market it in retail shops but I have never been very good at marketing. So I eventually went to a trade exhibition to see if I could find an outfit who might be interested in it for advertising display purposes.

I was attracted to one particular stand at the exhibition at Kensington Olympia, which had all sorts of wonderful high tech display units. I approached Living Images, and asked them if they would be interested in a display unit that would float anything from a cigarette box to a car in mid air? Brian Bain said well yes if you can indeed do that. Come and bring your device to our offices in Hampton.

That is when my relationship with Brian began. He got Spectrum in who had the contract for Ford or Vauxhall at the motor show. The idea was that we would put a large magnet under the roof of a Ford or a Vauxhall, and then float it 3 feet above the podium and 3 feet below the electromagnet on a bridge above the podium. It would have been a massive show stopper. Even today it would work really well especially for Tesla given their space conquering pedigree.

But in the end they were rather concerned that people with pacemakers might drop dead or that the car might fall down (only the latter turned out to be a valid concern in the end). So the largest device we made was a 5th scale model car for Vauxhall which we displayed at Monaco and a large oil barrel for Shell. The funny thing was that when the Japanese took photos of the levitator, the flash light would blind the infrared eye and the electromagnet would drop the object - which amused the Japanese even more!

Brian had spent 15 years in the Navy prior to his joining living Images and was especially interested in working with and managing people who could solve technical problems. I have never met a better motivator of men than Brian. He somehow makes you feel that you can do anything.

His character is so empowering and he is fearless if somewhat disorganised. In fact he is so disorganised that his girlfriend brought him a Samsonite briefcase in which to keep his personal organiser, in order to stop him losing it and to stop him dropping it on the floor and destroying it. Brian then proceeded to run over the briefcase in his car, destroying both the Samsonite case and the organiser! But he can make a team of people he has never met before work all night for him and thank him for the fun of it after 24 hours straight.

Eventually Living Images bit the dust and Brian and I went our separate ways. But in life there are people you will meet who make you feel that you can do anything and there are people who make you feel you can do nothing. It is truly incredible what effect other people can have upon you. We, Brian and I, inspire each other to acts bordering on total insanity with this completely unfounded belief that everything we do together will somehow work out fine - which it rarely does.

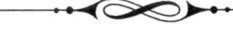

THE LIFE OF BRIAN

I was born on the 18/12/1947 in Mansfield and was brought up in Warsop with my brother and sister, who were twins.

1n 1962 when I was 15 I joined the navy. I got a train from Mansfield to Waterloo station in London where I was met by a variety of petty officers from the boys training centre in Gosport. There were 3 choices for a young naval cadet in those days. I could be trained as a JEM, a Junior Electrical Mechanic, a seaman or mechanical engineer, a stoker. The brighter ones became JEMs. So I decided to have a crack at that option.
We left on the train down to lee-on the Solent where I joined the Fleet Air Arm because, because that was where the JEMs went.

I did my first sea training on board HMS Wakeful which was a WW2 frigate.

From there I went to HMS Fitzguard in Tourpoint, which was not a sea going ship but rather a naval base in East Cornwall. That is where I started my 4/5 year apprenticeship as a CEA1 Control Electrical Artificer 1st class, in earnest! (Surface weapons)

The second night in barracks we decided to have a little pillow fight with the next door barracks. 37 seconds into the fight, I was punched on the nose by a Scottish boy - the first of many such communications.

In East Cornwall, studying for my apprenticeship, I managed to get back classed in the first term. I was forced to retake the whole term - all very embarrassing. I was warned that I would not be allowed to complete the course if it happened again. I found it quite a struggle because most of the boys I was competing with had O'levels whereas I had no qualifications at all. Also they were that bit older than me.

However, I was determined to do my best and make this into a career. After knuckling down to it my exam results were exemplary. In fact they were so good that I was presented with the Victor Ludorum Prize for the best course average! So although I most certainly started at the bottom of the boat, with no qualifications, I ended up on the captain's bridge as it were.

Here is a brief history of my assignments in the Navy in historical sequence

1. HMS FITZGUARD
2. HMS WAKEFUL
3. HMS GURKA - THE FIRST TOUR OF EUROPE
4. HMS SIRIUS - THE FIRST TOUR OF THE WEST INDIES
5. HMS ARIADNE - THE SECOND TOUR OF THE WEST INDIES AND BRAZIL
6. HMS ARIADNE - THE SECOND TOUR OF EUROPE
7. HMS COLLINGWOOD - ELECTRICAL SCHOOL IN FAREHAM
8. SHIP'S YARD PORTSMOUTH
9. SHIP'S DIVER
10. SHIP'S DIVING SUPERVISOR
11. SMA Ships Maintenance Authority DOCK YARD - Writing technical manuals in Portsmouth for Navy Ships

In 1967 I was assigned to the training ship HMS Wakeful. This was my first sea going experience. The gunnery officer on board was the appropriately named Commander Tricky. He introduced himself to me by shouting the words: Hey lad, you masquerading as a sailor - I did not flinch. Then I heard an even louder voice behind me saying 'am I hurting you lad' I replied 'no sir' to which he responded 'WELL I EFFING SHOULD BE AS I'M STOOD ON YOUR HAIR'. This was the standard Navy way of informing sailors that they needed a haircut.

My 3rd sea going assignment was aboard HMS Sirius in 1972. I remember it was a dark and dreary night, drizzling with rain when I boarded the boat. As I walked over the gangway I was conscious of a group of men looking down at the pontoon.

Out of the water came a diver, who hauled himself up onto that pontoon. Someone passed him a lit cigarette. This was a seminal moment in my life. The diver was Smudge Smith who was to become my lifelong friend, and ally.

I decided to take a ship's diver's course in Plymouth before returning to HMS Sirius for a European tour of duty.

On the course the diving instructor told us lads that only 20% of you will get through.

The course mainly consisted of diving into the freezing cold and inky dark waters of Plymouth Harbour, with no dry suit gloves or hoods permitted. Sometimes for a special treat we were taken outside the harbour to the sea, which was even worse especially when it had been snowing.

One day in the harbour, four of us were sent down together with a hammer and chisel each and told to cut through a massive iron mooring chain. We spent 4 weeks down there but never managed to chop that chain. We would take breaks together sitting on the mud below the jetty. I soon learnt to cover myself to keep myself warm. Unfortunately we attracted at 5th member to the party in the form of a giant eel which would come and bite us whenever we stopped working on the impossible to break chain.

On the second day I felt something on my right leg. Thinking it to be the eel, I hit it with my hammer and it retreated smartly. Then half an hour later when I surfaced one of the other divers was limping around. So I kept very quiet!

By the end of the diving course 10 people had dropped out and three were left.

The final exercise was jumping off the flight deck of an aircraft carrier into the sea below. When we went to jump I went from the front of the queue to the back in 10 seconds because I was crapping myself. We were wearing a water proof ring around our neck to keep the head free but keep the water out of the body part of the suit. We had have to hold the metal ring as we fell to prevent it from decapitating ourselves when we hit the water. As I gathered speed towards the water I made the mistake of looking down at the rapidly approaching water just at the moment I was about to enter it. This tipped my head and body forwards so that my face and belly took the full force of the 60 foot drop. This wounded me, caused my eye socket and my nose to bleed, and my tooth to go through my lip. Fortunately the clearance diver running the course did not ask me to do it again correctly. He confided in me that he hated that part of the test himself.

THE FIRST TOUR OF THE WEST INDIES IN HMS SIRIUS (1972-1973)

We arrived in Bermuda on December 7, 1972. I could not wait to dive in the crystal clear waters of the Caribbean. What a contrast it was when compared to the dark and cold waters of Plymouth harbour. This was a paradise by comparison. I dived just outside the sea wall in wonderful visibility, the sea was so warm and inviting, nothing like the cold waters of England. I had only been in the water 10 minutes when I found myself being dragged to the surface and then facing a large and very angry West Indian fisherman who asked me what I was doing diving on his lobster pots? I spluttered out a sorry and his beaming smile forgave me.

When we were just about to leave Bermuda the Governor of the island was assassinated. So we were asked to stay there a bit longer in order to act as the guard of honour at his funeral.

Next we went to Barbados arriving there on 28th December 1972. The first run ashore in Barbados was to the Pepperpot open air night club where I was amazed to see petty officer seaman Ted Perkiss doing the limbo underneath a suspended bar on top of the main stage. As I walked away from the bar my eyes landed on a girl wearing a blue angora catsuit. I went and asked her if she wanted to dance: She replied 'there is no way you are going to ball me tonight!' I was not sure what that phrase meant. So I enquired from the older crew with me in the night club and they explained that it meant sleeping with her.

After a few drinks I finished up in a Hotel with her. Bear in mind that I had not slept with any women for months having been stuck on the ship. She took me to a party in the hotel and presented me to the party goers there as her boyfriend. She then informed them all that we were to be married by the captain of the ship in the very near future. I spent the night with her (my Stag night) and in the morning there was a 3 piece calypso band outside our room welcoming the happy couple into imminent Holy Matrimony. Anne then flew back to Canada, sold her car and flat and returned to find me in the West Indies.

The next stop was Curacao in the Dutch Antilles. We had been in harbour for 15 minutes when I was called to the flight deck by a Dutch sailor who explained that there was a phone call for me in the office on the shore side. When I walked in to the office to take the call, there was Anne of the blue angora who had somehow got the ships program. Our next stop was Fort Lauderdale in Florida. Upon docking I was again informed that there was someone looking for me on the jetty. When I came up on deck, there was Anne with a pillow stuffed up her blouse shouting out: Have you got a Brian Bain on board. Then I took her into the mess on board. Women were permitted to come on board as guests for a short time. But could not stay overnight on the boat. Anne followed me around the West Indies for the entire 4 month tour.

I should mention that I was married at the time of this tour. But as a result of meeting Anne of the blue angora, I left my wife to further my relationship with Anne back in the UK. This went on for around 6 months. But it was doomed to fail because she did not want me to remain in the Navy. And the Navy was the focus of my working life, since I had signed up to it for 12 years. So I eventually went back to my wife and we had a daughter together.

I should mention that during my first European tour in HMS Gurkha a bunch of US and UK sailors decided to run the original Marathon course run by Pheidippides, from Marathon to Athens. Over 100 sailors took part and I won. On my second European tour in HMS Ariadne we had a race up the Rock of Gibraltar. I came second in that one. I was better on the flatter ground but quite a good athlete in the Navy. It is often the case the people with very active lifestyles who then cease training and become couch potatoes fall victim to Type2 Diabetes.

THE SECOND TOUR OF THE WEST INDIES IN HMS ARIADNE (1977)

This tour took in Belize, Puerto Rico, Brazil, British Honduras, Paradise Island and many other beautiful places.

By now I had reached the grand rank of chief electrical artificer responsible for the maintenance of surface weapons. I also was the ships diver. I found myself on Belize a beautiful island next to British Honduras in the Caribbean. One evening I decided to go to the shore. I left the ship in a Gemini diving boat (like an Avon inflatable dinghy) and an officer came with me to have a drink. The dock in Belize was a cross between the African Queen and Pirates of the Caribbean. All the houses dockside were built on wooden stilts and the whole dock was teaming with brightly coloured Caribbean fish.

I stopped at the first building that looked like a bar and went inside, whilst the officer stayed outside taking photographs. To my surprise I was confronted with two teenage girls screaming and shouting and one of the girls had a small knife in her hand. I raised my voice and told them to stop fighting and asked them what they were fighting over.

One of them whispered in my ear that the other girl had informed her that her 'privates stank'. With that my colleague, the naval officer entered the room in his full white tropical uniform. I asked if he would take part in a small trial to determine the veracity of said olfactory accusation. He agreed. So we sat him down and asked the accused girl to stand right in front of him. Then for entirely judicial purposes you understand, the officer started to sniff the accused teenager in the aforementioned region. His immediate reply was 'she smells like a rose'. I asked the two girls to hug each other and the small bar erupted into cheers !!

The two girls now took me on a tour of the town. We went to a local disco where I spent the night admiring all the lovely white teeth illuminated by the Ultra Violet Strobe lights. I must admit here that I fell for the rose scented Eliza. Furthermore I have no hesitation in confirming the findings of my officer, having made my own slightly more detailed analysis of the subject matter in question.

When returning to the boat with Eliza, a large goat appeared in front of me. So I went down on all fours and began to scrape the floor with one hand to say heel dear Goat. All of a sudden he charged at me and continually head butted me until I managed to get away by rolling into a monsoon ditch.

When I tried to get up I discovered that I had sprained my ankle. So with Eliza as my crutch, I made way to the liberty boat, which ferries the sailors to and from the shore. I missed the first one and therefore arrived late and was put on captain's defaulters, which meant that I had to appear before him to explain my tardiness.

Fortunately the captain was fair and good humoured. He had an unwritten code that if a defaulter made him smile he would be more lenient. When I appeared before him he asked 'what is it this time Chief 'at which I replied ' I have been goat wrestling sir' This brought a small smile to his face and he graciously let me off.

On the next occasion when I appeared before him for tardiness, his analysis of my behaviour was that my dick was charging around the West Indies whilst I was hanging on to my balls for the ride.

Later in the tour as a result of the trickle drafting system used by the Navy, the Captain was replaced by a less humorous officer. He stopped all my shore leave and prevented me returning to Bermuda, my favourite Caribbean Island.

So there it is. I went into the navy a boy. And I came out a man. I loved all the time I spent in the Navy. When I was getting close to the end of the 12 year term which I initially signed on for after 3 years of training (making a total of 15 years) I was seriously considering signing up for another 12 years. But Pete, a chef on the Ariadne, had agreed with me to start a business together. Also the next assignment for me was going to be a nuclear submarine. These things stay submerged for 6 months at a time. And my idea of a good time is not looking at the world through a periscope for 6 months solid.

CIVILIAN LIFE

So I entered into civilian life in 1977, the year after Gordon went up to Cambridge.

I settled down in Selling, in Kent, waiting for my business partner to leave the Navy. In the meantime I worked for GEC mechanical handling in Erith where I helped with the development of replenishment-at-sea systems (in voyage refuelling etc.). My first assignment was to Scott Lithgow on the Clyde. My second was to the Carg, which was in the Walker Yard on the Tyne (which by then had become Swan Hunter), which Maggie Thatcher had impounded until it was paid for by Iran. I come from the North East. So I was inundated after work by all my Geordie relations taking me to the pub. So much so that I had to pretend to be working somewhere else in order to sober up!!

My next assignment was Charleston South Carolina with GEC and with a team of engineers. We were to carry on testing a replenishment-at-sea system which was fitted on board a supply vessel. We checked into a small hotel at about 6.00 pm local time. Myself and another engineer decided to go to the nearest pub we could find - since we were gasping for a drink! I asked the taxi driver to take us to the nearest watering hole and was surprised when he asked me 'was it gay or straight' that we wanted? My reply was 'we don't mind we just want a beer'. I told my companion that I am not going to do a pepper pot here. I am just going to have some nice innocent fun.

Upon arrival, I went to order the drinks. But upon turning round I saw my chum being chatted up by a gorgeous woman. The barman said to me 'a word of advice, your pal is being chatted up by a dude!' So striding over to him I tried to pull him off only to be told to leave him alone as he was well in. Whispering to him I said: Check the Adams apple ….he did and discovered to his dismay that this was definitely a dude!!

I told him there was no hurry. We did not need to rush this. There are plenty of actual girls around!

I had been chatting to the barmaid and her boyfriend Leroy and being Americans I took a quick poll of everyone in the bar asking them if they had ever been shot or had shot anyone. All the arms went up together. There was no one in that bar who had no been involved in a shooting. Two days later during an electrical storm and heavy rain, I was in my hotel room and there was a knock on the door. When I opened it, there was the head barmaid, Ms Santos herself. She was standing there with my favourite drink - a white Russian. One thing led to another and she stayed the night.

When, we surfaced in the morning, I drove her to work. After travelling about a mile we heard a sudden bang, bang and I immediately thought of her boyfriend bad, bad Leroy Brown. Fortunately, it was merely a double puncture from running over something sharp in the road.

In 1979, I took a job with Marconi avionics working in Radlett on the new Nimrod control system for the UK equivalent of an AWACS aircraft. I spent nearly a year with them. My main recollection of that period is of playing practical jokes and making prank phone calls to electrical retailers, with a dialogue that went something like this...

Store: Good morning can I help you

Brian: I hope so I have a laptop that has stopped working
Store: Is it still in warranty?

Brian: Well….no it isn't. It has just gone out of warranty ..can I still bring it in?

Store: 50% would say bring it in but don't mention the warranty.

Brian: Thank you. There is something else I have got to tell you

Store: What?

Brian: I dropped it

Store: 50% would say: Well that invalidates your warranty!

But normally I would manage to convince the engineer to permit me to bring it in anyway - The art of the persuasion!

I would then deliver the punchline: There is something else I've got to tell you.

Shop: What………

Brian: I dropped it in the sea

When the engineer was fully exasperated I would say the following

Brian: The water was not very deep. So I washed it off in the bath when I got home, and I did get all the seaweed off of it. Even then some shops said come in anyway and others just hung up!

It took me several attempts before I could get through the whole spiel to deliver the punchline without giggling.

Further to this there was a crusty head of department at Marconi, who was always moaning about his telephone bill being too high. So we phoned him one day and this is how it went:

Brian: I am calling from BT [this was guaranteed to send him off into 5 minute tirade saying things like: I've been calling you lot for weeks my because bill seems far too high and I want a refund]

Brian: [managing to interrupt him] I'm phoning about the Busby awards because you have got the highest phone bill in the country

Crusty: [now in a screaming rage] I told you so. I've been saying it, haven't I been saying it?

Brian [calming him down]: Can I ask you a few questions about your bill first and then we can discuss it afterwards?

Crusty: Yes

Brian: is there anyone in your office with access to your telephone making calls either overseas or very long distance ones

Crusty: [angrily] No

Brian: What about your wife could she be seeing someone else?

Crusty went ballistic and the 8 people who were listening to this were hysterical with laughter as was I. But he was really belligerent so I told him that regrettably he had disqualified himself from the Busby award because his temper was too short.

After my year at Marconi, my business partner Pete was discharged out of the Navy and we bought a licence on a pub in Cheltenham. We ran it for 2 years and then Pete emigrated to the US, so we sold the place and took half each. I used my part of the proceeds to purchase the licence for Great Stukeley hall in Huntingdon. Our main clientele there came from the Americans at Alconbury air base, until the day came when my security staff got involved in a massive punch up with them outside the hall. As a result of that altercation the commander of the base then banned his personnel from coming to see us, for a minimum of two years. That ended the business. The weird thing is that Gordon is a descendant of John Stukeley, the grand father of William Stukeley (1687 - 1765) who was Sir Isaac Newton's biographer. He is Gordon Stukeley Ritchie.

HOMAGE TO STEVE MCQUEEN AND HIS GREAT ESCAPE

One evening I was coming home from a squash match having had a couple of drinks and driving a car belonging to one of my staff, who had borrowed my vehicle in order get himself to Heathrow. Suddenly a car pulled out in front of me. So I slammed on his brakes, which weren't as effective as those in my car, and failed to prevent me from running into the back of this car very gently. I went to check on the passengers inside it and they said they were alright. Worried that I had been drinking just a couple of beers I decided to get out of there and walk home! But before I could put 20 yards between myself and the accident, I was apprehended by a policeman, who asked if I had been involved in the accident. I said: No.

I knew it was only going to be a few minutes before he realised that I was lying and I had spent many years training with the Navy as a cross country runner. I was especially good at steeple chases. So I decided to take a short cut across the fields to run home in order to escape being breathalysed. It was only a few minutes later that I saw a car come into the field and then the dogs barking. I threw my sports bag up a tree and set off running. I hurdled a barbed wire fence, jumped across a small stream, jumped into the stream for 30 yards to lose the dogs and then reverted to jumping over the stream a number of times. I got home covered in blood and jumped straight into the bath, then to bed.

In the morning I reported the accident, and the policeman said he wanted to see me straight away I said I could not make it for a couple of days. So we agreed I would come in after 2 days. On going down to the station I was shown into a room where the policeman and a witness sat waiting to hear what I had to say.

I declared that I couldn't remember a thing. This was met with a howl of contempt - you must be able to remember something said the policeman. I just shook my head and said: No, but if you get rid of your witness, I might be able tell you something. He had already written up a charge of not staying with the car and reporting the crash too late. He was getting anxious for me to sign it.

After the witness left the room I immediately told him that he was right and I asked him if I could join the police running team and told him his dogs were a bit out of shape which gave him a good belly laugh. He said I can't believe the dogs didn't get you, because they were very close. I told him all about jumping the river, and hurdling the fence, and running through the water to lose the scent.

In the end I didn't get off scoot free. But I did escape a driving ban. Then I went to LKB Biochrome making Spectrophotometers at the Cambridge Technical Park. After only a few weeks with that firm, one of the directors there told me that work was drying up. So he would have to let me go. I said no worries I have an interview with Oric Computers. He said ah, well you might be meeting me again there! So we both left and joined Oric.

I started working for Oric as a temp in their small office in the same Cambridge business park as LKB. Whilst I was there I was told that I had an interview with members of the board of Oric in London. So I travelled to the Sheriton Skyline Hotel, together with the rest of the staff from the Cambridge office. The plan was to attend the interview at lunchtime and then go to the big staff party in the afternoon. I got the job as works manager in their new production facility in Hampton.

Later that evening I was sitting at my table surrounded by Oric angels [beautiful and promotional ladies] and feeling ready for a great night. Suddenly the doors opened and the directors appeared with an angel on each arm. We had dinner and then the music started and then one of the angels, who was an ex London Palladium Tiller girl, started dancing on the table. So I joined her. Then the coaches turned up to take the staff back. But I decided to stay on and in the early hours I went back to the company Mansion in Ascot near Wentworth with a troupe of directors and angels.

When morning came the PA to the directors appeared and kindly told me that she had arranged for a taxi to get me home from Ascot back to Cambridge. She told me that the MD was greatly unimpressed by my 1st day at the office because I had inadvertently whilst dancing up the table, stepped in a VIPs dessert. She herself however found the incident highly amusing.

In order to keep fit, I joined the nearby West Surrey Squash Club and then joined Colletts health and fitness club. A group of us from there formed the tea gang in 1991 to go on day long bike riding trips. These bike rides still go on today in 2021, 30 years later.

Oric eventually went bust in 1986 and I joined Living Images in Hampton, an advertising display company, which lasted until 1990 when it too went bust.

Then in 1987 we did took a display stand display at the point of sale exhibition at Olympia. Gordon came to the stand and offered us his Levitator.

Living images was full of very creative people. It was run by John Wimbourne, who had a very free management style.

The most prestigious job we did was the Garden Festival in Gateshead in 1990. One of the national papers did a two page spread on it and said that it was the most innovative and interactive display they had ever seen. As you approached it there was a talking puppet on a huge screen which would interact with the crowd. He was operated by a man out of sight. The festival was all about living a safer and healthier lifestyle. When one approached the tree of life exhibit, a man could be seen in the tree sawing off branch that he was sitting on. Eventually both he and the branch fell of the tree. This was supposed to teach people how to avoid accidents in the home and how not to destroy our environment.

Then we built a how to stop eating junk food area on a wibbly wobbly bridge with a bin crying out: Feed me, feed me! Next we had a 'packet in man' a very different version of Pacman persuading you to stop smoking and improve your lifestyle. the contestants would be unable to shoot using our infrared guns until they had answered some questions about how much they smoked, how much they drank and what was their diet. The better their lifestyle the more shots they got.

Many other displays were made for places all over the world including talking heads, wrestling bulls, 50 years of the BBC, the crusades exhibition in Winchester, Never neverland in Southend and many more.

1990-2010: GYMS, HEALTH CLUBS & HOUSE BOATS

Due to my experience in building theme parks with Living Images, I moved into Health club construction for David Lloyds and L.A Fitness.

In 1993 I had the privilege of working with downs syndrome children for 12 months. They were some of the most charming and loving people I have ever met.

In Japan in 1995 we built a part of a leisure centre. But shortly after we arrived there the Kobe earthquake occurred and our hotel in Nagoya shook dramatically. Meanwhile our shipment of parts was severely held up. The net result was that whilst there was an argument with the Japanese about them not allowing to being declared a force majeure, they gave the contract to us to build 4 more sights around Japan.

I split up with my second wife Michelle, in 2002, in the year before Rugby world cup in 2003.

I lived on various house boats moored in the Thames from the demise of Living Images in 1990 until I met Mandy and we moved to Lowestoft in 2014. Michelle got my last house boat in the divorce.

For the Millennium party, we took the houseboat down the Thames to see all the fireworks. We watched the fireworks with the cast of East Enders who had moored next to the boat and they came and joined us.

We decided to leave at 4 in the morning because there were 1000's of boats down the Thames and when we got to Teddington Lock we were one of the first to pass through and there was a rather grumpy lockkeeper who made me stop to get a river licence (which takes around 20 minutes to complete) to drive up the non-tidal part of the river. I explained to him there were too many boats behind us to waste time on that. But he insisted and by the time I got back there were already 20 boats bumper to bumper. So I think he saw that he was beaten and gave up with everyone after me.

FIRST DIAGNOSIS

I was first was diagnosed as borderline Diabetic in 2009/2010. I went dizzy in the boat in which I lived on the Thames at Thames Ditton. I called a friend of mine, Wilfe, who he took me to Kingston Hospital. They took my sugar and made the diagnosis. They suggested tablets. But I went for diet and exercise. I was playing a lot of squash at the health club and going on long bicycle rides with the tea gang. This kept my sugar reasonable.

2014-2018 LOWESTOFT

I met my present partner, Mandy, and went to Lowestoft with her in 2014May20. I was offered the opportunity to run a slipway and boat repair yard there. We took in barges and fishing boats to either service them or refurbish them-often bringing them up from London by the Thames and the North Sea.

I would often do maintenance on various sea based wind farms in the North Sea. When out at sea we had a visit from a friendly dolphin and a pilot whale which were swimming alongside the boat, knocking off the barnacles, and eating them. They stayed with us for about an hour.

On another occasion our assistant boat pilot took charge of the boat and was driving when I suddenly noticed he was heading towards the Dogger sand bank. So I told him to alter course. But it was too late and we ran aground upon it. We were stuck there for 12 hours with a colony of seals.

During this period I was taking Metformin and Glipizide and various other pills to mitigate the side effects of these anti diabetic drugs. But my sugar was getting progressively worse.

THE THAMES WITH SPACESHIPS 1ST STROKE

Mandy and myself and my assistant pilot, were navigating from Lowestoft back to Hampton Court in September 2017.

We went through the centre of London on the Thames. A mile out from Hampton Court, I started to hallucinate and saw a spaceship in the river. The spaceship was like a giant flying saucer hovering above the Thames. I had been awake for 24 hours solid prior to this. I then very gingerly moored the boat at Hampton Court. I did not discover that I had had a stroke until I went to hospital after my second stroke.

AIR FRANCE AND MY 2ND STOKE

Mandy and I flew to France in October 2017. I started hallucinating on the flight and after we had landed. I imagined I could see birds nesting upon the wing of the aircraft. After we landed I tried to drive and found myself mounting the pavement. I kept assuring Mandy that everything was OK.

I drove onto the central reservation and Mandy took over. Then in a friends house where we were staying I was seeing ghostly figures going up the stairs. Mandy was worried because I had no conception of the danger we were in. I thought that everything was fine but there were a few birds nesting on the wing of the aeroplane and a few ghosts running up and down the staircase. I told Mandy and expected her to take this on board as a totally normal state of affairs. Mandy had no idea how to deal with my condition or my attitude to it other than to have a few more glasses of French wine.

The hallucination stopped after about 48 hours. I felt a bit sick, but generally OK on the flight back. We went to St. George's Hospital on our return. And they confirmed that I had had two strokes.

By early 2018 my sugar was getting worse and the doctor recommended that I should up my Metformin dose from 2 tablets to 4 tablets and told me that this would buy me a bit of time before I would have to start taking insulin injections.

Given that I had already had two strokes caused by my diabetes, I began to realise that this disease was going to kill me in the near future if I did not do something radical. I was then taking around 12 different types of pills every day for the strokes, the diabetes and the side effects of the various medications. I knew that this was a one way ticket to oblivion and I needed to jump out of this box somehow. So I called Gordon, who had a website dedicated to curing Type2 because I knew that if anybody in my circle of friends could outthink this disease it was him.

GORDON GETS RELIGION

I gave up my desire to build a quadrocopter because I became a Jehovah's Witness and realised that mankind was in the End Times, and knew that Drones would not be used for good things. I actually had a vision of myself being killed by a drone with a machine gun mounted upon it. That vision was given me around 1990. So I gave up my dream (but only in this system). I made a deal with God and he never lets his sons down. I said I will fix your church if you give me another shot at my quadrocopter in the Kingdom of God.

I then proceeded to catch up with all the doctrine of the Watchtower and I saw much of it was correct and worked out how to improve it enormously (rather like I had done at Imperial College). It took me 3 years to catch up with their bible understandings and then came the day when I overtook them. But I never could have done that without the help of another friend of mine Massoud Vakili whom I met at Imperial College.

Massoud was working on a US government contract to research into the Harrier Jump Jet. He was very, very bright and we became close friends.

His father owned one of the largest banks in Iran. But his bank was stolen by the Shah of Iran just prior to the revolution. That theft actually saved his father's life because the revolutionaries saw him as a fellow victim of the oppression of the Shah. But Massoud and his family left Iran and like many other non revolutionaries, came to the UK and the US.

Massoud came with me to a few of the meetings at the Kingdom Hall with the Jehovah's Witnesses - Quite a shock for an Iranian infidel.

But Massoud was a very deep thinker. And one day following a business disaster which had led him into bankruptcy, he decided to read the bible for himself - the whole bible. He did this because he knew me. He knew if I was doing it, there must be something to it, and because he wanted to know about God. Being from the aristocracy in Iran he knew all about the hypocrisy of the Mullahs, buying plastic keys to 70,000 virgins in heaven from Hong Kong and giving them to soldiers before they were commanded to walk into the minefields of the Iran Iraq war. He read the entire book in 3 months. Then he rang me up and said come over. When I arrived at his flat in Hornton Street by Kensington Town Hall, there he was unable to pay his mortgage and living off cheese and biscuits. But as St. Paul said: When I am weak, then I am strong. So the conversation went something like this...

Massoud: You are brainwashed.
Gordon: Perhaps, but I am brainwashed by the true religion.
Massoud: What is a true religion?

Gordon: It is the religion to which God reveals the truth.
Massoud: So do you think that God can reveal the truth to you?
Gordon: No because I am not the true religion.
Massoud: So if God reveals the truth to me then would that make me into the true religion?
Gordon: Yes of course. But that will never happen.
Massoud: Oh really? Well, how about this interpretation of the 4600 days of Daniel8?

Massoud then gave me his interpretation of the greater meaning of the 4600 days of Daniel8. It sounded convincing (it was not correct actually). I then checked the Watchtower and they had NO understanding of Daniel8 at all. I thought to myself Massoud's understanding may not be correct BUT it is better than nothing. Massoud then said this...

Gordon I have known you for 10 years. You have a very, very good mind. I want you stop reading the bible with the eyes of a bunch of old men in Brooklyn (who run the Watchtower) and start reading it with your own eyes, with your own mind just like I have done for the last 3 months. I am telling you, you WILL see something that they have not seen. God will show you something.

Now I was a Scholar at Dulwich College, I was a mathematics Scholar at Cambridge. I won the Magdalene College maths prize, I got a single first in Maths. I came 20th in the UK national maths competition aged 17 without being in the maths stream at school (I was doing sciences). BUT NONE OF THAT WAS ANY DEFENCE AGAINST BEING BRAINWASHED BY THE WATCHTOWER.

It was Massoud that broke my mind free from that prison and I shall forever be grateful to him for it.

So I started reading the bible with my own eyes, with my own mind. and when I got to Leviticus 26 I saw a 2nd proof that the continuous Gentile Times ended in 1914, which was the fundamental doctrine upon which the Watchtower was built. I showed this proof to my Study Conductor, Clifton Turner, who was an enlightened JW. He said: You could start a whole new religion with that interpretation my brother. I said: The last thing the world needs is another religion.

To cut a long story short, I took that understanding and found it to be one element of a symbolic bible code. NOT the equidistant letter skip code of the now deceased Michael Drosnin. But the true bible code, the symbolic and numerical and cryptic code that God's book is written in.

This code was first seen secularly by Philo Judaeus, a contemporary of Jesus Christ and the Apostles. It was lost in the dark ages as a result of Catholic Persecution of the 2nd true church, the Gnostics of St. Paul. But a part of it is preserved in the Gospel of Philip which was found with the Nag Hammadi scrolls hidden in an urn in the ground

The church I eventually founded, the Lords Witnesses, had independently worked out most of the doctrine in the Gospel of Philip before we actually came across that Gospel.

The Code was rediscovered in part by Sir Isaac Newton who almost drove himself mad with despair, thinking himself to be an Elijah (calling out in a wilderness of faithlessness and ignorance), knowing that all England was worshipping a logically non existent Trinity rather than the one almighty God, Jehovah. Newton refused to Sign the attestation to the Trinity which was required for all the fellows of Trinity College Cambridge at that time. He appealed to King James (who authorised the King James Bible). The King determined that if Sir Isaac could convince him that the Trinity was a false doctrine, then he would wave the attestation for Sir Isaac by Royal decree. Newton succeeded in convincing the King, who issued the decree and Sir Isaac became a fellow of Trinity College Cambridge and then became the Lucasian Professor of Mathematics there.

Newton knew the danger to his position and life that a public declaration of his heretical religious interpretations would have posed. So he arranged for his insights to be published posthumously, His book: Observations on the Prophecies of Daniel and the Apocalypse of St. John is still in print today - *http://www.historicism.com/Newton/newton.pdf*

I have found in this life that if you wish to advance any subject you have to be a bit of a heretic. Because mankind always manages to get himself stuck on tram lines going in the wrong direction.

So, I then decoded several more accounts and sent 12 copies of the results of the decoding to the 12 members of the Governing Body of the Watchtower on September 11 1992. Massoud actually personally delivered them to Brooklyn. They were astonished and I very nearly overturned the entire church. An emissary from the Governing Body came to see me in 2003 and told me that had I pushed it a bit harder I would have overturned them. But at the end of the day they chose to throw me out just like Imperial College did, rather than advance their understandings which would also have changed the church and the world for the better. But would also have empowered me and worried them.

So I ended up indeed forming the very church that I did not want to form. And it was just another sad lesson in politics over academic truth. Politics is today and has always been the enemy of truth. It is of course, the art of formulating and selling the lie.

Here is the choice that every man and more so every woman gets wrong.

HIGH STATUS LIES VERSUS NEGATIVE STATUS TRUTHS (CONSPIRACY THEORIES)

Eve was blinded by the status of Satan, who offered her the status of a God, deciding for herself right from wrong, in return for eating the fruit. She was thoroughly deceived according to Paul...

14 And Adam was not deceived, but the woman being deceived was in the transgression. *(1 Timothy 2 KJV)*
14 Also, Adam was not deceived, but the woman was thoroughly deceived and came to be in transgression. *(1 Timothy 2 NWT)*

Things are not so different today. Notice that the scripture does not say Eve, was deceived. So in the greater meaning, today the woman, women actually are still being deceived by the serpent. But they are wising up. And when the modern woman sees through to the truth, the serpent will be toast.

Here are some of the more masterful high status deceptions and zero status truths. Status is the means by which a lie is sold.

High status lie: The twin towers were knocked down by two aeroplanes
Negative status truth: It was a controlled demolition by the deep state.

High status lie: Coronavirus evolved in bats and then escaped from the BSL4 lab in Wuhan 1500 miles away from the bat cave where it evolved.
Negative status truth: COVID19 was gene spliced by demon possessed members of the US/Chinese military and deliberately released to force vaccination.

High Status lie: You have to take an emergency use vaccine because there are no other efficacious treatments for COVID19.
Negative Status Truth: The UK banned the parallel export of and did NOT licence Hydroxy Chloroquine for prescription on March 13, 2020 just before the COVID pandemic became a problem. It was necessary for all alternative COVID treatments to be pooh, poohed in order for an emergency use vaccine authorisation to be granted by the FDA.

Efficacy of all the other Drugs for COVID

Early Intervention	Improvement	Studies	
Proxalutamide	92%	2	
Fluvoxamine	89%	2	
Budesonide	82%	1	
Povidone-Iodine	82%	4	*(Aquafresh mouthwash is good too)*
Bromhexine	79%	2	
Ivermectin	78%	23	
Vitamin D	78%	3	
Bamlanivimab	75%	3	
Casiri/imdevimab	68%	3	
Hydroxychloroquine	66%	29	
Nitazoxanide	49%	5	
Zinc	42%	2	

Favipiravir	38%	3
Vitamin C	18%	1

https://twitter.com/robinmonotti2/status/1403215093253480448 - Dr Nyjon Eccles is one of the most respected Integrated Medicine physicians in the UK. He holds a raft of medical and academic qualifications, including the MBBS, and is a Member of the Royal College of Physicians (MRCP). He also holds a PhD in Pharmacology (London).

https://rightsfreedoms.wordpress.com/2021/05/29/covid-19-early-treatment-real-time-analysis-of-659-studies/

High Status lie: You must wear a face mask and refuse to visit your friends and relatives and socially isolate your self for you own health and for the health of others.
Negative Status truth: Face masks have a negligible effect on virus transmission when new and are bad for your health after 24 hours. UK lockdowns save 1 person today at the expense of killing 2 people in the UK tomorrow and 10 people in the third world. They reduce the strength of your immune system. The purpose of ALL COVID legislation is the destruction of love between humans because mankind will later this year (on 2021Tishri4 - 2021September12/13) enter into the love test of the sheep and the goats of Matthew25. If you fail that test you will go to Hell. If you pass you will go into the Kingdom of God.

High Status lie: The Kingdom of God either does not exist or is in your heart or is in your mind or is exclusively in heaven.
Negative Status truth: The Kingdom of God is the next administration of this planet. It has already been installed in a clandestine way. It becomes more and more obvious over the next 14 months until 2022August13/14 (2022Ab14), when it is fully established.

High Status lie: Type 2 Diabetes is not curable
Negative Status truth: Sugar numbers are reversible with a Ketogenic diet and exercise (that is known). But actually it is fully curable with prebiotic antifungal paleo ketogenic diet and exercise, once you know the cause, which is a gut flora overgrowth.

High Status lie: Satan persuades Eve to sin saying 'you will have the status of a God'
Negative Status truth: I will be the progenitor of the human race through you rather than Adam who you are going to kill.

High Status lie: Judas complains about Mary washing Jesus' feet with expensive perfumed oil.
Negative Status truth: Why was it this perfumed oil was not sold for 300 denarii and given to the poor people? Judas was a thief who had control of the money box and used to steal the money in it. He wanted his percentage of the 300 denarii. (John 12).

High Status lie: US/UK Coalition invades Iraq because of the WMD threat and link between Saddam and Bin Laden.
Negative Status truth: Perhaps Oil security, perhaps Israeli security, perhaps keep the war on terror going for political advantage to the incumbent administration, perhaps pay Saddam back for attempting to kill Bush Senior etc. etc.

High Status lie: Many Fundamental Churches tell their followers that they will burn in hell unless they stay in the church. The bible teaches that those not in our church will burn in hell.
Negative Status truth: They wish to rule their flock by fear in order to get more out of the flock for themselves. And they wish to scare people into staying under their control in the church.

High Status lie: US/UK Coalition invades Iraq because of the WMD threat and link between Saddam and Bin Laden.
Negative Status truth: Perhaps Oil security, perhaps Israeli security, perhaps keep the war on terror going for political advantage to the incumbent administration, perhaps pay Saddam back for attempting to kill Bush Senior etc. etc.

High Status lie: Microsoft launch Windows XP to give the user an enhanced computational experience.
Negative Status truth: Maintain their monopoly position in order to make more money for their shareholders.

High Status lie: Robert Mugabe (President of Mugabeland) bulldozed 250,000 houses to clear out rubbish.
Negative Status truth: Persecute his political opponents so that only those who vote for him feel secure.

High Status lie: Tabo Mbeke (President of South Africa) did not buy any AIDS drugs for his people as HIV does not lead to AIDS.
Negative Status truth: He loves money more than he loves his people, 25% of whom now have AIDS.

High Status lie: Catholic Church bans condoms as contraception is against God's law.
Negative Status truth: The main method of generating more Catholics is through procreation by Catholics. Hence the huge number of Catholic schools.

High Status lie: Catholic Church propounds the false trinity doctrine, knowing that Jesus Christ was the angel Michael (Michaelmas = Christmas) God is 3 co-equal co-eternal beings yet is only one being. And his son Jesus Christ was uncreated.
Negative Status truth: If we can get them to believe this (to abolish the number 2 and to have a son that was not created by his father) then they have abandoned both numeracy and literacy. So we know they are brainwashed. So we can allow them into the congregation without any danger that they will expose us as frauds and we can play God to them and get whatever we want from them. The trinity is a brainwash-ometer!

High Status lie: Boeing prevented Concorde from landing in the USA, when it was first built as the sonic boom breaks stained glass windows in American churches and makes American men impotent.
Negative Status truth: Kill any supersonic competition to their subsonic aircraft.

High Status lie: Fox News asking if deep throat was a hero or a traitor as they are interested in public opinion.
Negative Status truth: They wish to manipulate public opinion to the point where their viewers believe that a traitor is not someone who betrays his country, but is rather someone who betrays the Republican Party.

High Status lie: The EU draw up an EU constitution to run things a bit more smoothly.
Negative Status truth: Form a 21st century empire by soft power rather than hard power. Take away the sovereignty of 27 nations. Throw away the sacrifices of 30 million people made in two world wars fought to prevent a European Superstate run by the Germans with the collaboration of the French.

DIABETES

In 2001 the love of my life left me due to my misunderstanding of the magnitude of the damage done to her by her controlling husband and due to my and her love being not strong enough to overcome that abuse.

Actually the whole world is heading for disaster due to mankind's misunderstanding of the scale of the damage done to our morality and our love by control freak politicians. Those who disguise their attacks on the moral majority as defences of various ethnic or religious or sexual orientation minorities. But they are not interested in those minorities. They are interested in controlling the majority by invalidating them, their identity, their gender, their rights, their individuality, their ancestry, their nationality, their history, their culture, their family, their family relationships, their authority over their own children, their sexuality, the sexuality of their children and their love for their friends and family.

I can see it so clearly in 2021 with the world. But I failed to see it so clearly with the love of my life in 2001.

I asked her if she wanted to marry me. She said: I will do anything you want.

I said: I did not ask you what I wanted: I asked you what you wanted.

She had just made me the absolute best possible offer that a victim of a control freak can ever make (she had not known or done very much that she herself wanted to do for 20 years. She had spent 20 years trying to please a control freak, which means doing what he wanted).

But I, in my naivety, wanted her to say: I want to marry you. She was not in a position honestly to say that, Although she had agreed to marry me several times before that awful day.

In my defence she left her abuser before she married him and we fell in love and she agreed to marry me and told her abuser. Then when her abuser saw that I had upped the anti, he divorced his previous wife with whom he had several children and married her. He was impotent and she wanted a family. But she made the mistake of expressing her desires to him, which he then frustrated completely - knowing that he could not provide her with a family.

I never had any sisters and went to an all boys school and all male college at Cambridge. So I love women and find women fascinating but really am slow in understanding them. I am really good at understanding things of the mind. But understanding women is a thing of the heart. The tragedy of our demise lead me to binge drink Coca Cola and set up a software company, HyperOs Systems, to compete with Bill Gates.

I eventually stopped drinking Coca Cola when my teeth started to hurt all the time. But my desire for sugar had by that time taken a hold of me and I replaced the Coke with fruit juice, chocolate and cake.

In 2012, I was running a Hotel in Central London and eating half a chocolate cake, one bar of Cadbury's whole nut and drinking one litre of fruit juice every day. I had been very, very thirsty for a year previously and had developed a frozen toe on my right foot, which felt like it was stuck in a ski boot the whole time.

Then I got this terrible pain in my left ball. It felt like a knitting needle had been pushed through it. The pain was unbearable. It got slightly better when stood naked in front of a fan. But I could not do that all day. I had not had a medical check-up for 20 years because my father, who was a Professor of Surgery, had died in 1992 and he used to act as my GP.

So reluctantly I went to see a private GP. He did a blood test and my blood sugar came back as 23 mmol/L (414 mg/dl). He told me I was badly diabetic. Normal sugar is 4.5 mmol/L 81 mg/dl.

Then a truly wonderful thing happened to me, I got sent to this enlightened diabetic specialist at the London Bridge Hospital. He saw me at a cost of some £400 and at the end of the consultation (during which my sugar was 18.0 mmol/L) he said well yes you are badly diabetic. I said what should I do expecting to be given a nice brochure detailing all the foods I should eat and all the foods I should not eat and all the exercises I should do and all the exercises I should not do. Instead he just said to me: Don't eat sugar!

£400 for don't eat sugar? You would think this guy was the worst diabetes doctor on the planet. Actually he was and is in my opinion the best. Because he said: Really I should prescribe you with some Metformin and some Glipizide (a sulphonylurea which turns on the pancreas).

I replied that I want to try some diet and exercise and see what I could do myself because I reasoned that lifestyle had certainly got me into this mess. So perhaps lifestyle change could get me out of it. He said: Go ahead, but I will give you the prescriptions anyway in case your diet and exercise routines do not work.

I then went for a long walk and my sugar came down to 12 mmol/L (216 mg/dl). I spent the next two weeks doing 2 hour walks every night and eating less carbs in my diet. After two weeks my sugar was around 7.5 mmol/L (135mg/dl). But it was very had work and my heels were starting to fall off from all the walking I was doing.

So I ran up my spectacularly loquacious diabetic specialist for a couple more words of his great and learned wisdom. I said: I cannot continue with this exercise regime. It is too knackering and I have only managed to get my sugar down from 18 to 7.5 mmol/L (324mg/dl to 135 md/dl). He said: No, you have done really well. Believe me, the prescriptions I gave you would not achieved that within 2 weeks. Whatever you are doing keep doing it and I don't want to hear any more about 7s and 8s I want to hear and 5s and 6s.

That advice was worth way more than £400. So I carried on walking and got my sugar slightly lower but all the time my frozen toe was getting worse. And my balls were still hurting a lot.

One night I was lying in my bed and I could not sleep due to the diabetic neuralgia in my foot (frozen toe syndrome). If the sheet just touched my foot it felt like my foot had been hit on the funny bone. I had already devised a frame to keep the bed sheet off my foot whilst I slept. But things were not getting any better. They were getting worse.

So I said to myself: Why are you lying here not able to sleep? Go for a walk and walk and walk and walk until you can bloody sleep. I don't care if you have to walk all night. Do the work. So I embarked on a 3 hour walk and when I got back to the hotel my foot no longer hurt from the neuralgia. It hurt from the walk - which was a big improvement. I slept like a log. That was really my first victory over type2. My aching ball was better too.

So then I decided to become professional, having had my first taste of victory over this impostor. I purchased a treadmill and the most padded trainers on the planet (Skechers) and put 2 layers of impact absorbing insoles in both of them (Sorbothane and Noene as used by the Swiss Army). I realised that my feet were a crucial weapon against Type2 and I felt that Type2 kind of knew this and was therefore attacking my feet.

So the battle ground for this fight was my feet. I found that walking upon the treadmill was more effective than walking upon the pavement by around 30% in time terms. But that it was not as good for the skeleton. So a bit of pavement walking was included too.

Then I made the mistake of reading the work of Professor Taylor of Newcastle University. He recommended a really, really low calorie diet and propounded the theory that diabetes is caused by fat in the liver and that drastic weight loss was the only chance to fix the disease. So I went on a crash diet and my weight fell from 13 stone to 10 stone 6. I became so weak that I could not open a door. I was thinner than the super models amongst my hotel cleaning staff with whom I would hold belly competitions to show them what fat cows they were.

Losing all that weight did not improve my blood sugar at all. It destroyed the very muscles in which my sugar was being stored. It destroyed my health and it made my diabetes worse.

It was at this point that I reached the terrifying conclusion that mainstream medicine had absolutely no clue about what caused type2 or how to cure it.

But having learned how not to cure type2 I was of course one step nearer to learning how to cure it! So I then read the work of Drs Bernstein, Feinman and Westman on low carb diets and soon realised this was a better route for a type2 cure. The seminal paper on this is...

Low Carb Diabetic Cures

http://www.nutritionandmetabolism.com/content/5/1/9 (Dr Bernstein, Dr Feinman, Dr Westman and 18 others in desperate plea to use carbohydrate restriction as the primary intervention in Type2)

Other papers are...

http://www.diabeteshealth.com/read/2009/01/13/6044/extremely-low-carb-ketogenic-diet-leads-to-dramatic-reductions-in-type-2-bg-levels-medications/

http://www.dietdoctor.com/category/health-problems/diabetes?mod=visa-kategorier (Low Carb News)

http://www.dietdoctor.com/new-study-low-carb-diet-intermittent-fasting-beneficial-diabetics (Low Carb Diets are best for diabetics)

http://medicalxpress.com/news/2012-05-high-fat-diet-lowered-blood-sugar.html

http://www.bodybuilding.com/fun/keto.htm (Good description of the benefits and drawbacks of Ketosis from Ketogenic diets) *http://www.nutritionandmetabolism.com/content/3/1/16 (LOBAG diets - shows 20% carb or 40gm carb per day works fine too)*

http://www.nutritionjrnl.com/article/S0899-9007(14)00332-3/fulltext (Low Carb Ketogenic diet is way better than a Low Calorie diet for diabetics)

http://www.nutritionandmetabolism.com/content/5/1/36 (Dr. Westman Low Carb Ketogenic diet is way better than Low Calorie Low Glycaemic Index diet for diabetics)

http://www.cbn.com/cbnnews/healthscience/2014/february/dump-sugar-eat-fat-and-cure-diabetes/ (Dr Westman Low carb high fat diabetic cure)

More recently Tom Watson, the Labour minister, reached the same conclusion and reversed his sugar numbers with a low carb rather than a low calorie diet. Low carb diets are sustainable, you can stay on them as long as you like. Low calorie diets are not. You starve to death if you remain on them for too long. So going low carb but keeping the calories up to maintain a reasonable body weight became the next mission.

The problem is this. There are 3 types of food, protein (4 kcals per gram) carbs (4 kcals per gram) and fat (9 kcals per gram). Actually there are 4 if you include alcohol (7 kcals per gram) which is metabolised differently to the other 3.

So if you cut out the carbs you are eating protein and fat. The temptation is to eat a lot more fat. There are essentially 4 types of fat. Saturated fat (butter, cheese etc), Omega9 monounsaturated fat (avocado, olive oil etc.), Omega6 polyunsaturated aft (corn oil, sunflower oil etc) and Omega3 polyunsaturated fat (fish oil, chia seed oil, flax seed oil).

I did a huge amount of research into all of these fats and their effect on your metabolism. This research can be found on my website www.cureddiabetes.com.

There is a theory that type 2 is caused by eating too much Omega6 polyunsaturated fat which is inflammatory and increases your insulin resistance, and too little Omega3 polyunsaturated fat which is anti inflammatory and decreases your insulin resistance. The theory roughly states that your cell walls become made entirely out of inflammatory Omega6 fats and then the insulin cannot cross over into your cells properly to store your blood sugar. I put this to the test. And by putting this to this test I mean I really went for it. I stopped eating any and all Omega6 fats and ate huge amounts of fish oil and started making bread out of ground up flax seed and later added ground up WHITE chia seed (not the black stuff which causes kidney ache).

Eskimos eat around 15 grams of EPA and 15 grams of DHA per day, which are the two main Omega3 fats. I decided to go 1/3 Eskimo in circumstances where the Mayo clinic and standard mainstream medicine recommend no more than 3 grams of fish oil per day and undistilled fish oil is only 1/3 DHA and EPA. So I ended up taking the equivalent of 30 grams of fish oil per day. This is 10x what mainstream medicine recommends. The danger of taking too much fish oil is that your blood could in theory become too thin. But there is no clinical evidence to support this that I could find. Indeed women on large fish oil doses (above what mainstream medicine recommends), were having Caesarean sections and bleeding no more profusely than normal, because fish oil manages to thin the blood without reducing blood clotting. It is well known that a high fish oil diet, such as the traditional Japanese one, reduces the incidence of heart attacks very significantly. In fact Eskimos on their traditional diet do not get heart attacks at all or type2.

But heart attacks and other cardiovascular problems are one of the main causes of death from type2. So I reasoned that main stream medicine was too conservative, and the numbers they recommend are probably determined by committees of lawyers rather than professors of nutrition.

Also I was looking for a result. I did not want to spend 6 months experimenting with few drops of fish oil. So I became 1/3 Eskimo and my sugar became much easier to control. I did not have to do nearly as much exercise on the treadmill to get it down to normal levels (around 2 hours per day instead of 3 hours).

I should say that initially when first diagnosed, I needed 3 hours per day walking on concrete outside to get my sugar down to 7 mmol/L (126mg/dl). Then once I purchased a treadmill I could get down to 5 mmol/L with 3 hours per day of exercise on the treadmill. But after going 1/3 Eskimo. I only needed 2 hours per day for the first 7 days. But then slowly the type 2 fought back and once again I needed 2.5 hours per day for perfect sugar.

So Omega3 was a help but it was not the full answer.

My favourite experiment with Omega3 was to take 30 Jarrow MaxDHA pills (you are supposed to take only 2) and then get on the treadmill. Wow! For the first time since I was diagnosed I felt like I wanted to sprint on that machine! I felt like Superman. It also gave me very vivid dreams (DHA is the main constituent of brain tissue). Women do not need as much DHA as men because they manufacture it for babies (who have a large head containing a large brain and a tiny body). I then got a nose bleed. So I realised I had taken too much DHA. So I reduced the dose down to the level which did not cause a nose bleed (1/3 Eskimo - around 7 MaxDHA tablets and 5 Holland and Barrett triple strength fish oil tablets (950 mg of EPA/DHA).

So Omega3 was really the first dietary success that I had with Type2 but it was almost completed negated by some kind of fight back which I did not understand but which I found hugely depressing. However it did not dampen my desire to kill Type2 before it killed me.

Then an amazing thing happened. As a type 2 you learn that every meal puts your sugar up. The ridiculous thing is that even a small meal can put it up almost as much as a large meal. So one way to deal with this is to eat only once, or at most twice, a day, and to stop snacking.

But this particular evening I went for a curry at the Bombay Palace in Bayswater near to the Hotel I was running. I left the hotel with a blood sugar of 7.0 mmol/L (126 mg/dl) I had a lovely curry, and I returned to the hotel with blood sugar of around 6.6 mmol/L I could not believe it. I had eaten a meal and my blood sugar had actually gone down. It was a fascinating piece of the puzzle. But I did not know where to place it at that time.

I commented on my post prandial sugar drop on a restaurant review website and got a response from a fellow diabetic who told me that red wine prevents sugar from going up too. I tried this out and found it to be true for red wine but not for spirits. So it was not the alcohol in the red wine which was keeping my blood sugar low it was something else - another piece of the puzzle which I did not yet have a place for.

By 2013 I had got my HbA1c, which is a 2 month blood sugar average, down to around 5.3% which is the equivalent of an average sugar of around 6.2 mmol/L. This is a non diabetic number. So I had successfully REVERSED by diabetes, in the sense that I had reversed my sugar numbers. But they would only stay that way if I ate no carbs, ate shed loads of Omega3 and exercised for 50 + 50 + 50 minutes every day on my treadmill. I had stopped the disease progressing. I had stopped the disease damaging me further. But I had to give it 150 minutes per day to achieve that.

So I said to a close friend of mine: I can't win. Either I lose 10% of my life by dying early or I lose 10% of life by exercise. His response was. No you are still alive when you exercise. He was right. All that exercise is very good thinking time and it helped me with all sorts of problems in my life.

The next piece of the puzzle was curcumin, the active ingredient in the yellow Indian spice turmeric. I tried taking some curcumin tablets and for 7 days my sugar improved and I could get away with 90 minutes exercise rather than the normal 2 hours. But after 7 days type2 fought back and I returned to nearly 2 hours per day of exercise whilst continuing to take the curcumin.

LIFE OF BRIAN PART 2

In the meantime Brian had also become diabetic. But he had followed the mainstream medicine route. This led to him taking all sorts of diabetic pills, and then all sorts of further pills to treat the side effects of the diabetic pills. But he took no Omega3 and did not do much exercise. So he had 2 strokes and was hardy able to walk by the time we met up. His doctor told him that he might have to go on insulin injections.

Incidentally bad diabetic doctors tell their patients that so long as they keep their sugar in single figures, less than 10 mmol/L (less than 180 mg/dl) they will not do themselves much damage. This is false for many people. There are some diabetics who can take sugar up to 15 mmol/L (270mg/dl) for long periods. But many of us get serious damage above 8 mmol/L (144 mg/dl)

Brian knew that he was not going to last long unless he did something. So he contacted his old friend Gordon. This was difficult for him to do because I had become a full on biblical prophet and was spouting end times prophecies all of which were incorrect. So I did not have a huge amount of credibility in the eyes of most people. But Brian knew me better than that and he read my website www.cureddiabetes.com and saw that I could offer him an alterative path to the one he was on which he knew was not working.

When we reconnected Brian could hardly walk and was on over a dozen types of pills. So this is what I did. We took his sugar - it was around 8.4 mmol/L - and I took him out on a walk. It was very straightforward. I said I don't care how slowly you walk and I don't care how long this takes. But we are not going home until your sugar is 6 mmol/L (108 mg/dl). We are going to walk and walk and walk until you hit that number. Brain said: OK but how do you know that will happen? I said it is the laws of physics Brian. You have finite supply of sugar and we are going to burn it all off.

Fortunately Brian was living by the river Thames in London. So we had a nice slow walk along the side of the Thames. After an hour we took his sugar. It was 7.5 mmol/L (136 md/dl) not a dramatic improvement. But it was an improvement. Then we walked for another hour and Brian started getting tired. I told him one thing I learned from all the hours and hours of walking I had done. Legs are amazing. The more you use them the better they get. There were times when one leg was damaged and in pain. But somehow the other leg would compensate keep me walking. Humans are designed to walk. It is the best therapy our bodies can have. So I persuaded him to continue and the miracle began. Firstly his sugar went down to 6.5 mmol/L (117mg/dl) secondly he started to loosen up a little bit. We finally got him down to 6.0 and we went home. At that point Brian became a believer.

The thing was that he used to be in the Navy running team. Brian was no stranger to exercise training - he liked it. He just never realised how powerful a device it was in treating type2. He asked his girlfriend to bring him all his tablets. He then asked me which ones he should throw out. I said all of them except Metformin. I am not a doctor, but I did do a year of cell biology at Cambridge before I changed to Maths because my father insisted that I keep the door to medicine open. I had read the papers on the results of his various medications. The trouble with glipizide is that it can cause hypos with too much exercise. And in any event I knew from my hyper verbose diabetic doctor, that diet and exercise were more powerful than all the drugs in reducing sugar numbers.

So we changed Brian's diet and he started exercising by walking and rowing on his rowing machine and I got him a spin bike. After a few weeks his sugar had improved and we took his Metformin dosage down from 4 tablets per day to 2 tablets per day. Not only that but he could bend down and actually get into his car again. His whole body had loosened up and he felt great.

He found that lifting up heavy batteries sent his sugar flying up from 6 mmol/L (108 mg/dl) to 13 mmol/L (234 mg/dl). But the worst thing was eating a stale ham sandwich. That put it up from 6 mmol/L to 14 mmol/L. Yet another piece of the puzzle. By now both Brian and I were wearing the Freestyle Libre continuous Glucose monitors. These were to prove critical to eventually finding the cause and therefore the cure to Type2.

Brian and I would talk everyday and both learn from each other's dietary mistakes and successes. Basically eating takeout food was a disaster (unless extremely high quality) and eating low carb veggies and protein and flax and chia seed bread with plenty of butter worked very well.

But try as we might we could not get Brian's sugar down to totally normal levels - where mine was. So we decided to terminate his Metformin altogether. This initially put his sugar up and made it quite volatile. But after a week it settled down to the normal low level where mine was. At this point Brain could no longer resist going to see his doctor. He had his HbA1c taken and it came back normal. His doctor asked him what tablets he was taking now. Brian answered: None. A big smile appeared upon his GPs face. He said that he had 2 other patients who had managed the same feat and that doctors were beginning to recognise the power of diet and exercise in curing type2.

So by late 2018 Brian had completely loosened up. He could walk perfectly and he was very fit. Both he and I had normal sugar but we still had to do 2 hours of exercise per day and eat very low carb zero Omega6 fat diets to achieve it.

At this time I realised that I would have to spend the rest of my life exercising for 2 hours per day unless I did something dramatic. Incidentally I had also by now lost my potency. I could climax (just) but my nob would only rise up to about 60 degrees. I could not even get 90 degrees. I told this to Brian and he said: That's nothing mate, I can get 360!

I wanted to get back with the love of my life. I did not want to have to do 2 hours of exercise per day as I had been doing for 6 years. I had categorically proven that eating the right type of polyunsaturated oil (Omega3 rather than Omega6) helps, but does not cure type2. I had categorically proven that losing so much weight that I became skinnier than a Super Model did not fix type 2. I had categorically proven that going to a perfect dietary lifestyle with a huge amount of exercise does reverse your sugar numbers, and does prevent the disease from progressing. But it had become apparent that it did not as I had at first hoped, put the disease into regression. No you could stop losing but you could not win.

Incidentally, I had also discovered that Vitamin D helped quite a bit. Diabetics are often deficient in vitamin and proper Vitamin D levels help the immune system. And another theory was the Type 2 was some kind of autoimmune disorder.

But still Brian and I needed something more. We were breaking even. We were not winning.

THE BIG BREAK

Then I read a paper by Herapath Bird written in 1850 for the precursor to the British Medical Journal. The result is best explained by my revised letter to the editor of that Journal quoted here below...

Madam,

I write to disclose the causes of Type 2 diabetes and the permanent cure for them and to attempt to correct various misunderstandings which have plagued the clinical treatment of this condition in recent years and prevented mankind from getting to the true cause of the condition.

On March 25th, 1854 W Bird Herapath (MD London FRS Edinburgh) gave a paper read at the Quarterly meeting of the Bath and Bristol Branch of the Provincial Medical and Surgical Association. His paper was published in the Association Medical Journal LXIX April 28, 1854 page 374 This Journal I understand to be the predecessor to the BMJ.

Bird, treated a severe case of Type2 diabetes with 2-3 tablespoons per day of the yeast termed at that time "Torula Cerevisiae". The names of yeasts have been changed several times since then but as far as I can ascertain the modern name for that yeast is Candida Robusta, which is a common food fungus Mycobank has Torula Cerevisiae being referred to in 1840 in France as being Candida Robusta - *http://www.mycobank.org/BioloMICS.aspx?TableKey=14682616000000067&Rec=107064&Fields=All*)

Bird reasoned that the yeast would convert excess glucose which he believed to be present in his patient's intestines into alcohol or lactic acid and thereby improve his condition. In those days blood sugar was estimated from the grains of sugar per imperial pint of urine! His patient went from 850 grains per pint to 300 grains per pint within 2 days of the treatment and was fully cured in 6 weeks.

This case fascinated me because I had never seen a full cure of Diabetes Milletus before. Bird accepted in his article that he was presenting his singular result too early for concrete clinical conclusions to be drawn. But this candour convinced me that his findings were genuine,

I have been type 2 diabetic for 7 years and was managing my sugar exceptionally well with a low carb high good fat (Omega3 and dairy fat) low bad fat (Omega6 and Omega9 and animal meat fat) high fresh protein low preserved protein diet and exercise routine. My HbA1c has been 5.0%-5.2% (30-34 mmol/mol) for the last 6 years. Furthermore my insulin resistance is normal (HOMA IR1 is 1.2%). So having fixed both my fasting sugar levels and my HbA1c and my insulin resistance, I should in theory have cured my diabetes. But I am still diabetic having to do around 80 minutes of carb burning exercise per day on a low carb diet to keep my sugar at normal levels. However for 5 years I would go to sleep with sugar around 4.5 mmol/L and wake up with sugar around 4.5 mmol/L

So I decided to try this cure myself. I ate 100 grams of Young's Active Dried Yeast (manufactured by Lesaffre) over 4 days. The result was that my diabetes became uncontrollably bad. My sugar would shoot up after a meal and no amount of exercise would bring it back down again. I would burp and fart regularly and I smelt like a brewery. I postulated that since I had eaten beer yeast, perhaps wine would stop it. So I took 2 glasses of Chilean Merlot. That stopped the burping and farting and enabled exercise to bring my sugar back to normal. So for a week my condition improved and I was able to return my sugar to normal after my meal due to adding actually a bottle of red wine to the menu each day. But my sugar no longer remained static at night. It would rise and I would wake up initially at 6.0 and then 5.5 and then 5.2 mmo/l (during those 7 days).

The wonderful thing about my condition was that the burping and farting would physically tell me the level of activity of the yeast. And whenever they started I knew my sugar would rise. It became very obvious that this yeast was the cause of my much worse type2 and that it was setting my base/fasting sugar level not me.

Then I investigated what it was precisely in the wine that was inhibiting the yeast. I thought perhaps it was the alcohol. But brandy had very little effect. A diabetic friend of mine (Brian Bain) who also took this yeast and had precisely the same results as myself, tried some French Fitou and his condition improved just as mine had done. So we knew that something in the wine has inhibiting the yeast but it was not the alcohol.

This led me to believe that it was the Sodium/Potassium Metabisulphite (E223/224) or Potassium Sorbate (E202) that is put in most wine to prevent re-fermentation and preserve the vintage and stop it going mouldy. So my friend and I both made up a solution of wine preservative in the same ratio as one would use for wine (88mg/L of the Metabisulphite and 200mg/L of the Sorbate) and we drank a litre of it on January 25th. My results were stunning. My sugar went from 84 mg/dl to 59 mg/dl according to my brand new abbot freestyle continuous glucose monitoring sensor. These instruments underestimate sugar by around 20 mg/dl for the first 8 hours of use. So in truth the wine preservatives (E202 and E224) took my sugar from around 104 to 79 mg/dl.

This categorically proved that the yeast was setting my sugar levels. Of course the farting and burping stopped after having taken the Es. So I continued taking more of these Es which was a really, really bad idea, because they stun the yeast and then it comes back after about 6 hours. When the yeast came back, my sugar was worse than before because the Young's dried active yeast is more resistant to the inhibitor than the other yeasts in my gut. However here again was absolute proof that the yeast was setting my sugar level. If I drank the inhibitor the sugar level would fall actually to the level that it would be at if I was not diabetic. Then after the inhibitor wore off, my sugar levels would climb back to diabetic levels.

After 4 days of this treatment I had done significant damage to my gut flora and I terminated the treatment and went back to the Merlot and the Fitou. Then I became more diabetic than I have ever been before by a long way. My sugar rose at night, and during the day, even if I ate nothing all day. However the Merlot and the Fitou were having have less and less effect too (on January 27th I needed 2 bottles of Fitou and 140 minutes of spin biking per day to fix my post prandial sugar) which means that it must have been the combination of the Sulphites and the alcohol in those wines which inhibited the yeast.

So then, in order to prevent myself and Brian both becoming alcoholics, I terminated both taking the sulphites and the sorbate and wines containing them.

I should say here that all the way through this voyage of discovery, Brian and I would talk several times a day on the phone and compare notes. In this way were we able to determine which factors were affecting both of us and were therefore likely to be significant, and which factors were only affecting one of us and were therefore likely to be incidental.

I have been cavalier with my health. But in doing so I have found one of the causes of type 2. It is caused by at least one and probably more than one yeast.

One type of diabetes results from having more bad yeast than good yeast in the gut essentially, as my body has just demonstrated.

So now we can see what perhaps happened with Bird's patient. The Torula Cerevisiae he took in such large quantities was replacing the pathogenic diabetes causing yeast that his patient was suffering from.

Certainly we have now solved riddle of why certain wines are great for type 2 but alcohol per se is not. It is the combination of the alcohol and the sulphites and the sorbate that inhibits the diabetic yeast. We know this because it stops our burping and farting and our sugar returns to non diabetic levels. At least it did in my case until the yeast developed resistance to the inhibitors.

At present we have found that wine in small doses works very well (one small or large glass is best). But large quantities of wine or of the inhibitor do not.

Finally I went to see Prof Hay at the London Bridge Hospital and he prescribed Itraconazole. The minute I took the first capsule at noon on January 29th (not with a meal) my sugar shot down from around 126 mg/dl to 86 mg/dl within one hour. This was precisely the same effect that I had already seen with both red wine and the inhibitor. But the Itraconazole effect lasted for 15 hours. Then the sugar started climbing again and the farting and the burping recommenced.

I was on one 100 mg capsule per day, which was insufficient. So I took 2 glasses of wine and then took the 2nd pill at 6 am the next day, January 30th, after my once daily meal. Again my sugar came down and my gut felt a whole lot better.

But I was extremely scared given the rise after the 15 hours and I knew the dosage was too low, but was not interested in any more self medication. So I went to the absolutely wonderful St Thomas's A&E. They saw me very rapidly and upped the dosage to 100mg twice per day for both myself and my friend Brian Bain who had also eaten the yeast. This essentially cured Brian. But I had more of the yeast and more of the inhibitor. So I went back to A&E and the dose was doubled once more to 200 mg twice per day. That fixed the yeast infection. But then my original diabetes got markedly worse and became equally unmanageable.

This was fascinating. My diabetes became the most aggressive at maximum Itraconazole concentration 4-8 hours after taking the tablets. So this was not the yeast which was under maximum suppression during that period. Actually it was the toxic effect of the Itraconzazole, which although killing the yeast was also stressing out my guts and my liver. It is a very powerful antifungal drug.

On the 9th day of treatment I reduced the dosage in the morning with the meal to one 100mg tablet and kept the 2x 100mg at night which were taken without a meal and were therefore only 60% effective. This made my sugar much more manageable at peak Itraconazole level between 10:30 and 14:30 (4-8 hours after taking the capsules at 06:30). Brian was taking 100 mg with a meal twice a day.

So this ghastly strain of Saccharomyces Cerevisiae which the lab eventually identified as bog standard Saccharomyces Cerevisiae, has led us to the cause of the majority of type 2 diabetes cases. It is a type of yeast, which has the capability to set your fasting sugar level when overgrown and active in sufficient quantity.

Regards
Gordon Ritchie

At the height of my war against this yeast I honestly thought that it might kill me. I had to do 6 hours on a spin bike every day to keep my sugar at normal levels and I did not think my legs would hold out. I lost a stone in 4 weeks. I was doing 2/3 of a stage of the tour de France everyday on my spin bike aged 61. After the 14 day course of Itraconzaole my sugar remained unmanageable for a further 26 days. Towards the end of this period I was desperate to discover some other means of reducing my sugar numbers. The good news was that I knew the gut was where it was all happening and I knew that yeast was the cause. I read that curcumin was strongly anti fungal and almost as good as Itraconzaole and Fluconazole at killing yeast So I tried a new brand of curcumin with piperine in it from Oxford Vitality. It had the curcumin from 2500mg of Turmeric and it had 10mg of piperine (the active ingredient in black pepper). And it had no capsule so was very fast absorption and affected the stomach and the upper gastro intestinal tract. This helped a bit.

I also knew I should take a probiotic. But I was not going to eat any more microbes. That mistake was what put me in trouble in the first place. So I decided to go instead for a prebiotic (food for a probiotic). I found Bimuno a galacto oligosaccharide and Orafit Inulin a fructo oligosaccharide. These are not probiotics, but prebiotics, which are supposed to feed the good bacteria in your gut. I needed something to fight the yeast so I tried large quantities of these. I went for 1 and a third sachets of Bimuno per day and 12.5 grams of Orafti inulin. I also stopped drinking red wine.

Almost immediately things started improving. Then I tried different meats, measuring the post prandial trajectory of my blood sugar on my continuous glucose monitor, and found that Turkey was by far the best, presumably because it is the driest meat and so the least affected by fungi.

Then it was that the first breakthrough occurred. Around the 2nd week in March 2018 all of a sudden I only had to do three 25 minute exercises a day for normal sugar. Then 2 days later it was only 2 exercises per day. Then 2 days later only one exercise per day. Then 2 days later it was NONE. My sugar went up after my meal and then came down all by itself. I was astonished and elated and in a state of total disbelief.

What had happened was that the toxic effect of Itraconzaole had worn off. The body had recovered and the Itraconazole had left my system, it remains for a few weeks after the course has finished. But in addition to that, the good bacteria were winning out over the diabetic yeasts in my gut. I could watch my sugar go up after the meal and then come down like a normal person but without any exercise at all. In fact I would burp when my sugar went up and fart when it came down. The good bacteria were residing in the lower intestine (hence the farting) and the bad yeast in the upper intestine (hence the burping). the oligosaccharides were feeding the good guys and they were winning.

My second delivery of Orafti inulin tasted different to the first and did not work. After 3 days on this second batch my sugar stopped going down after meals and instead just sat there. So

I went to a new supplier: *www.hellenia.com* and their batch worked fine. This showed me that the oligosaccharides were critical in fully curing my condition. Regular inulin does not work. Orafti inulin (from beneo in Belgium) does work and I do not know why. You can tell if it is working because you will fart a lot a few hours after ingestion (at first).

All the way through this sorry tale of sheer panic on my part, the yeast would declare itself by burping, which would lead instantly to a rise in sugar. But then the cavalry would declare themselves by farting leading instantly to a fall in sugar. I have never loved farting so much!

So there I was, cured totally, as was Brian. We neither of us had to do any exercise for perfect sugar. I used to run around my bed at night not knowing what to do with my legs.

But in the back of my mind I was worried about a recurrence. So Brian and I both continued to wear our continuous glucose monitors. Then on the very same day that I starting burping a lot and my sugar started rising. Brian rang me and said the same thing had now happened to him. The yeast had grown back after the Itraconazole had gone and we were both diabetic all over again.

The only weapons we now had were the Bimuno the Orafti Inulin and the curcumin. So I put Brian on two curcumin tablets per day and took 3 myself having had the larger yeast infection. That stopped the burping and things retuned to normal for Brian who 3 months later stopped burping altogether and was fully cured both from the brewer's yeast infection and from type2. He no longer had to do any exercise. But I continued to burp and had to take more and more curcumin. I now know why, but I did not know at the time.

I was so scared, I lost my mojo. The only thing that pulled me through was my faith in God. I prayed to him and asked him to fix me if he willed, or if not to show me how to fix myself. He chose the latter path and I could not be more grateful to him.

The reason that Brian recovered from his yeast infection and I did not was that I could not take a bath due to my aching ball. In 2015 I got the correct diagnosis for the pain in my ball. It was Diabetic Erythrasma. The cure was supposed to be Erythromycin or Clarythromycin or just scrubbing with surgical standard anti bacterial scrubs such as Povidene or Chlorhexidine. The trouble is that I am actually no good with erythromycin. It causes me to come out in spots when applied topically. And to cut a long story short none of the standard treatments for Erythrasma ever worked on me and so I could not take a bath or a shower because Erythrasma loves water and I would be in agony afterwards. So my whole body was actually covered in fungus on the outside and my immune system was too busy fighting that to be able to win the battle against the yeast on the inside of my skin in the intestine.

I know that because when I started swimming in a chlorinated pool thanks to better.org, my skin cleared up and my burping stopped. This was because I reduced the fungal load on my immune system from my external skin so that it could concentrate all its resources on my internal skin, lining my gut, and beat the yeast.

But before I started swimming I was fighting the yeast infection by taking more and more curcumin tablets. I started off with 3x 2500 mg (the curcumin produced by 2500 mg of turmeric) per day and ended up taking 67 of them each day. This was not a good idea. Curcumin although antifungal is equally antibacterial. So it does inhibit the yeast but it also inhibits everything competing with the yeast. So the net effect is probably around zero especially in very large doses. The same actually is true of Oregano oil in large doses.

I also tried Nystatin, but it was not powerful enough and the yeast eventually become resistant to it somehow.

Infectious diseases at St Thomases suggested that I should try taking curcumin without piperine because the piperine caused the curcumin to be absorbed into the blood stream rather than to lie in the gut where the yeast was. I felt that advice was incorrect but followed it anyway because it was logical. That made my type2 a lot worse. It seems that the piperine puts the curcumin into the bloodstream and that helps kill the yeast, because this yeast feeds from sugar in the blood. Curcumin without piperine does not help. Curcumin with piperine does.

So I needed another tablet that selectively attacked the yeast but not the beneficial bacteria. I was in the classic Candida yeast overgrowth situation, which is yet another malaise for which mainstream medicine has no solution.

I found that tablet in the form of Candaway anti Canddia tablets from Lamberts or Nature's Best (the same company).

I have to say that I found them to be the best and you can take as many as you like no problem. They recommend taking 2 per day. I recommend 2 when you get up 2 before and after each meal and 2 before bed. Taking Candaway fixed my yeast overgrowth after around 6 weeks and fixed my type 2 diabetes to the point where I did no exercise actually for 3 months and I now have an HbA1c of 5.0%.

There is one further thing that really helps and that is cloves. I got that idea from Gwyneth Paltrow's GOOP website. Cloves are a strong antifungal. If you fry up some turkey and leave it in the pan for a day it starts to smell. If you add 5 cloves to it and leave it for a day - there is no smell. So I take one whole clove (as if it were a pill) with every Candaway tablet now.

So here I am 8 years after diagnosis. I can eat as many roast potatoes as I want. I can eat chocolate cake again. I can even eat rice. I no longer have to do any exercise and my sugar is better than most at my age. My peripheral neuralgia in the toe on my right foot has all but gone. I can walk around barefoot no problem. This is because God showed Brian and myself the cause. It was a damn yeast overgrowth.

In fact if you dose up on Candaway tablets and cloves and then eat chocolate cake and then take more candaway tablets and cloves you knock out any diabetic yeast you may have in your stomach before the chocolate cakes hit your guts and your sugar will not go up.

What happens when a diabetic eats sugar is NOT that the sugar goes into his bloodstream. No it feeds the yeast and the yeast multiplies and releases some kind of toxin into the blood stream or stresses out the gut and the immune system sends out an alarm to the rest of the system and that puts up your sugar. So now we can put all the pieces of the puzzle together as follows...

1. The reason my sugar went down after I ate the curry at the Bombay Palace was that the spices in a curry are antifungal. Indeed the purpose of using spices in a hot country is not only to improve the taste of the meat, but also to stop the meat going off.

2. The reason that drinking a glass of wine with a curry prevents blood sugar going up is that wine contains Potassium Sorbate which is a fungal inhibitor, which prevents the wine from going mouldy when stored in a cellar for 10 years. The inhibitor stops the diabetic yeast

overgrowth which causes type2 from operating which you are digesting the curry. So you feed your body rather than feeding the yeast.

3. The reason that curcumin can stop sugar gong up is that it is s strong antifungal.

4. The reason that type2 has the capability to fight back when you find an effective treatment (as was the case with Omega3 and curcumin) is that it is a living organism not a passive cellular condition.

HOW TYPE2 WORKS

When we eat carbs, the yeast becomes more active and overgrows more and that drives up your fasting sugar. We can see the sugar go up on our continuous glucose monitors and we can hear the yeast causing us to burp when it is active. The burping and the sugar rise are coincident. The burping is the Carbon Dioxide from the fermentation process. If we control the yeast with a mild antifungal then eating carbs does not push our blood sugar up much if at all.

The whole premise of type2 is that it is caused by insulin resistance. Well certainly type 2 causes insulin resistance but insulin resistance is not the cause. It is a gut microbe which when it is fed with carb, multiplies, and then irritates the gut and that puts up the fasting sugar. This was very obvious with the active brewers yeast. It is more clandestine with whatever is the main cause of type2 which is presumably a bacteria/yeast/microbe that infects rotten red meat (given how much an old ham sandwich will put up the blood sugar of a diabetic).

Whatever the microbe is, it is very prevalent in rotten red meat. **DO NOT EAT REHEATED red meat. RECOOK IT!**

Here is the logic that led us to a red meat eating gut microbe as the causative agent for type 2 diabetes.

1. If you eat a fresh steak your sugar will go up a bit. It you eat fresh steak mince or a steak burger it will go up a lot more. That is because mince has a much larger surface area for steak eating microbes to colonise and grow upon. So you are eating a lot more of the rotten meat eating microbes.

2. If you eat pork or beef sausage your sugar will go up a lot more than if you eat roast beef or roast pork. This is because you are eating old, non fresh, preserved, very large surface area, and ground up meat. So the meat eating microbes have had time to grow and plenty of surface area to grow on

3. If you eat roast lamb your sugar will not go up much. If you eat reheated roast lamb the next day (not re roasted - just reheated) then it will go up more. This is because there are more meat eating microbes on reheated lamb than there were on the original lamb. The worst possible example of this is a doner kebab. The writer (Gordon) used to buy a large lamb doner and eat half of it. Then he would leave the other half in the fridge and reheat it and eat that the next day. There is what gave him type2. He was eating 99% bacteria and 1% lamb!

4. If you eat freshly cooked roast pork your sugar does not go up much If you eat a ham sandwich which has been lying around in a shop for days, then your sugar goes bonkers. This again is due to the diabetes causing microbes present in the preserved old ham in the sandwich.

Here is the logic that led us to yeast overgrowth in the gut as being the fundamental cause of Type 2 Diabetes:

1. We ate 100 grams of live active Brewers Yeast (Saccharomyces Cerevisiae) and our type 2 diabetes became almost uncontrollably bad. Every time the yeast became active - detected by the most obvious burping and farting of fermentation gasses from the upper (burping) or lower (farting) intestine - our sugar would go up. And then when the burping and farting stopped, the sugar would go down. It could not have been more obvious.

2. If a type 2 diabetic drinks some wine with a meal, his sugar does not go up as much as normal. Whereas if he drinks whisky, there will be no effect on his sugar rise due to the meal. This is because wine contains the antifungal agent, potassium sorbate, a mould resister. It is put into wine to stop it going off, since it is generally stored for years. Most type 2 diabetics know that a large glass of wine helps with their sugar. We discovered why. It is because Type2 is caused by a yeast, a mould, which the sorbate inhibits. We actually used potassium sorbate to fight the yeast infection. We took a gram off potassium sorbate in water. DO NOT DO THIS. It worked the first time, reducing our sugar to normal levels. The second time it worked less effectively. The 3rd time it did not work at all. The brewers yeast became resistant to the very large quantities we were eating. **THIS DAMAGED OUR GUT FLORA. DO NOT TAKE POTASSIUM SORBATE.**

3. The husband of Gordon's true love, was non diabetic and never liked sweet things in his life until the age of 63, when he went mad for Stinking Bishop, the mouldiest cheese in the world. You can smell the stuff in the kitchen when you open the front door to your house. He ate huge amounts of it for a year. Then he went on holiday to a place where you could not get stinking bishop and his wife noticed that he started craving ice cream and sweet things which he had never done before in his life. He was always thirsty and drinking water like a fish. He was diagnosed as Type 2 diabetic when he returned home. He died of complications from Type 2 diabetes in 2018. He was killed by the mould in that cheese. The particular mould in the cheese may not be the precise causative agent for type 2. But all mould helps the moulds in the gut beat the bacteria and other microbes with which they compete. So his diabetic causing yeast started to overgrow, whilst his immune system was fighting the stinking bishop yeast.

4. Any type2 diabetic who has successfully managed to improve his sugar with a new supplement or dietary regime, will have found that the diabetes will fight back and after around 7 days he will be back where he started. That means type2 is not caused by a passive condition such as insulin resistance - which has no capability to fight back. It is caused by a living organism, which can fight back.

5. The writer has been eating way more Omega3 fat than Omega6 for over 7 years (triple strength fish oil and massive amounts of flax seed and chia seed bread and a small amount of rape seed oil). This helps but does not cure type 2. So type 2 is not caused by your cell membranes being made up of the wrong type of fat. For more on this see - Insulin Resistance

6. **THIS IS A CAST IRON MATHEMATICAL PROOF.** But nobody has any confidence in maths these days.

If a moderately to severely diabetic person eats 200 grams of sugar his blood sugar will go up say from 1 gram per litre (100 mg/dl) to 2 grams per litre (200 mg/dl). This means that each litre of his blood will contain twice as much sugar as normal. It will contain 1 gram more sugar than normal. So his entire body (which has 5 litres of blood), will contain 5 grams more sugar than normal. One teaspoon of sugar is all that it takes to double your blood sugar! But this means that the type 2 diabetic has successfully stored 195 grams of sugar, and has failed to store only 5 grams of sugar.

If that same diabetic eats only 100 grams of sugar, then his blood sugar will go to say 1.5 grams per litre (150 mg/dl). So he has failed to store 2.5 grams of sugar (and extra 0.5 grams per litre in 5 litres) and successfully stored 97.5 grams of sugar. But we know from the thought experiment above (or indeed from a real experiment) with 200 grams of sugar, that he has the capacity to store 195 grams of the stuff. So his sugar is NOT rising due to a lack of sugar storage capability. Neither is it rising due to insulin resistance, because he has enough insulin even with his level of insulin resistance to store 195 grams of sugar. He is simply not producing that insulin and not storing the sugar by metabolic choice. This shows that insulin resistance does not cause type 2. It is a result of type 2. The cause of type 2 is a hack of the body's sugar regulation mechanism by a yeast which eats sugar. The diabetic yeast is a true parasite. It turns you into a sugar factory for its benefit.

We know that viruses hack our DNA or RNA to turn our cells into virus factories. Well, now we see that yeasts hack our metabolism to turn our cells into sugar factories!

If you feed your yeast overgrowth with 100 grams of sugar, it produces enough toxin to put your sugar up to 150 mg/dl. If you feed your yeast overgrowth with 200 grams of sugar it produces enough toxin to put your sugar up to 200 mg/dl. The way to pass an oral glucose tolerance test (eating 150 grams of sugar in the form of Lucozade, is to dose up on antifungal first, to suppress the yeast, then drink the Lucozade, then take some more antifungal. This prevents the yeast overgrowth being fed by the sugar and your blood sugar will not go up as much.

7. The writer (Gordon) has completely cured his type 2 by taking antifungals and oligosaccharides, His HbA1c is now 5.0% and he does not exercise at all and eats potatoes, bananas and chocolate cakes etc. Gordon and Brian have shown that moderate to severe type2 can be reversed (sugars number returned to normal) by diet and exercise. Yes, but that is not a cure. It can be cured (the yeast overgrowth eradicated) by strong antifungals and the correct prebiotics within 3 months.

Itraconazole cured it temporarily (for 6 weeks after a 2 week course of 2x 100mg per day) but the yeast bounced back 6 weeks after the end of the course.

CANDEX helped initially a lot. But was not able to finish the job (It is worth taking for perhaps 4 weeks at most).

CANDAWAY and cloves finished the job

The cure is to feed yourself, NOT the diabetes causing gut microbes! So you must take antifungals before and after each meal to prevent the yeast overgrowth from getting any of your food.

8. It is known that low carb diets are more effective than low calorie diets (and more sustainable) in putting type 2 into remission and reversing sugar numbers (neither can cure Type 2). This is because yeasts eat carbs, not fat and not protein.

9. My girlfriend suggested in 2013 that I read a book called: The fungus link to diabetes - Doug A Kaufman 2003. She did this because I was diabetic and was prone to fungal infections. She was wondering which one was the cart and which one was the horse. I read the book which theorised that fungal infections had something to do with type2 but did not go as far as proving it. The author's latest post in 2013 can be found at: *https://knowthecause.com/diabetes-and-the-fungus-link/*

Thiazolidinediones such as Actos® and Avandia®, are used in the treatment of type2.
"An Indian study in 2011 proved that some of these thiazolidinediones exhibited remarkable Antifungal activity, while a 2011 Tennessee study declared that these drugs showed an ability to inhibit fungal growth comparable to Diflucan."

THE CURE

Duration: 8 weeks Turkeytarian

Permitted food:

1. Eat one large or two medium meals per day and no snacking at all.
2. No Vegetable oil at all except a small amount of organic rapeseed oil (the best vegetable oil for type 2 - rich in Omega3: Omega6:Omega3 is 2:1).
3. No Nuts at all. No sugar at all.
4. No Dairy at all except butter. No animal fat except a small amount of turkey fat with your fried or roasted turkey.
5. 2 thick slices of flax seed and white chia seed bread per day
6. Eat 25-50 grams of spreadable butter which is butter with a small amount of rapeseed oil (such as Lurpak spreadable). Do not eat butter containing any other type of vegetable oil.
7. 33 grams of WHITE chia seed, salba seed (not black chia seed), roasted at 105 centigrade for 80 minutes, then ground and mixed with 300 grams of water into a porridge. Then drink 200 grams of water with it. Store the white chia seed in a cold place (not the fridge). Only purchase it from retailers who store it cold such as Tesco or Sainsbury. Do not purchase it from Amazon or Ocado. Chia seed is like fish (very high Omega 3). It should be kept in the fridge (it is vegetable fish oil essentially). Take the Orafti Inulin and the Bimuno supplements below mixed into the ground chia seed of the porridge.
8. Eat FRESH Turkey meat (least fat). And fry it or roast it well to remove most of the fat. Eat 300 - 500 grams per day of it. Eat no other meat. Do not eat tinned or smoked or otherwise preserved turkey meat. Do not eat turkey Bacon.
9. Eat at least 400 grams of spinach per day (for Vitamin A etc.)
10. Eat no raw food (it contains mould)

11. Permitted cooked vegetables are:
    Spinach
    Chard
    French beans
    Mange tout
    Tomato
    Cauliflower
    Broccoli
    Broccoli spears
    Courgettes
    Marrow
    Sprouts
    Spring onion
    Rocket, Parsley, Mint, Coriander (cooked only)

EAT NO OTHER FOOD

Permitted drinks
Green Tea
Water
SUPPLEMENTS

When you get up:
4 grams EPA from molecularly distilled triple strength fish oil (it is important to limit the amount of other carrier oils in the pill which will be full of Omega6)

4 grams DHA from molecularly distilled triple strength fish oil

5,000 IU Vitamin D3

The curcumin from 2500 mg of Turmeric (with 10 mg of black pepper). (Oxford vitality is by far the best but is stored is awful cardboard pouches. Best to buy the small pouches and restore in small make up jars with screw tops.

400 mg Magnesium (we recommend Swanson premium triple magnesium complex - it stops all muscle cramps)

9 grams precisely of Orafti ST Inulin, which is available from www.hellenia.co.uk and manufactured by Beneo.com in Belgium (not insulin but inulin which is a fructo-oligosaccharide)

1 sachet of Bimuno (galacto-oligosaccharide) every day with the chia seed porridge. The oligosaccharides feed the good bacteria which bring your fasting sugar level down. You will notice the difference after 4 days.

2 Candaway tablets (Nature's best)

3 Cloves

500 mg of citric acid in a small glass of water (to remove traces of alcohol in the gut from yeast fermentation). Yeast loves Alcohol and makes it. We must eliminate it from our guts to beat the yeast.

Before each meal
2 Candaway tablets (Nature's best)

3 Cloves

500 mg of citric acid in a small glass of water (to removed traces of alcohol in the gut from yeast fermentation)

After each meal
2 Candaway tablets (Nature's best)

3 Cloves

500 mg of citric acid in a small glass of water (to removed traces of alcohol in the gut from yeast fermentation)

When you go to bed
The curcumin from 2500 mg of Turmeric (with 10 mg of black pepper). (Oxford vitality is by far the best but is stored is awful cardboard pouches. Best to buy the small pouches and restore in small make up jars with screw tops.

400 mg Magnesium (we recommend Swanson premium triple magnesium complex - it stops all muscle cramps)

2 Candaway tablets (Nature's best)

3 Cloves

500 mg of citric acid in a small glass of water (to removed traces of alcohol in the gut from yeast fermentation)

Exercise starting 2 hours after each meal.
30-45 mins on spin bike (comfortable pace)
OR 30 mins on rowing machine (low intensity)

OR 45-120 mins walk outside.

Alternate exercises as much as possible. Do not do the same one 3x in a row.
After 8 weeks you should be clinically non diabetic - in our experience. The writer can now eat what he wants and does not have to do any exercise at all. the yeast overgrowth that caused his type 2 had gone.

Things to buy

0. Abbot Freestyle Libre Continuous Glucose Monitoring system (or other CGM system). You cannot fight something that you cannot see - https://www.freestylelibre.co.uk/libre/
1. Cheap but good rowing machine. Amazon do one by Viavito for £199 with free postage - *https://www.amazon.co.uk/Viavito-Sumi-Folding-Rowing-Machine/dp/B0153NKCZG/* and by JLL for £179 plus postage - *https://www.amazon.co.uk/JLL-R200-Adjustable-Resistance Advanced/dp/3251464140/*
2. Cheap recumbent spin bike Amazon do one by JLL for £129 - *https://www.amazon.co.uk/JLL RE100-Recumbent-Exercise-Resistance/dp/B00QFNGBJK/*
3. Access to a treadmill or get a treadmill
4. Kenwood chef kitchen mixer
5. Cheap but effective modern kitchen blender (or coffee/spice mill) - *https://www.amazon.co.uk/Andrew-James-Nutri-Fit-Smoothie-Processor/dp/B01M5GE53B/*
6. White chia seed. This is the most effective anti diabetic food.

You will need to bake our flax seed and chia seed bread - it is really easy. On the first day I would eat nothing all day until dinner and then have the following: Typical 1 meal a day daily menu

2/3/4 thick slices of flax seed and chia seed bread, with spreadable butter, or pureed vegetable spread.

THEN

300-500 grams of turkey (breast or leg) fried in butter or roasted and tomatoes with fried Spinach or with steamed broccoli or with steamed sprouts or with steamed/fried Swiss Chard.

THEN

33 grams of roasted then ground WHITE chia seed (not black chia seed) with 300 grams of water mixed together into a porridge. Add the oligosaccharides to the porridge and mix them in. Then drink a further 200 grams of water with it. Store the white chia seed in a cold larder.

Do not take more than 50 grams of raw white chia seed per day (with 500+300 grams of fluid). A Clinical trial showed no ill effects from 40 grams of white chia seed per day for 12 weeks. Black chia seed will give you kidney pain at a much lower intake. White chia is the most Omega3 rich food there is and by far the better choice.

THEN

Wait for 2 hours to give your body a change to absorb some sugar, like a normal metabolism. Then do 30 minutes on the recumbent spin bike pedalling at just below the point where you have to breathe through your mouth. Then at least a one hour gap, then do it again. Then do it as many times as necessary to bring your sugar down to the desired level.

ALTERNATIVELY walk upon the treadmill as a brisk pace in the same pattern.
ALTERNATIVELY row SLOWLY for 250 strokes 3x with a 10 minute break between the rows and then do 2x 24 minute sessions on the spin bike. This deploys all of your muscles.

If you are using a treadmill you may have to walk (at a comfortable speed stretching yourself but not stressing yourself, just under the point where you have to start breathing through your mouth rather than your nose - this will be 50% of VO2 max) for 3 hours on the first day to get your sugar numbers to be half decent. Get the most impact absorbent trainers you can and use impact absorbing insoles inside then. I use 2mm Noenes in addition to Sorbothane pro insoles, PROTECT YOUR FEET. If your feet get blisters or sores they will heal very slowly due to type2. Your feet are your main weapon against type2. And it is as if type 2 knows this. It will mercilessly attack your feet.

You have a choice
1. Recumbent spin bike - just slower than or at the point where you have to breath through your mouth
2. Rowing machine - SLOWLY
3. Treadmill - just slower than or at the point where you have to breath through your mouth

Those are the only exercises (other than walking outside) that have a large effect in our experience)

If you use a rowing machine then row slowly not quickly. Rowing quickly puts sugar up. Rowing slowly brings it down. This is not the case for the bike or the treadmill. They will reduce sugar even at a medium pace. Whereas a medium pace row will not reduce sugar. This is because rowing increases the blood supply to the guts which helps the yeast is done to vigorously!

This has something to do with power muscles in the arms and legs verses endurance muscles of the core. Endurance muscles should be exercised slowly and repeatedly. Power muscles should be worked much harder. Toning your endurance muscles in your core appears to be the best strategy for type 2. It reduces sugar without burning too many calories. It is not stressful to do.

CONCLUSION

It took us 8 years to discover the cure but we can explain it in the following dietary intervention and exercise tables

1. Low calorie diet - only of use if overweight.
2. Low carb diet - better
3. Ketogenic diet (very low carb and high protein) - better
4. Paleo Ketogenic (+ high Omega3:6 + high fibre) - better
5. Antifungal Paleo Ketogenic diet (+candaway +cloves +citric acid) - better
6. Oligosaccharide Antifungal Paleo Ketogenic diet (+Bimuno +Orafti Inulin) - better
7. Supplemented Oligosaccharide Antifungal Paleo Ketogenic diet - best

There will be a probiotic which helps - we have not discovered it yet.
One meal per day is best. Two meals per day with no snacking will get you there a bit more slowly.

Never give up (Churchill)
Keep asking questions (Einstein)
Keep on asking and ye shall be answered (Jesus Christ)

1. 45-120 minute walk on level ground at a reasonable pace
2. 45 minutes on a spin bike at a stretching but not stressful pace
3. 30 minutes LOW INTENSITY rowing machine at a slow comfortable pace (least effective)
4. Start exercising one hour after the meal.
5. Do not do the same exercise twice in a row

6. Leave one hour between each exercise.
7. Keep exercising until your bedtime sugar is below 6.0 mmol/l (108mg/dl)
Exercise should be done an hour after the meal (to give your insulin a chance to do some work too.

Rowing increases blood flow to the gut which is not a great idea. Rowing will drop your sugar nicely but one does not want to increase blood flow to a gut which has a diabetic overgrowth. So if you row too fast, which is easy to do, it will not be so effective because you are feeding the bad guys in your gut which eat the sugar from your blood.

Exercising for 20 minutes is no good because the first 10 minutes has a release of adrenalin which puts sugar up and needs to be burnt off.

The aim is to exercise every different muscle that you can. We wish to deploy all our muscles in the war against type 2.

Whilst rowing it is a good idea to exercise the neck, and do shoulder rolls, and generally try to exercise the muscles that other regimes do not reach.

FINAL ADVICE AND TIPS

Please do not be scared of Type2. You can conquer it. It is just a gut overgrowth of bad diet microbes. It does not matter how old you are. It does not matter how ill you are. Go antifungal, go prebiotic, go low carb, go paleo, and walk, and spin bike, and road bike and swim your way down to below 6.0 mmol/L (108 mg/dl) every night before bed.

If your sugar gets stuck in one place for a long time do 5 minutes of higher intensity exercise to dislodge it. Either a jog, or an uphill cycle ride, or reasonably fast on a spin bike.

Keep up the protocol and in our experience the day will come when you can eat what you like (in moderation) and keep a normal HbA1c with a 45 minute walk twice a week.

1. The trouble with natural antifungals is that they are not quite strong enough. The trouble with prescription antifungals such as fluconazole and Itraconazole, which are strong enough, is that they are quite toxic and so can only be taken for short periods, and they suffer from bounce back. So our solution is to take as much natural non-antibacterial antifungal supplementation as you possibly can and over a prolonged period. Oregano oil is antifungal but too antibacterial so does not help much. Curcumin with pepper and vitamin C is strong antifungal but also fairly antibacterial. So only take a limited amount of that. Feel free to try other natural antifungals

2. Garlic oil is a good antifungal and not too antibacterial. It works well. You can add high strength garlic oil supplementation to the regime (after each meal). If you find any other natural antifungal which is not too antibacterial it may also help. Check its effect with a glucose monitor.

3. Please consult your doctor about our dietary and exercise routines.

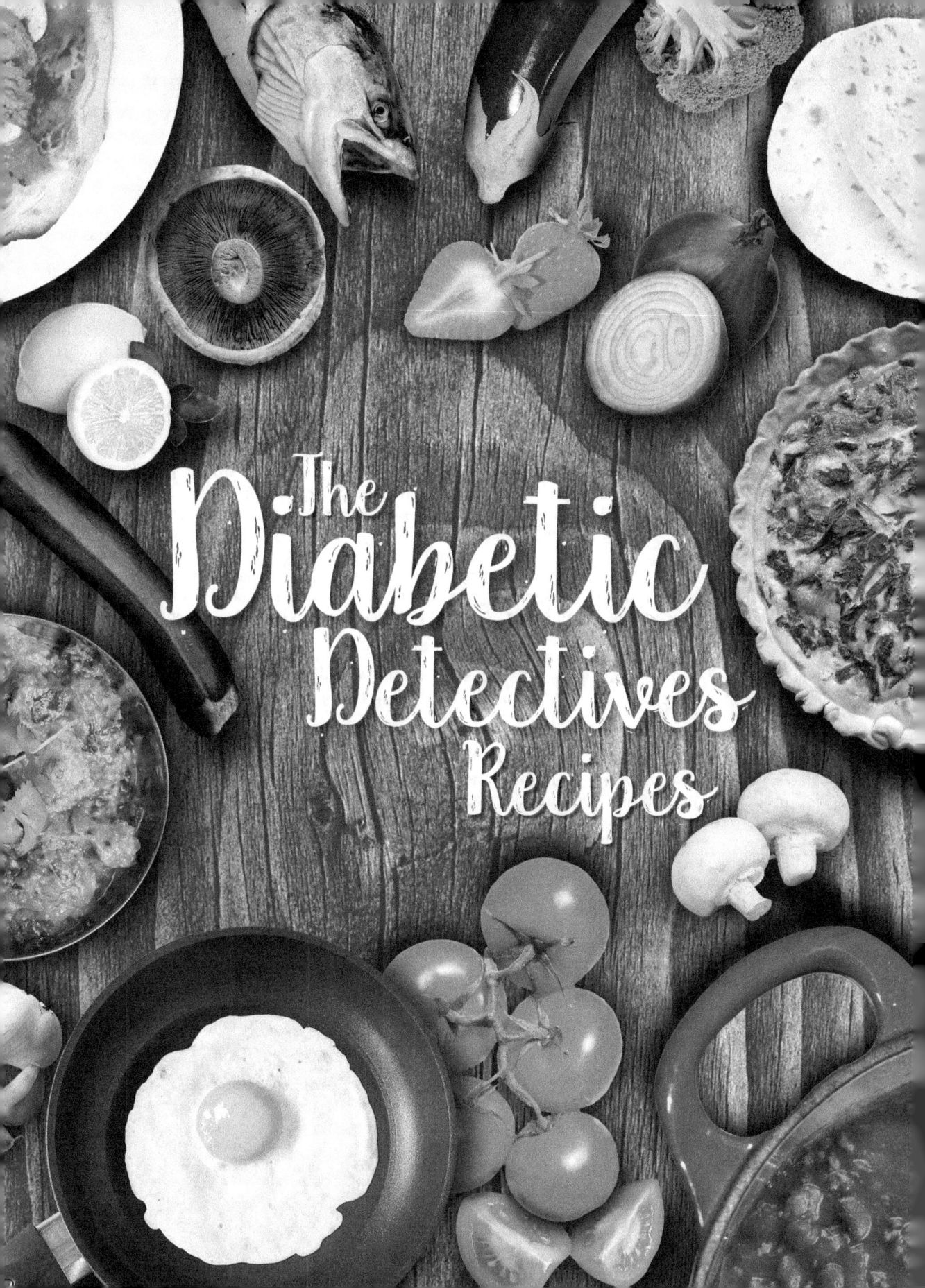

Introduction

Welcome to the Diabetic Detectives Recipe section of the book. Our dishes are categorised as easy, simple and medium difficulty {each recipe has a black circle with a number in it to give you the difficulty of the recipe to cook. 1 - Easy, 2 - Simple and 3 - Medium) ; although even an inexperienced cook can achieve a decent result with the more difficult recipes, it's easier than you think!

In most cases there maybe only one person who is diabetic in a household, but that doesn't mean that the rest of the family cannot share the dishes in this book, they are designed to be tasty and they are healthy for non diabetics as well. It was tempting to do dishes for one, but the flavours can be severely diminished as it's nigh on impossible to use, for instance, a quarter of an egg in a recipe and the subsequent wastage that would inevitably occur. In a family it would also mean that two meals would have to be prepared, which is time consuming and in most cases would cause problems in the average kitchen especially if everyone wanted to eat together. Instead, we felt that in would be better to create larger dishes that the whole family can enjoy together. However, if it is the case with you that either you are alone or that the family just can't get used to the new flavours that this book introduces, we felt it better that you make a larger dish that you either place in the fridge and eat within a couple of days or that you freeze that which you do not consume.

We've given all the recipes' ingredients weights, e.g. teaspoons, tablespoons and even a bay leaf but these small weights don't have to be strictly adhered to, just use a teaspoon or a tablespoon or one bay leaf etc as per the recipe. All timings are guidelines based on our kitchen, so when we say - "Bake until it's golden brown", we are giving flexibility to our timings. In my opinion, and let's face it, it's one of life's little mysteries, there can be no predetermined time for achieving this. The key thing is to be engaged in the act of cooking and the rule is that you just have to keep checking, on everything. The more time and love that you put into cooking a meal, the more love you transmit to those that eat that meal.

Just be aware that these recipes were constructed and produced in a particular place and to particular palates, your physical environmental conditions and your palate are different. I made the White Tuscan Pie (on page 111) for some friends and I was a little liberal with the herbs and I found that, for me, the herbs overpowered the dish. My friends disagreed, they loved the herbs! So the lesson was, keep experimenting with any recipe until it suits you and those you are cooking for, just remember you won't please everyone. The secret is to get a feel for a recipe and adapt it accordingly, the recipe isn't sacrosanct. Don't worry if things go wrong, learn from the mistakes. Some good rules to follow are: when making a sauce or dough (as in our bread and pastry), or adding any liquids to your dish, measure the required amount, but gradually add the liquid to the dish until the desired consistency is reached (even add more if needed). When adding spices or herbs, measure the amount and gradually add them, leave for a few minutes, then taste to see if it is right for you and add more if you'd like a stronger flavour (especially important with hot spices).

When it comes to our low carb breads, pizzas, pastry and Yorkshire puddings, these are delicious alternatives to the traditional products. The traditional foods are high in carbs and contain unbalanced fats. Our recipes are low carb, balanced fat, good fat recipes that are great for diabetics. Most low carb bread recipes that are available contain Almond flour or Coconut flour etc. but these fats are inflammatory and should be avoided.

For US readers we've added a section at the back of the book of the most common differences in food names and a conversion guide for grams to cups and metric to imperial. We've also included a glossary

Introduction

of the most common cooking terms. All cooking oven temperatures (gas mark, °C and °F) are based on a fan assisted oven. For conventional ovens add 20°C (40°F) and use conversion guide for the gas mark equivalent using the adjusted +20°C.

Note: Most of the nutritional data for our recipes is per serving and not per 100 g (some are per recipe, i.e. Dill Pickled Gherkins on page 169), no 100 g of food is above 15 g in carbohydrates.

Thank you for reading, and enjoy our low carb, balanced fat diet. Happy cooking!

Gordon Ritchie

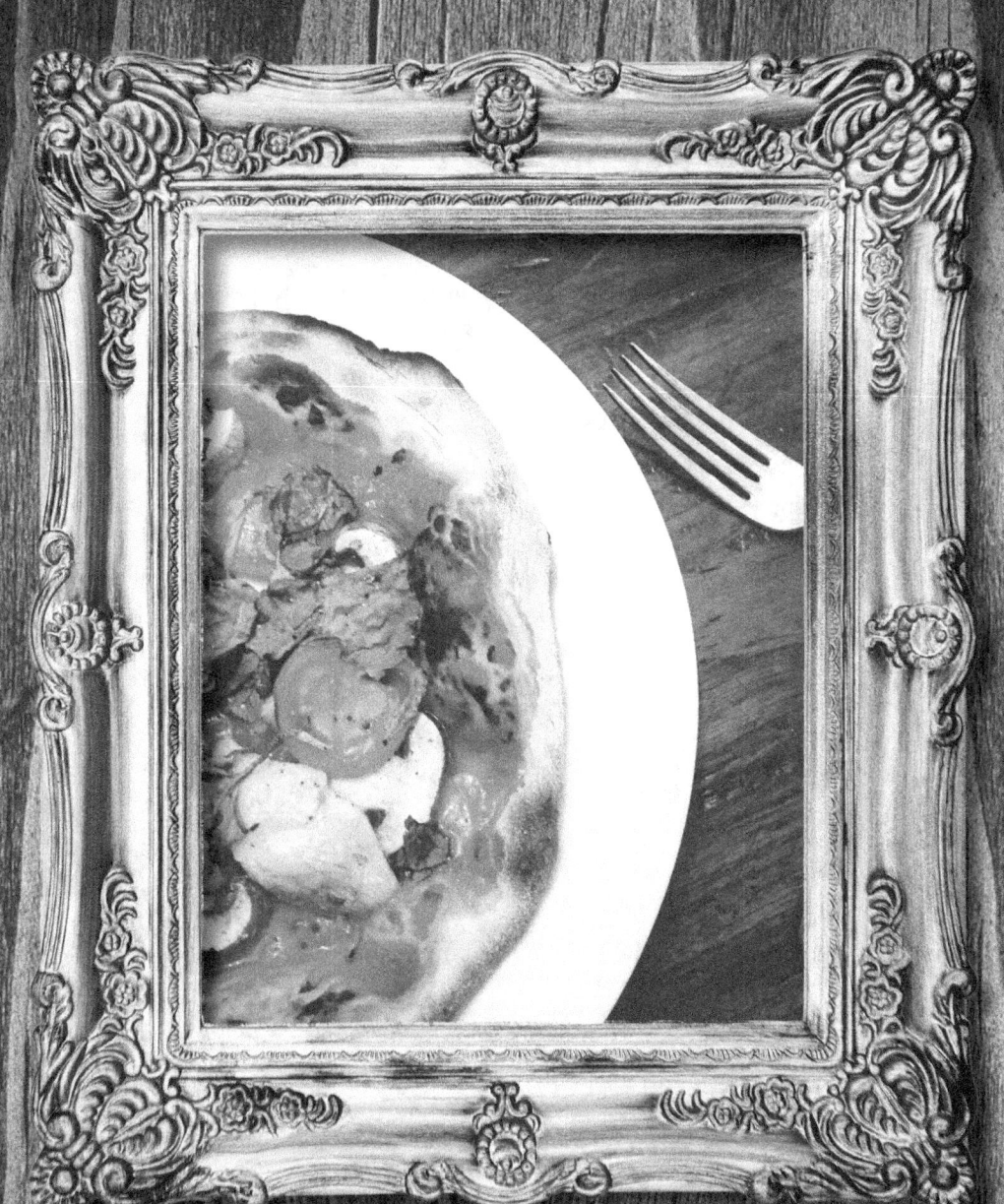

Bread & Pizzas

Flax & Chia Seed Bread

Regular bread is around 9% protein, 40% carbohydrate, 3% fat and 4% fibre (by weight). This recipe has 20 times less carbohydrate, 4 times more fibre, 2 times more protein and 6 times more fat (seed fat) than your regular loaf. This bread is wheat free, gluten free and egg free and has high amounts of Omega 3, fibre and protein - and no appreciable carbohydrates, only 1¼ g per slice.

Makes a 1 kg loaf - 16 slices (1 cm thick)

INGREDIENTS
266 g Flaxseed, ground into flour
133 g white Chia (Salba) seeds, ground into flour
40 g Psyllium Husk, ground into powder
40 g Rice Protein
12 g Baking powder
750 ml water

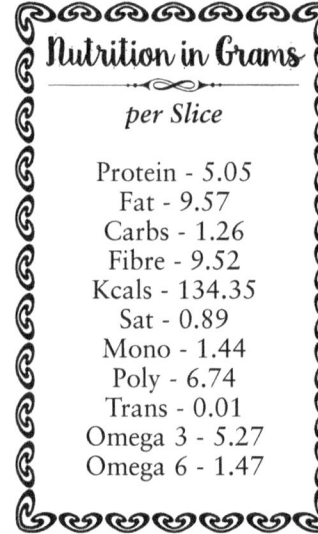

Nutrition in Grams per Slice

Protein - 5.05
Fat - 9.57
Carbs - 1.26
Fibre - 9.52
Kcals - 134.35
Sat - 0.89
Mono - 1.44
Poly - 6.74
Trans - 0.01
Omega 3 - 5.27
Omega 6 - 1.47

Grind the Flaxseed and Chia Seeds into a fine powder in a Cuisinart spice mill or a coffee bean grinder or a powerful blender or best of all in a NutriBullet with the milling blade (this makes wonderful flour). Grind the Psyllium Husk into powder. Add all the powders together with the rice protein and mix together well (using a Kenwood chef or a similar device with a dough hook).

Pour in the water and mix with the Kenwood Chef on a fairly fast setting for around 1½ minutes until the dough sticks to the mixing attachment and not to the side of the bowl. The dough should now have the consistency of putty. Scoop the dough out and slap it with your hands until all the cracks have gone and a subway type shape is achieved. If the dough sticks to your hands a lot then you have used too much water.

Pre-heat the oven to gas mark 8 - 210°C (410°F). Put the dough in the 900 g/2 lb loaf tin. Bake for 1 hour and 10 minutes in the centre of the oven. The great thing about this loaf is that it hasn't enough carbs to attract the bacteria, consequently it will stay fresh in the fridge for a couple of weeks.

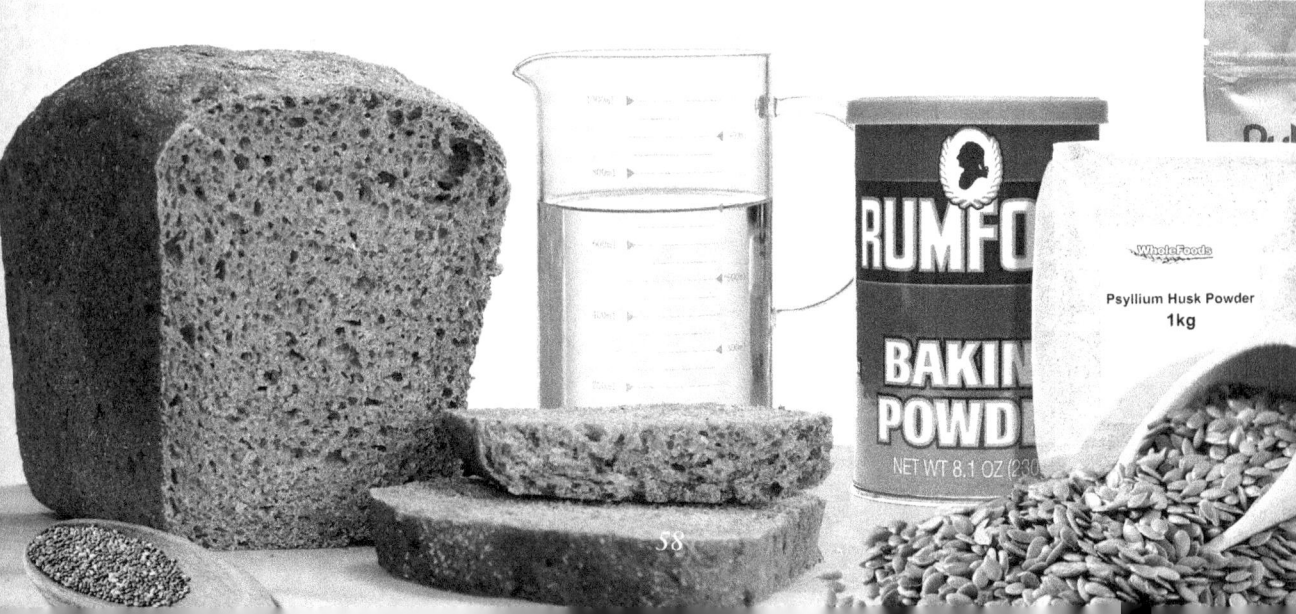

Bread & Pizzas

Low Carb Buns
Makes 4 Buns

INGREDIENTS
100 g Flax seed, ground into flour
50 g white Chia (Salba) seeds, ground into flour
19 g Psyllium Husk, ground into powder
15 g Rice Protein
5 g Baking powder
280 ml water

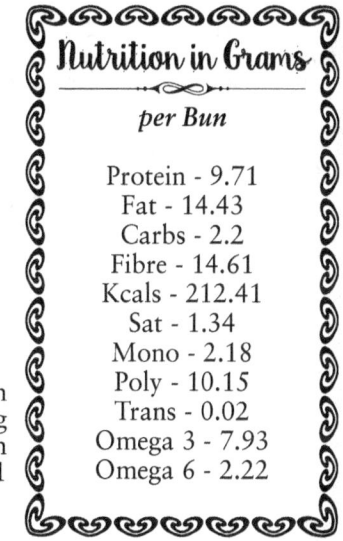

Nutrition in Grams

per Bun

Protein - 9.71
Fat - 14.43
Carbs - 2.2
Fibre - 14.61
Kcals - 212.41
Sat - 1.34
Mono - 2.18
Poly - 10.15
Trans - 0.02
Omega 3 - 7.93
Omega 6 - 2.22

Follow the recipe for the Flax and Chia Seed Bread, but split the dough into 4 equal bun shaped parts. Place the 4 dough in an indented baking tray with 4 indents 10 cm/4 inches in diameter and roughly 1 cm/½ inch in depth. Pre-heat the oven to gas mark 8 - 210°C (410°F). Bake for 1 hour and 5 minutes in the centre of the oven.

Low Carb Tortillas
Serves 2

INGREDIENTS
50 g ground Flaxseed
25 g white Chia (Salba) seeds
9 g Psyllium Husk Powder
7½ g Rice Protein
2 g Baking Powder
5 ml Olive oil
140 ml water

Nutrition in Grams

per Serving

Protein - 7.85
Fat - 7.25
Carbs - 1.5
Fibre - 7.61
Kcals - 120.65
Sat - 0.68
Mono - 1.1
Poly - 5.08
Trans - 0.01
Omega 3 - 3.96
Omega - 1.12

Preheat the oven to gas mark 6 - 200°C (400°F). Grind the seeds in spice/nut mill, coffee bean grinder or a powerful blender. Pour all the seed flours into a bowl. Add the Psyllium, rice protein and the Baking Powder and mix together well with a dough mixer (i.e. Kenwood Chef).

Pour in the water and olive oil and mix with the Kenwood until the dough sticks to the mixing attachment and not to the side of the bowl. Remove the dough out and separate into two equal amounts. Slap the 4 dough with your hands until all the cracks have gone and a nice smooth ball of dough is made. Flatten the dough onto a baking tray either by slapping it with your hands or by rolling it out as thin as you can. Bake for 25 minutes in the centre of the oven.

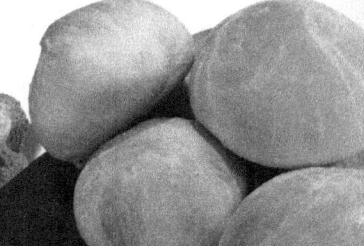

Bread & Pizzas

Garlic Bread

This delicious Low Carb French stick bread can be served as an appetizer, a side dish or as large croutons for a soup. It's crispy on the outside, soft on the inside and has a lovely flavour thanks to the garlic butter.

Serves 8

INGREDIENTS

1 portion of Low Carb Buns dough (see page 59)

Garlic Butter

100 g Low fat (light) Spreadable Butter with rapeseed or olive oil (or both)

2 Garlic cloves (12 g), crushed

2 tablespoons (30 g) fresh Parsley, finely chopped

½ teaspoon (2½ g) salt

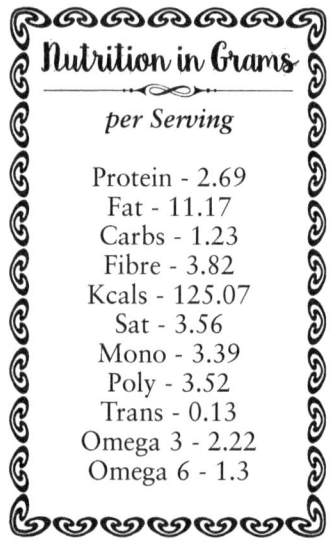

Nutrition in Grams

per Serving

Protein - 2.69
Fat - 11.17
Carbs - 1.23
Fibre - 3.82
Kcals - 125.07
Sat - 3.56
Mono - 3.39
Poly - 3.52
Trans - 0.13
Omega 3 - 2.22
Omega 6 - 1.3

Prepare the bread dough as per the instructions previously. Preheat the oven to gas mark 5 - 175°C (350°F). Roll the dough into a large sausage shape about 2 inches in diameter. Grease a baking tray with a little spreadable butter, place the dough onto it and put into the centre of the oven. Bake for about 40-50 minutes, or until it has risen well and is crusty on top. Remove the bread and let it cool on a rack.

You can make the garlic butter while the bread is baking. Just simple mix all the ingredients together in a bowl until it's a smooth paste and put it in the fridge until you ready to spread it on the bread.

Turn your oven up to gas mark 9 - 225°C (425°F). When the bread has cooled down, cut it evenly with a bread knife into 1 inch thick slices. Take the garlic butter out of the fridge and spread it over one side of each slice. Place the bread slice onto the baking tray butter side up and bake for 15 minutes, until golden brown and crispy.

Low Carb Naan Bread

These are a great accompaniment to our Chicken and Spinach Balti recipe or for that matter, any curry dish, replacing the rice.

Serves 2

INGREDIENTS

50 g ground Flaxseed

25 g white Chia (Salba) seeds

9 g Psyllium Husk Powder

6 g Baking Powder

Bread & Pizzas

7½ g Rice Protein

7½ g Olive oil

140 ml water

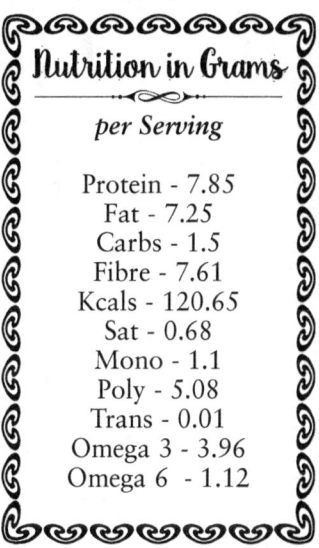

Nutrition in Grams

per Serving

Protein - 7.85
Fat - 7.25
Carbs - 1.5
Fibre - 7.61
Kcals - 120.65
Sat - 0.68
Mono - 1.1
Poly - 5.08
Trans - 0.01
Omega 3 - 3.96
Omega 6 - 1.12

Preheat the oven to gas mark 7 - 200°C (400°F). Grind the seeds in spice/nut mill, coffee bean grinder or a powerful blender (e.g. NutriBullet with a milling blade). Pour all the seed flours into a bowl. Add the Psyllium, rice protein and the Baking Powder and mix together well (Kenwood chef).

Pour in the water and olive oil and mix with the Kenwood until the dough sticks to the mixing attachment and not to the side of the bowl. Remove the dough out and split into 2 equal amounts. Slap each half with your hands until all the cracks have gone and a nice smooth ball of dough is made. Flatten the 2 dough onto a baking tray either by slapping it with your hands or by rolling it out to about 1 cm/½ inch thick. Place in the top half of the oven and cook for 25 minutes.

Low Carb Pizza Base

The secret to an ultra Low Carb Pizza is simply an ultra Low Carb pizza bread base. Here are some recipes for a 30 cm/12 inch pizza.

Serves 4

Nutrition in Grams

per Serving

Protein - 7.85
Fat - 9.75
Carbs - 1.5
Fibre - 7.61
Kcals - 143.13
Sat - 1.04
Mono - 2.93
Poly - 5.28
Trans - 0.01
Omega 3 - 3.98
Omega 6 - 1.31

INGREDIENTS

Pizza Base

100 g ground Flaxseed

50 g white Chia (Salba) seeds

19 g Psyllium Husk Powder

12 g Baking Powder

15 g Rice Protein

15 g Olive oil

240 ml water

Grind the seeds in spice/nut mill, coffee bean grinder or a powerful blender (e.g. NutriBullet with milling blade). Pour all the seed flours into a bowl. Add the Psyllium, rice protein and the Baking Powder and mix together well (Kenwood chef).

Pour in the water and olive oil and mix with the Kenwood until the dough sticks to the mixing attachment and not to the side of the bowl. Remove the dough out and slap it with your hands until all the cracks have gone and a nice smooth ball of dough is made. Flatten the dough onto a baking tray either by slapping it with your hands or by rolling it out.

Pizza Toppings

Margherita

One portion of the Low Carb Pizza Base (see page 61)

INGREDIENTS

50 g Passata
100 g grated Mozzarella
3 large fresh Tomatoes, sliced (150 g)
1 teaspoon dried Basil (5 g)

Pre-heat the oven to gas mark 6 - 200°C (400°F). Spread the Passata evenly over the pizza base and sprinkle the dried basil over the top. Add the grated Mozzarella all over the pizza and place the sliced tomato evenly over the cheese. Cook in the top half of the oven for 25 minutes.

Nutrition in Grams
per Serving including base

Protein - 12.2
Fat - 23.29
Carbs - 3.9
Fibre - 14.24
Kcals - 309.15
Sat - 5.33
Mono - 6.19
Poly - 10.64
Trans - 0.22
Omega 3 - 7.99
Omega 6 - 2.64

Anchovies or Tuna with Capers 1

One portion of the Low Carb Pizza Base (see page 61)

INGREDIENTS

50 g Passata
100 g grated Mozzarella
1 clove finely chopped Garlic (6 g)
150 g sliced Tomato
160 g or 1 tin Tuna in brine/Olive oil but not in Sunflower oil or
100 g or 2 tins of Anchovies in brine/Olive oil but in Sunflower oil
1 heaped teaspoon small capers (8 g), rinsed if salty

Nutrition in Grams
per Serving including base

Protein - 21.7
Fat - 23.67
Carbs - 4.25
Fibre - 13.86
Kcals - 350.97
Sat - 5.39
Mono - 6.21
Poly - 10.76
Trans - 0.22
Omega 3 - 8.07
Omega 6 - 2.65

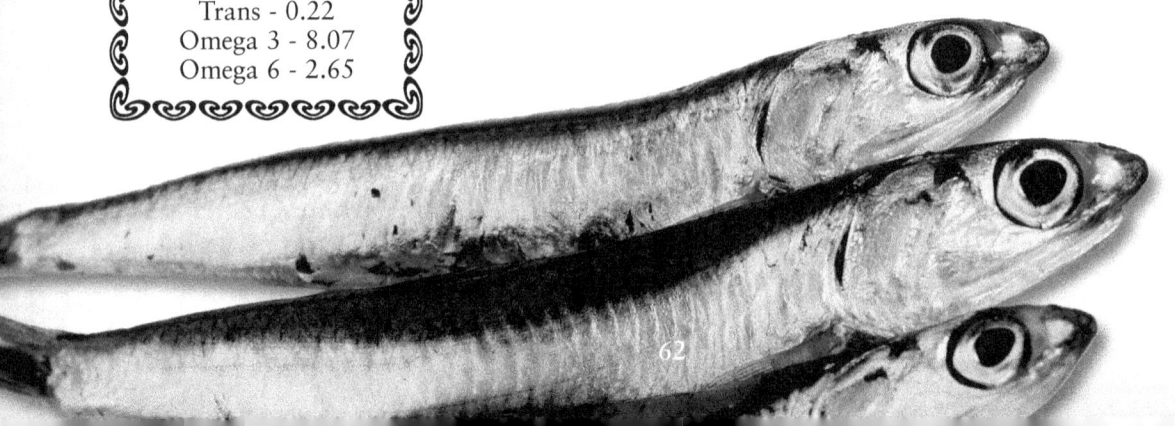

Bread & Pizzas

Pre-heat the oven to gas mark 6 - 200°C (400°F). Spread the Passata evenly over the pizza base and sprinkle the chopped garlic on top. Add the grated Mozzarella all over the pizza and place the sliced tomato evenly over the cheese. Place the anchovies or the tinned tuna randomly or creatively across the pizza. Cook in the top half of the oven for 25 minutes.

Barbecue Chicken

One portion of the Low Carb Pizza Base (see page 61)

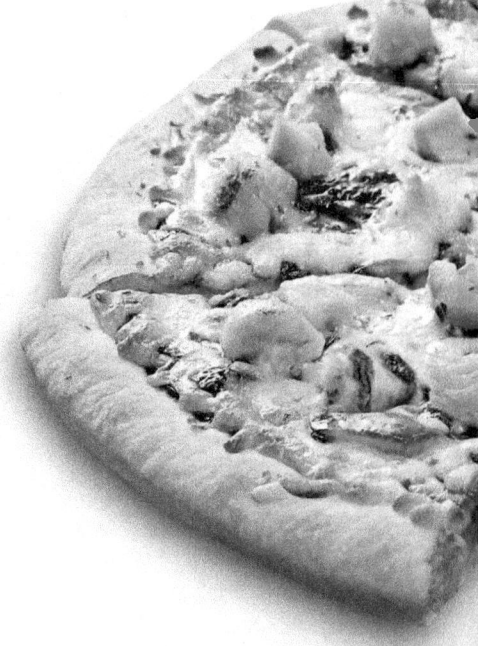

INGREDIENTS
400 g Chicken breasts
1 small Red Onion (150 g), finely chopped
100 g grated Mozzarella
A handful of fresh Coriander to garnish (30 g)

Barbecue Sauce
½ teaspoon (2½ g) Olive oil
30 g Red Onion, finely chopped
100 g Tomatoes, chopped
½ garlic clove (3 g), finely chopped
½ teaspoon (2½ g) Stevia
1 teaspoon (5 ml) Red Wine Vinegar
1 teaspoon (5 ml) Worcestershire sauce (see page 94)
½ teaspoon (2½ g) Tomato Purée
1 teaspoon (5 ml) Macadamia oil or Rapeseed oil for frying

Nutrition in Grams

per Serving including base

Protein - 34.92
Fat - 27.81
Carbs - 8.42
Fibre - 14.43
Kcals - 461.25
Sat - 6.15
Mono - 8.35
Poly - 11.14
Trans - 0.23
Omega 3 - 8.03
Omega 6 - 3.07

First, make the barbecue sauce. Pre-heat the oven to gas mark 6 - 200°C (400°F). Heat oil in a frying pan and add the onion. Cook over a low heat until softened and translucent. Add the remaining ingredients, season and mix. Bring to the boil, then reduce the heat and simmer for 25 minutes, until thickened. For a smooth sauce, simply pour the mixture into a food processor or a blender and blend for a few seconds.

Put the chicken breasts in an ovenproof dish, season with a little salt and pepper and brush with a little of the barbecue sauce mixture. Put it in the centre of the oven and bake for about 20 minutes or until the chicken flesh is white (just stick a knife in it and if it is still pink, carry on cooking - checking every few minutes - until it is white). When cooked, remove from the oven and leave to cool, and then cut the breasts into 1 cm/½ inch cubes.

Spread the remainder of the barbecue sauce evenly over the pizza base and cover with the mozzarella cheese. Evenly spread the chicken cubes over the cheese, followed by the red onions. Cook in the top half of the oven for 25 minutes and when done garnish with coriander and serve.

Bread & Pizzas

Beef & Basil ①

One portion of the Low Carb Pizza Base (see page 61)

INGREDIENTS
300 g Lean Beef mince (5% fat)
100 g Mozzarella cheese, grated
1 medium Onion, finely chopped (200 g)
2 cloves of Garlic, crushed (12 g)
1 teaspoon dried Basil (5 g)
Some fresh Basil leaves (10 g)

Nutrition in Grams

per Serving including base

Protein - 29.72
Fat - 26.41
Carbs - 7.4
Fibre - 14.56
Kcals - 423.07
Sat - 6.68
Mono - 7.44
Poly - 10.79
Trans - 0.32
Omega 3 - 8.04
Omega 6 - 2.75

Pre-heat the oven to gas mark 6 - 200°C (400°F). Fry the onion and garlic in a little rapeseed oil on a low heat until the onions are soft and translucent. Add the minced beef and dried basil and fry over a higher heat for 5 minutes, stirring constantly, until the meat is browned all over. Spread Passata over your base. Top with the mozzarella cheese, the beef mixture and the sliced tomatoes, in that order. Cook in the top half of the oven for 25 minutes. Sprinkle with some fresh basil leaves and serve.

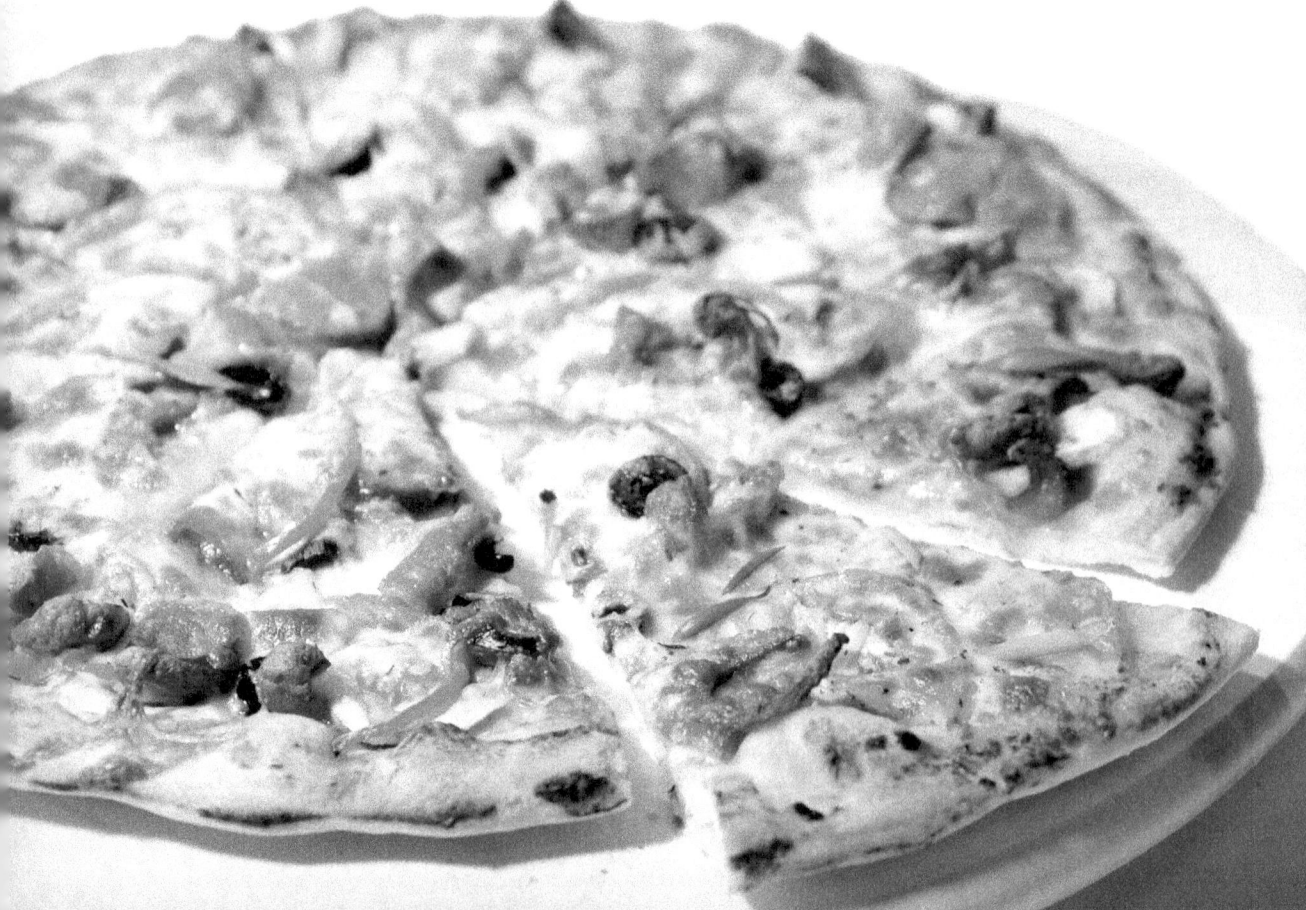

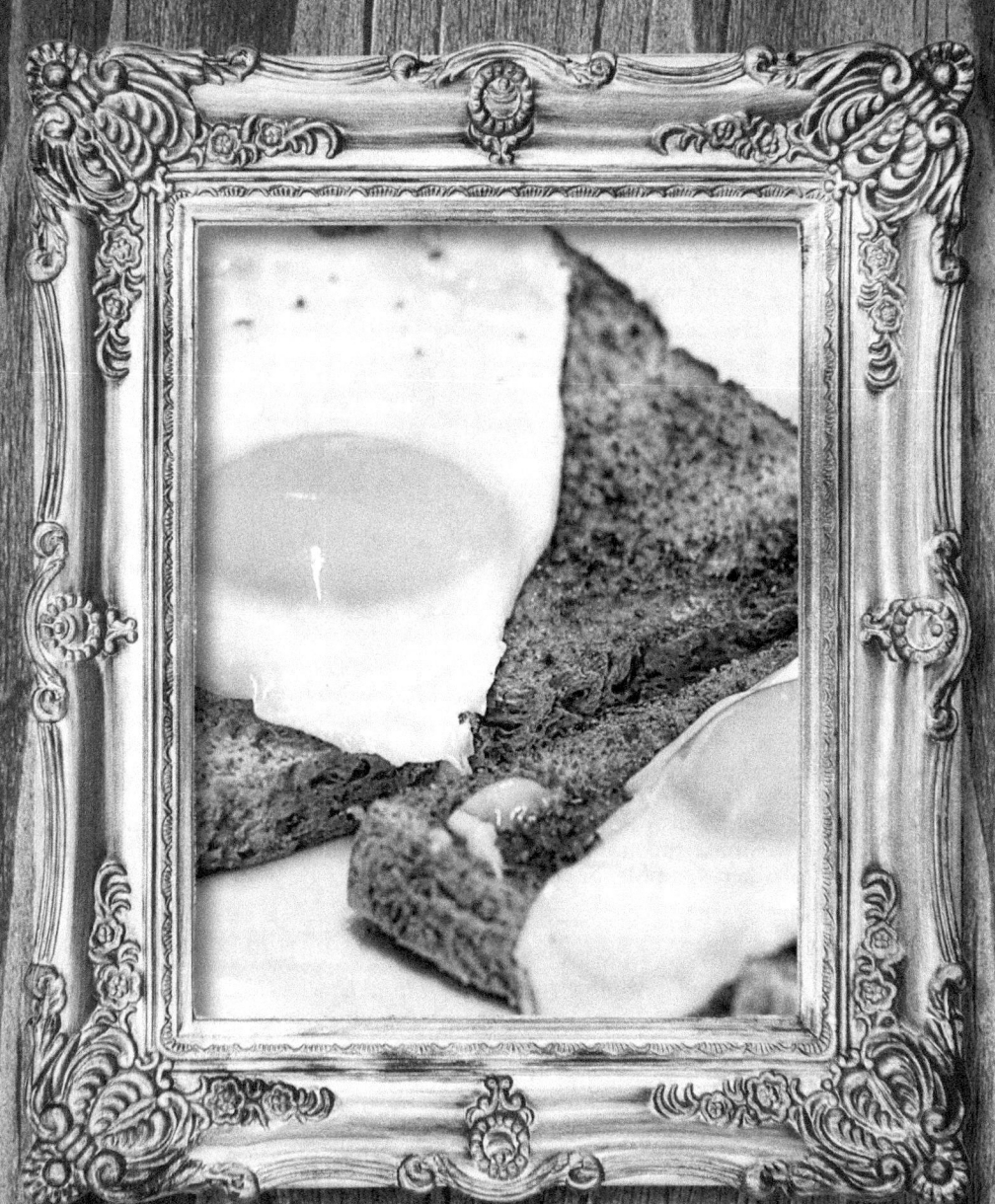

Breakfasts

Breakfasts

Flax Porridge
Serves 1

INGREDIENTS
70 g Flaxseed

210 ml of Water

80 g of whole or semi-skimmed milk

Salt to taste

Grind the flaxseed in a nut mill, coffee bean grinder or other kitchen blender. Add the water and mix with a fork or with a kitchen mixer until a smooth porridge is formed. Microwave for 90 seconds at 900 watts. Add salt or Stevia to taste. Add hot or cold milk.

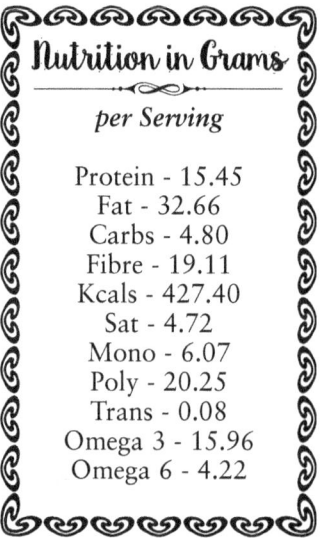

Nutrition in Grams
per Serving

Protein - 15.45
Fat - 32.66
Carbs - 4.80
Fibre - 19.11
Kcals - 427.40
Sat - 4.72
Mono - 6.07
Poly - 20.25
Trans - 0.08
Omega 3 - 15.96
Omega 6 - 4.22

Classic Full English Breakfast for Two

The full English breakfast is a tradition that dates back to the early 14th century. It evolved with the Victorians, who gentrified the tradition and, as was their want, made strict rules regarding the preferred ingredients to create a national phenomena. You can usually find an English breakfast being served wherever you find British people. Obviously, with a fried breakfast there's quite a lot of oil involved, so you need to minimise the amount of frying you need to do, so although you can fry the egg, it would be better to either scramble, or better, to poach the eggs.

MENU FOR TWO
(Combine any 5 of the following)

1. Pork Chops or Roast Pork Slices
2. Fried Eggs or Scrambled Eggs or Poached Eggs or Soft/hard-boiled Eggs
3. Bubble & Squeak
4. Turnip or Cauliflower Hash Browns
5. Spicy Baked Kidney Beans
6. Low Carb Fried Bread
7. Garlic Button Mushrooms
8. Fried Tomatoes

Keep the cooked food on a plate in the centre of the oven at gas mark ¼ - 100°C (215°F) while you finish the rest of the breakfast. Make sure that you cook the eggs last, as these spoil if left or warmed in the oven.

Pork Chops or Roast Pork Slices

To avoid cured bacon, you can use either pork chops or the left over pork from a roast (see the recipe on page 129).

Serves 2

INGREDIENTS
2 Pork Chops or Roast Pork slices (140 g)

Breakfasts

Preheat a grill pan. Season the pork chops well and then grill for about 5 minutes on either side, depending on the heat of your grill. Pork can easily dry out and become hard, just make sure that they are not pink inside. Do the chops at the end of preparing the rest of the breakfast while you are cooking the eggs.

Poached Eggs

Serves 2

INGREDIENTS
2 medium Egg (130 g)
A little malt Vinegar

Nutrition in Grams per Serving

Protein - 15.40
Fat - 6.23
Carbs - 0
Fibre - 0
Kcals - 117.60
Sat - 2.24
Mono - 2.59
Poly - 0.77
Trans - 0
Omega 3 - 0.07
Omega 6 - 0.70

Nutrition in Grams per Serving

Protein - 8.19
Fat - 10.53
Carbs - 0.19
Fibre - 0
Kcals - 126.75
Sat - 2.17
Mono - 6.34
Poly - 0.85
Trans - 0.01
Omega 3 - 0.10
Omega 6 - 0.75

This is easy if you have an egg poacher. If not then firstly, make sure your eggs are really fresh. Boil a saucepan of water with at least 8 cm/3 inches of water; turn the heat down so the water is gently simmering. Add a few drops of vinegar. Crack eggs individually into a cup. With a spoon create a gentle whirlpool in the water to help the egg white wrap around the yolk. Slowly, but in one movement, tip the egg into the water, white first. Leave to cook for 3 minutes for a soft egg, 5 minutes for a harder one. Remove with a spoon. Drain onto kitchen paper.

Scrambled Eggs

Serves 2

INGREDIENTS
2 medium Eggs (130 g)
10 g Low fat (light) Spreadable Butter with rapeseed
or olive oil (or both)
10 ml semi-skimmed Milk

Nutrition in Grams per Serving

Protein - 8.38
Fat - 8.71
Carbs - 0.46
Fibre - 0
Kcals - 113.05
Sat - 2.89
Mono - 3.48
Poly - 1.17
Trans - 0.06
Omega 3 - 0.18
Omega 6 - 0.99

Lightly whisk the eggs, milk and a pinch of salt together until all the mixture has an even consistency. Heat a small sauce pan for a minute on a low heat. Add the butter and let it melt, being careful not to brown it. Pour in the egg mixture and let it sit, without stirring, for 20 seconds. Stir with a wooden spoon, turning the mixture over and over. Let it sit for another 10 seconds then stir again. Repeat until the eggs are softly set and slightly runny in places, then remove from the heat and serve.

Breakfasts

Soft or Hard Boiled Eggs

Serves 2

INGREDIENTS
2 medium Eggs (130 g)

Make sure that your eggs are at room temperature and not straight from the fridge. Bring a saucepan of water (enough to cover the eggs by about a centimetre) to the boil and when it produces large bubbles, quickly but gently lower the eggs into the water, using a tablespoon. Now switch your timer on and give the eggs exactly 1 minute's simmering time. Then remove the saucepan from the heat and put the lid on it and set your timer again, depending on what sort of egg you like.

6 minutes will produce a soft, liquid yolk and a white that is just set, a soft boiled egg.

7 minutes will produce a firm creamier yolk with a white that is completely set.

9 minutes will produce a yolk with a white that is completely set, a classic hard-boiled egg.

Nutrition in Grams
per Serving

Protein - 8.19
Fat - 5.53
Carbs - 0.19
Fibre - 0
Kcals - 82.55
Sat - 1.49
Mono - 2.31
Poly - 0.77
Trans - 0.01
Omega 3 - 0.08
Omega 6 - 0.69

Nutrition in Grams
per Serving

Protein - 8.19
Fat - 10.53
Carbs - 0.19
Fibre - 0
Kcals - 126.75
Sat - 2.17
Mono - 6.34
Poly - 0.85
Trans - 0.01
Omega 3 - 0.10
Omega 6 - 0.75

Fried Eggs

Serves 2

INGREDIENTS
2 medium Eggs (130 g)
2 teaspoons (10 ml) of Macadamia oil
or Rapeseed oil

Pour a little into a frying pan on a low heat for about 20 seconds. Then gently crack the shell of the egg on the side of the pan and from about an inch from the frying pan pull the shell apart with your fingers and let the egg drop into the pan, this way you can keep the yolk intact. Fry for a few minutes until the egg white has turned white. With a spatula flick the oil over the top of the egg including the yolk until the egg white is completely cooked and the yolk has a whiter appearance. If you want a more solid yolk, when the egg has cooked well underneath, turn the whole egg over with a spatula and cooked for a couple of minutes more.

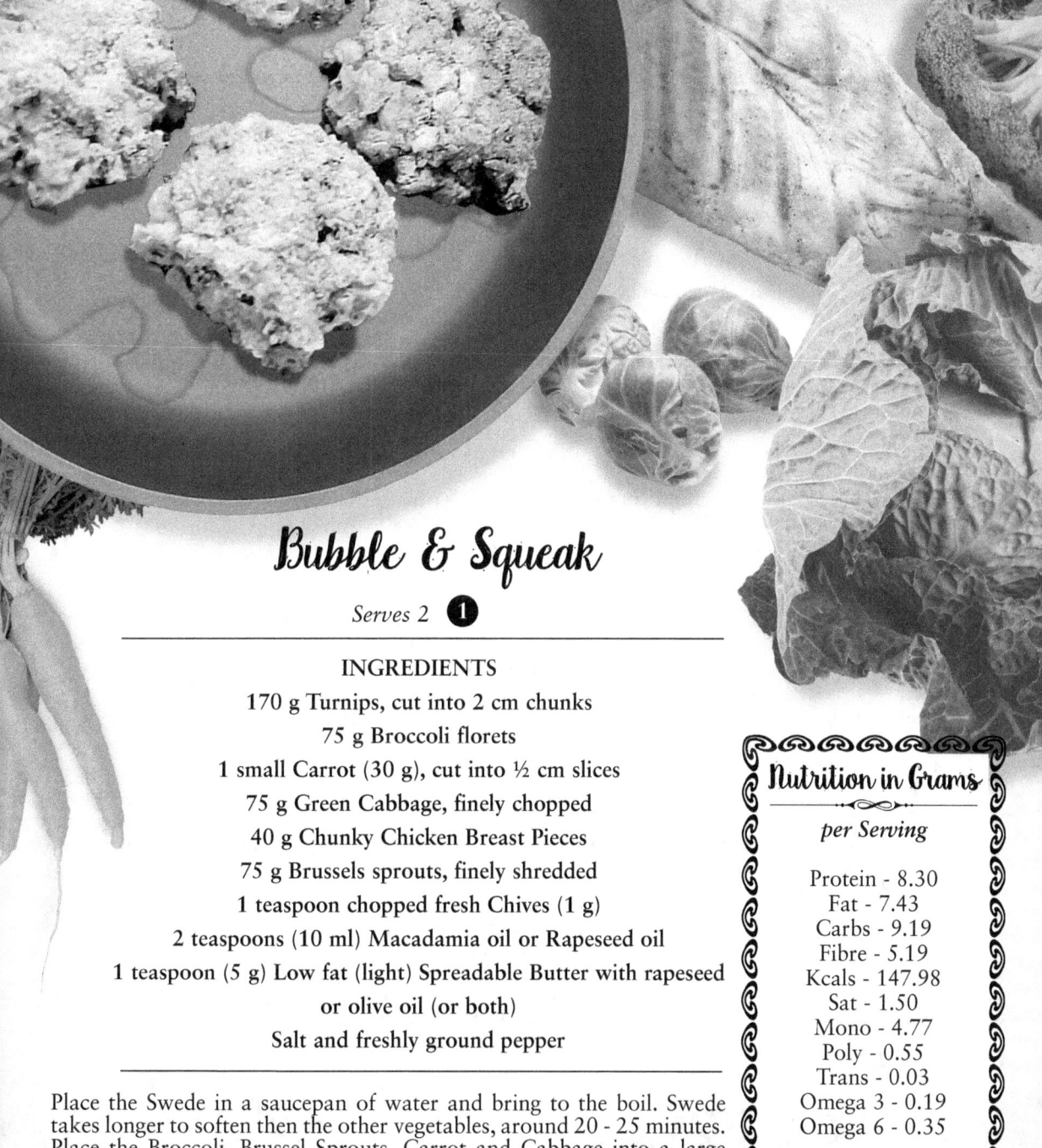

Bubble & Squeak

Serves 2 ❶

INGREDIENTS

170 g Turnips, cut into 2 cm chunks

75 g Broccoli florets

1 small Carrot (30 g), cut into ½ cm slices

75 g Green Cabbage, finely chopped

40 g Chunky Chicken Breast Pieces

75 g Brussels sprouts, finely shredded

1 teaspoon chopped fresh Chives (1 g)

2 teaspoons (10 ml) Macadamia oil or Rapeseed oil

1 teaspoon (5 g) Low fat (light) Spreadable Butter with rapeseed or olive oil (or both)

Salt and freshly ground pepper

Nutrition in Grams
per Serving

Protein - 8.30
Fat - 7.43
Carbs - 9.19
Fibre - 5.19
Kcals - 147.98
Sat - 1.50
Mono - 4.77
Poly - 0.55
Trans - 0.03
Omega 3 - 0.19
Omega 6 - 0.35

Place the Swede in a saucepan of water and bring to the boil. Swede takes longer to soften then the other vegetables, around 20 - 25 minutes. Place the Broccoli, Brussel Sprouts, Carrot and Cabbage into a large saucepan and boil them until soft, about 15 minutes. Drain both saucepans and put all the vegetables into a colander and leave them for a few minutes so that they are thoroughly drained. Transfer to a large saucepan, add the spreadable butter, season and mash roughly, leaving some large chunks.

Add the chunky chicken breast pieces to the mixture (you can get these from most supermarkets). Mix well and divide the vegetables and chicken into 2 equal individual servings or cakes.

Heat the oil in a frying pan over a medium heat. Cook the cakes until the bottom turns golden brown, around 5 minutes, and then turn them over and cook until the second sides are crisp and golden brown. Add a little more oil if needed. When they are done put them onto a plate. Serve topped with the chopped chives.

Breakfasts

Garlic Mushrooms
Serves 2 ①

INGREDIENTS

200 g of Button Mushrooms, chopped in half

2 Garlic Cloves (12 g), crushed

14 g Low fat (light) Spreadable Butter with rapeseed or olive oil (or both)

Melt a little spreadable butter in a frying pan on a very low heat. Add the crushed garlic and fry for about 30 seconds, being careful not to burn them. Add the mushrooms and coat them with the garlic butter. Cook for a few minutes on a slightly higher heat (still low), stirring constantly until the mushrooms are heated through thoroughly (the best way is to determine this is to taste a little). The mushrooms will juice a little which will prevent them from burning.

Nutrition in Grams
per Serving

Protein - 3.60
Fat - 4.59
Carbs - 3.29
Fibre - 1.13
Kcals - 66.65
Sat - 1.85
Mono - 1.59
Poly - 0.72
Trans - 0.07
Omega 3 - 0.14
Omega 6 - 0.58

Fried Tomatoes
Serves 2 ①

INGREDIENTS

3 large fresh tomatoes (400 g), sliced in half

2 teaspoons (10 ml) Macadamia oil or Rapeseed oil for frying

Heat a little rapeseed oil in a frying pan, on a low heat. Cut the tomatoes in half and place them in the oil cut side down. Fry on a low heat for a couple of minutes or until they are slightly browned. Flip them over and repeat (don't worry that they are now on the rounded side and some of the skin is not touching the pan, the main thing is that they will warm through. Now flip them again and cook for about another minute, then serve.

Nutrition in Grams
per Serving

Protein - 2.00
Fat - 5.20
Carbs - 4.80
Fibre - 2.40
Kcals - 74.20
Sat - 0.68
Mono - 4.03
Poly - 0.08
Trans - 0.00
Omega 3 - 0.01
Omega 6 - 0.07

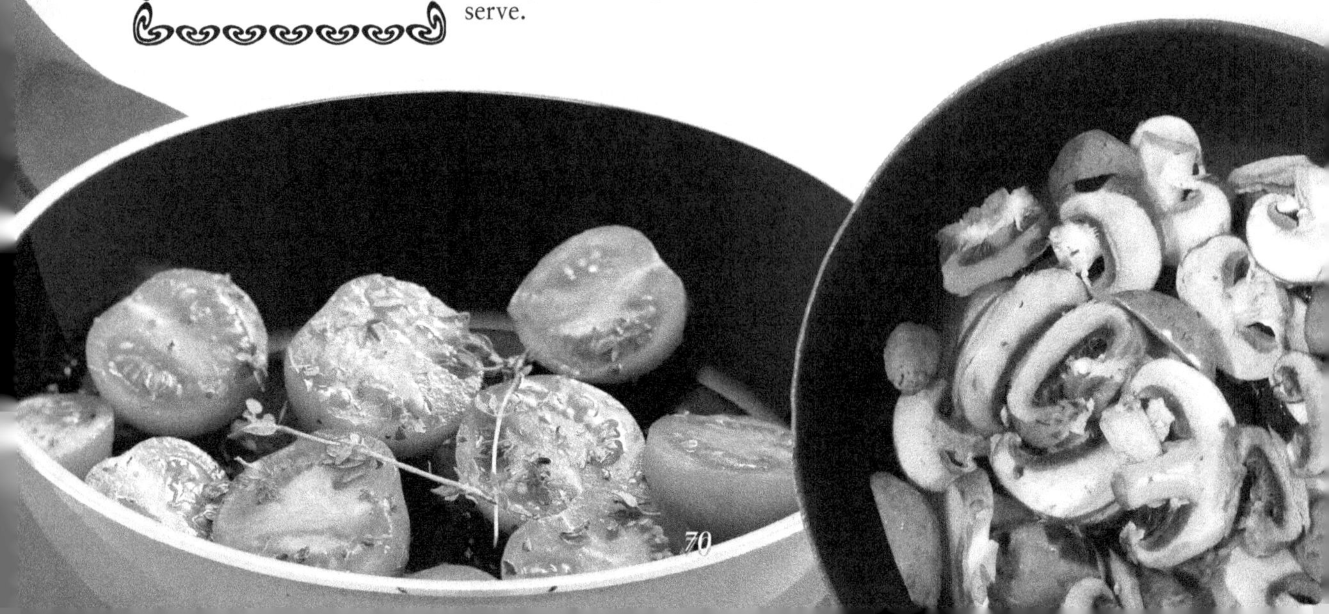

Breakfasts

Spicy Baked Kidney Beans

This a great alternative to canned baked beans which are usually high in carbs, sugar and salt and are in what basically amounts to a fake, processed tomato sauce. The chilli gives an edge to the sauce that makes these beans delicious on toasted Low Carb bread or as part of a breakfast, or you can leave the chilli out for a regular baked bean sauce. For a richer flavour you can substitute the Classic Tomato Sauce with the Red Wine version. This can be a breakfast or a snack on its own on 4 slices of Low Carb bread.

Serves 2

INGREDIENTS

20 g Kidney Beans, canned or dried (see below)

1 third portion of Classic Tomato Sauce (see page 91) or 1 portion of Red Wine and Tomato (see page 92)

A pinch (2 g) of Chilli powder (depending on preference)

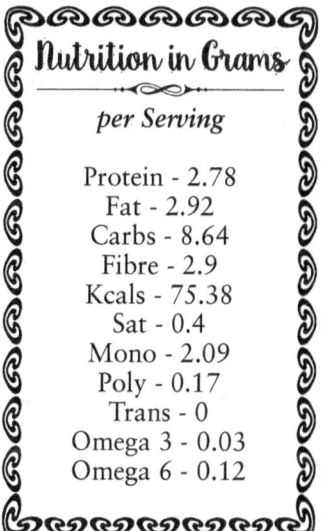

Nutrition in Grams

per Serving

Protein - 2.78
Fat - 2.92
Carbs - 8.64
Fibre - 2.9
Kcals - 75.38
Sat - 0.4
Mono - 2.09
Poly - 0.17
Trans - 0
Omega 3 - 0.03
Omega 6 - 0.12

Once you have cooked the tomato sauce, let it cool and pop it in a blender or food processor until it is nice and smooth. Put it back in the frying pan and sprinkle in the Chilli powder. Add the cooked beans you soaked or the canned beans and cook on a medium heat until warm throughout (if using the canned beans, taste the beans to see if they have warmed through completely). Meanwhile, toast your Low Carb bread, butter and pour a quarter of the mixture over 2 slices of bread four times and serve immediately for a delicious breakfast or lunch.

If you are using dried beans you need to prepare them as below.

Soaking Method
Soak the beans overnight in plenty of cold water. This process helps the beans to swell so that the final cooking time is reduced, and also helps remove some of the agents which cause flatulence and indigestion. Drain the beans and wash them under a running tap. Bring them to the boil in plenty of fresh water. Fast boil the beans for at least 10 minutes. This is because there are toxins on the outside skin of beans, which are destroyed by the soaking und cooking process. After fast-boiling the beans, turn the heat down to simmer, partially cover the pan and continue cooking them until they are soft. Do not add salt to the cooking water as this toughens the outside skin. When the beans are cooked, drain off the liquid.

Quick Cooking Method
Wash the beans and bring them to the boil in plenty of fresh water. Boil them fast for 3-5 minutes. Turn off the heat and let them soak in that water for one hour. Then drain off the liquid and re-boil them in fresh water as described in the soaking method. The first quick boil and one hour of soaking are a substitute for the long overnight soak.

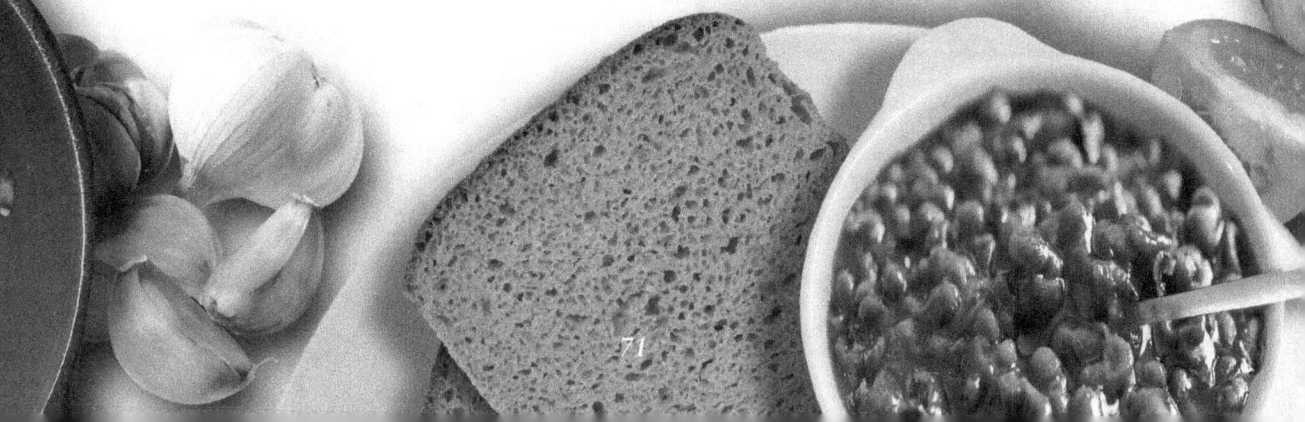

Breakfasts

Low Carb Fried Bread

Serves 2

INGREDIENTS

2 tablespoon (30 g) Macadamia oil or Rapeseed oil
2 Slices Low Carb Bread (see page 58)

Heat 1 tablespoon of the rapeseed oil in a frying pan and heat up on a low heat for about a minute. Place the two slices of Low Carb bread in the pan, turn the heat slightly up and fry for about 5 minutes (the oil will be absorbed by the bread but don't be tempted to add any more, just turn the heat down to continue browning the bread). Keep checking whether the underside has browned and when done to your liking, remove from the pan and place on a plate and heat up the remaining oil in the pan for a minute. Return the bread to the pan the other side up and repeat. Serve immediately.

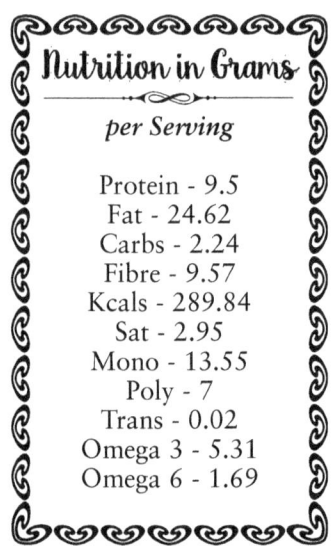

Nutrition in Grams

per Serving

Protein - 9.5
Fat - 24.62
Carbs - 2.24
Fibre - 9.57
Kcals - 289.84
Sat - 2.95
Mono - 13.55
Poly - 7
Trans - 0.02
Omega 3 - 5.31
Omega 6 - 1.69

Cauliflower or Turnip Hash Browns

These are delicious turnip or cauliflower hash browns that you can enjoy by themselves or with homemade mayonnaise, a hearty salad or serve as part of a breakfast.

Serves 2

INGREDIENTS

225 g Turnips, grated or 225 g Cauliflower, grated
2 small Eggs (100 g)
¼ large Onion (65 g), grated
Salt and freshly ground black pepper to taste
1 teaspoon (5 g) Macadamia Oil or Rapeseed oil, for frying

Grate the turnip or cauliflower on the largest setting on your grater (typically about ½ cm wide). Use the same setting for the onion. In a large bowl, mix the eggs thoroughly with a fork (don't whisk). Add the grated turnip/cauliflower with the grated onions, salt and black pepper in a bowl and let sit for about 10 minutes.

Pour the macadamia oil into a large frying on a medium heat. Place 4 portions of the turnip or cauliflower mix in the frying pan and flatten them carefully until they measure about 3–4 inches in diameter. If you haven't got a large enough frying pan, you can do these in batches, keeping the previous batches in the oven at gas mark ¼ - 100°C (215°F). Lower the heat and fry the hash browns for 5 minutes on each side or until they have browned nicely. Be careful not to burn them. Don't turn them over too soon (until they are browned) or they can fall apart.

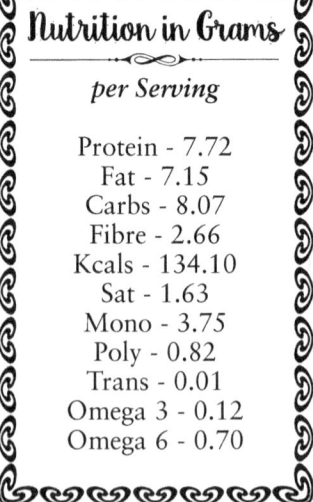

Nutrition in Grams

per Serving

Protein - 7.72
Fat - 7.15
Carbs - 8.07
Fibre - 2.66
Kcals - 134.10
Sat - 1.63
Mono - 3.75
Poly - 0.82
Trans - 0.01
Omega 3 - 0.12
Omega 6 - 0.70

Breakfasts

Bubble & Squeak with an Egg

This dish goes back to the 18th century Britain and traditionally was fried meat and cabbage, most commonly the leftovers from the previous night's roast dinner. The dish's name comes from the fact that the cabbage makes bubbling and squeaking sounds when cooked. Today it has morphed into fried potatoes and other vegetables, usually Cabbage, with no meat and is commonly used as a side dish to a roast or breakfast. In this recipe, Turnips, Cabbage and Brussel Sprouts stand in for the traditional base but you can use any vegetables in this fried mash.

Serves 6

INGREDIENTS

500 g Turnips, cut into 2 cm chunks

225 g Broccoli florets

1 large Carrot (80 g), cut into ½ cm slices

225 g Green Cabbage, finely chopped

120 g Chunky Chicken Breast Pieces

(you can get these from most supermarkets)

225 g Brussels sprouts, finely shredded

6 large Eggs (450 g)

1 tablespoon chopped fresh Chives (3 g)

2 tablespoons (30 ml) Rapeseed oil or Macadamia oil

1 tablespoon (15 g) Low fat (light) Spreadable Butter with rapeseed or olive oil (or both)

Salt and freshly ground pepper

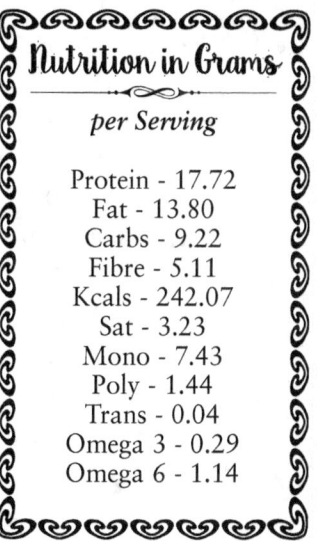

Nutrition in Grams

per Serving

Protein - 17.72
Fat - 13.80
Carbs - 9.22
Fibre - 5.11
Kcals - 242.07
Sat - 3.23
Mono - 7.43
Poly - 1.44
Trans - 0.04
Omega 3 - 0.29
Omega 6 - 1.14

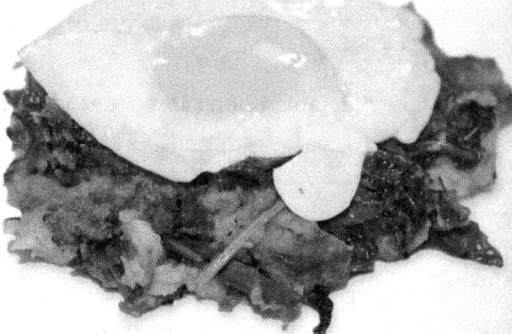

Place the Swede in a saucepan of water and bring to the boil. Swede takes longer to soften then the other vegetables, around 20 - 25 minutes. Place the Broccoli, Brussel Sprouts, Carrot and Cabbage into a large saucepan and boil them until soft, about 15 minutes. Drain both saucepans and put all the vegetables into a colander and leave them for a few minutes so that they are thoroughly drained. Transfer to a large saucepan, add the spreadable butter, season and mash roughly, leaving some large chunks.

Add the chunky chicken breast pieces to the mixture. Mix well and divide the vegetables and bacon into 6 equal individual servings or cakes.

Heat 1 tablespoon of the oil in a large frying pan over a medium heat. Cook the cakes in batches until the bottom turns golden brown, around 5 minutes, and then turn them over and cook until the second sides are crisp and golden brown. Add a little more oil if needed. When they are done put them onto a plate.

Heat 1 tablespoon of the oil in a large frying pan, again over a medium heat. Crack the shells of the eggs and gently pour the contents into the frying pan, being careful not to break the yolks. Fit as many of the eggs you can in the frying pan. Fry until the whites are set and flick some of the oil over the yolks to seal them in, while keeping the yolk runny. When they are done, sprinkle with a little salt and pepper and place an egg on each of the cakes. Serve topped with the chopped chives.

Breakfasts

Huevos Rancheros with Minced Beef

Huevos Rancheros is a popular breakfast dish consisting of eggs served in the style of the traditional fare on rural Mexican farms. Basically, it's a spicy twist on an English breakfast that warms you up for the day ahead.

Serves 4

INGREDIENTS

200 g Minced Beef (5% Fat)

1 green Chilli Pepper (45 g), deseeded and finely chopped

2 Cloves Garlic (12 g), crushed

2 Red Peppers (330 g), deseeded and finely sliced

1 teaspoon (5 g) Chilli Powder

1 x 400 g tin of chopped tomatoes

¼ teaspoon (1 g) Cumin

¼ teaspoon (1 g) fresh Oregano or ½ teaspoon (2 g) dried Oregano

6 medium Eggs (390 g)

100 g Extra Mature Cheddar Cheese, grated

A handful of fresh Coriander (54 g)

4 Low Carb Tortillas (see page 59)

1 tablespoon (15 g) Macadamia oil or Rapeseed oil for frying

Salt and freshly ground Black Pepper to taste

Nutrition in Grams

per Serving

Protein - 27.94
Fat - 33.91
Carbs - 7.76
Fibre - 16.22
Kcals - 486.95
Sat - 7.69
Mono - 11.35
Poly - 11.92
Trans - 0.22
Omega 3 - 8.15
Omega 6 - 3.81

Prepare the Tortillas, and place them on the plates you are going to serve them, in the oven on a very low heat to keep them warm, about gas mark ¼ - 100°C (215°F). In a large frying pan, fry the bacon with a little oil until they are cooked how you like them. Lay one rasher of Bacon on top of each of the Tortillas in the oven. Put a little more oil in the frying pan on a low heat and add the Garlic and fry for about a minute, being careful not to burn it.

Add the minced Beef and stirring continually, brown the mince all over, about 5 minutes. Add the tomatoes, chillies, chilli powder, cumin, oregano, salt and pepper. Cook for 5-10 minutes on a low heat to blend all the flavours. Remove the plates from the oven and pour a quarter of the beef mixture over the bacon and return to the oven. Add a little more oil and crack the eggs into the pan and fry them how you like them, turning them over if you like the yolks done (you can also use scrambled or poached eggs). Remove the plates from the oven and place an egg on each plate. Sprinkle with the grated cheese and chopped coriander.

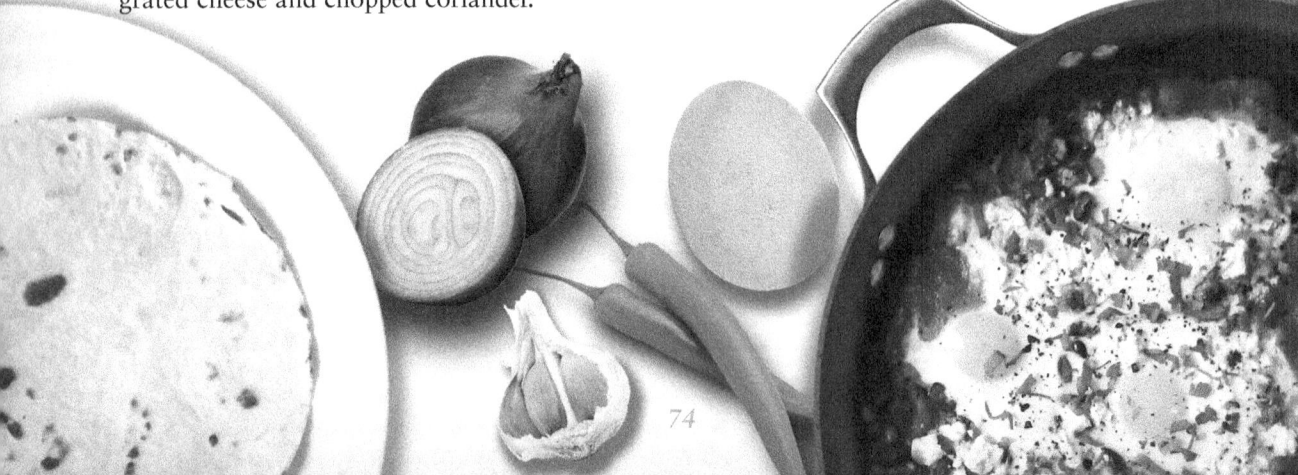

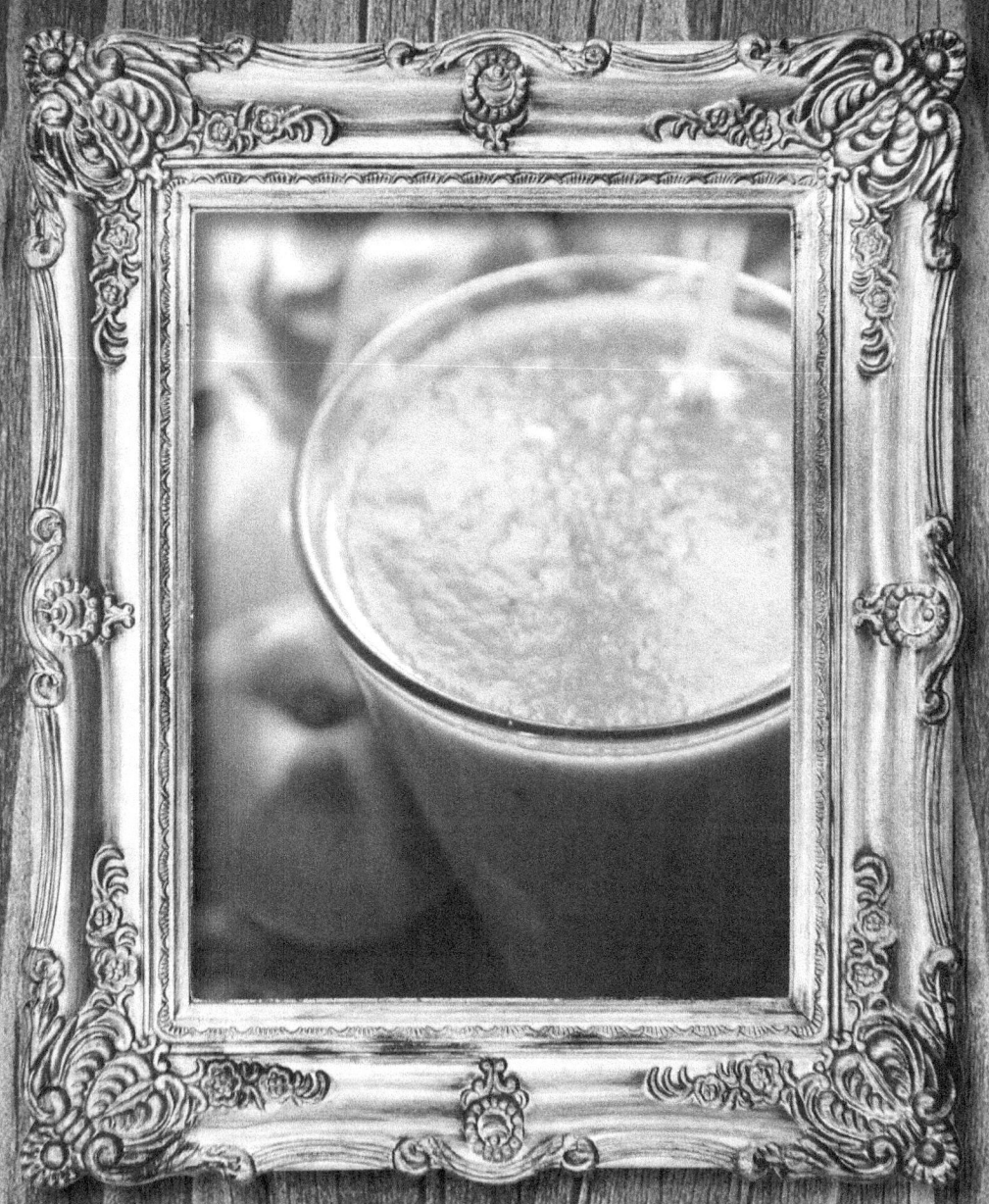

Smoothies

Smoothies

These are great healthy alternative for breakfast. Just put all the solid ingredients into a blender or food processor. Add the fluid base to fill the cup up to the Max Line. Blast the mixture until it is really smooth (20 or so seconds).

Asparagus Anthem ❶

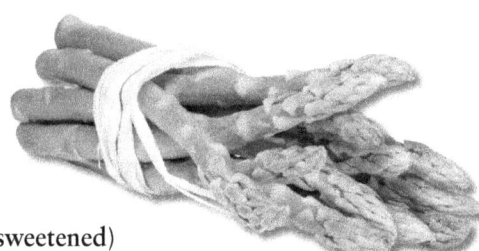

INGREDIENTS

80 g Swiss Chard

60 grams Raspberries

60 g sliced Asparagus

150 ml Almond Milk (Unsweetened)

Nutrition in Grams

per Smoothie

Protein - 3.96
Fat - 2.61
Carbs - 12.51
Fibre - 7.68
Kcals - 106.78
Sat - 0.22
Mono - 1.28
Poly - 0.77
Trans - 0
Omega 3 - 0.24
Omega 6 - 0.53

Nutrition in Grams

per Smoothie

Protein - 2.76
Fat - 2.56
Carbs - 11.64
Fibre - 6.20
Kcals - 94.40
Sat - 0.19
Mono - 1.27
Poly - 0.73
Trans - 0
Omega 3 - 0.24
Omega 6 - 0.50

Tomato Twist

❶

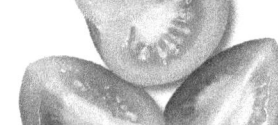

INGREDIENTS

80 g Swiss Chard

60 g Raspberries

60 g sliced Tomato

150 ml Almond Milk (Unsweetened)

Nutrition in Grams

per Smoothie

Protein - 3.91
Fat - 2.51
Carbs - 12.14
Fibre - 4.34
Kcals - 92.80
Sat - 0.28
Mono - 1.27
Poly - 0.68
Trans - 0
Omega 3 - 0.27
Omega 6 - 0.35

Green Breeze

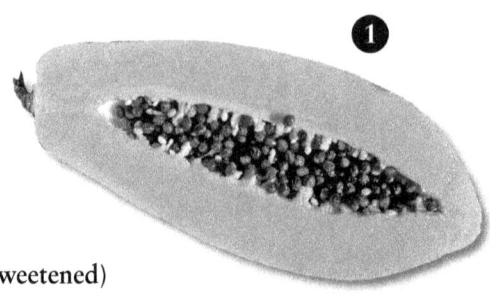

❶

INGREDIENTS

80 g Spinach

60 g Papaya

60 g sliced Asparagus

150 ml Almond Milk (Unsweetened)

Smoothies

Nutrition in Grams
per Smoothie

Protein - 4.18
Fat - 2.64
Carbs - 15.38
Fibre - 6.82
Kcals - 116.60
Sat - 0.26
Mono - 1.25
Poly - 0.81
Trans - 0
Omega 3 - 0.31
Omega 6 - 0.51

Fruity Boost

INGREDIENTS

80 g Broccoli Florets
60 g Blackberries
60 g diced Beetroot
150 ml Almond Milk (Unsweetened)

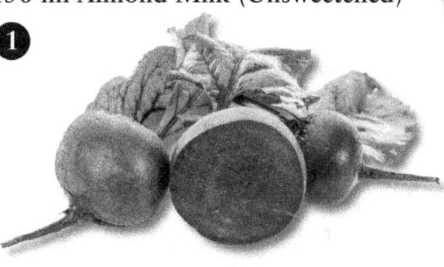

Bok Choy and Broccoli Collection

INGREDIENTS

40 g Bok Choy
40 g Broccoli Florets
60 g Apple slices
150 ml Almond Milk (Unsweetened)

Nutrition in Grams
per Smoothie

Protein - 2.37
Fat - 2.23
Carbs - 12.59
Fibre - 3.68
Kcals - 84.00
Sat - 0.17
Mono - 1.21
Poly - 0.52
Trans - 0
Omega 3 - 0.20
Omega 6 - 0.32

Nutrition in Grams
per Smoothie

Protein - 2.94
Fat - 13.87
Carbs - 6.95
Fibre - 4.74
Kcals - 170.20
Sat - 2.20
Mono - 8.82
Poly - 2.03
Trans - 0
Omega 3 - 0.28
Omega 6 - 1.68

Watercress & Advocado Gala

INGREDIENTS

40 g Watercress
40 g Red Cabbage
60 g sliced Avocado
150 ml Almond Milk (Unsweetened)

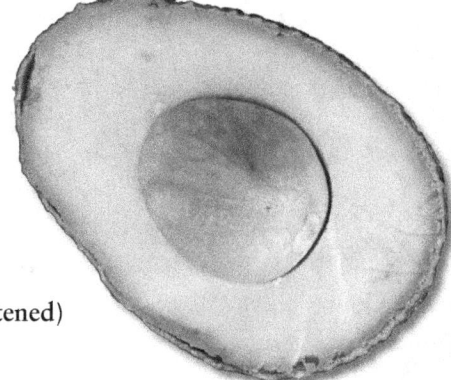

THE DIABETIC DETECTIVES

Green Lagoon

1

INGREDIENTS

40 g Black Kale de-stemmed

60 g Raspberries

60 g sliced Asparagus

150 ml Almond Milk (Unsweetened)

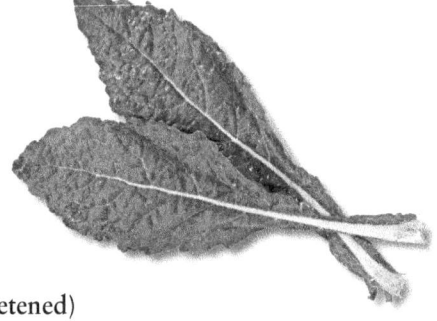

Nutrition in Grams

per Smoothie

Protein - 3.36
Fat - 2.69
Carbs - 10.44
Fibre - 6.98
Kcals - 96.60
Sat - 0.23
Mono - 1.24
Poly - 0.91
Trans - 0
Omega 3 - 0.23
Omega 6 - 0.55

Rocket Loves Orange

1

INGREDIENTS

40 g Rocket/Arugura Lettuce

60 g Orange segments

60 grams sliced Asparagus

150 ml Almond Milk (Unsweetened)

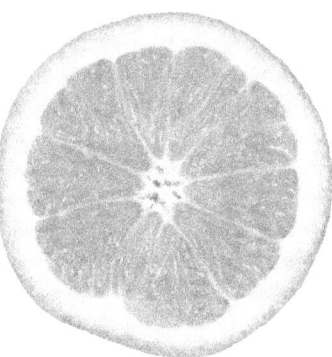

Nutrition in Grams

per Smoothie

Protein - 3.14
Fat - 2.28
Carbs - 10.72
Fibre - 3.56
Kcals - 80.40
Sat - 0.21
Mono - 1.22
Poly - 0.59
Trans - 0
Omega 3 - 0.16
Omega 6 - 0.44

Orange & Asparagus Refrain

1

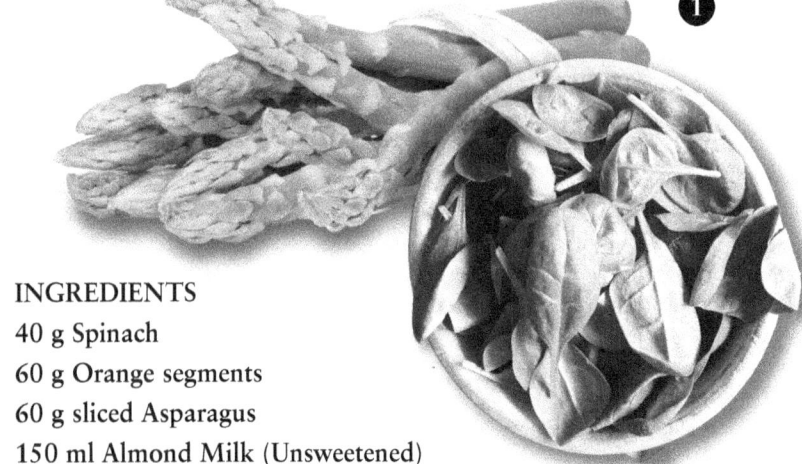

INGREDIENTS

40 g Spinach

60 g Orange segments

60 g sliced Asparagus

150 ml Almond Milk (Unsweetened)

Nutrition in Grams

per Smoothie

Protein - 3.00
Fat - 2.24
Carbs - 11.21
Fibre - 3.52
Kcals - 82.40
Sat - 0.20
Mono - 1.20
Poly - 0.55
Trans - 0
Omega 3 - 0.21
Omega 6 - 0.34

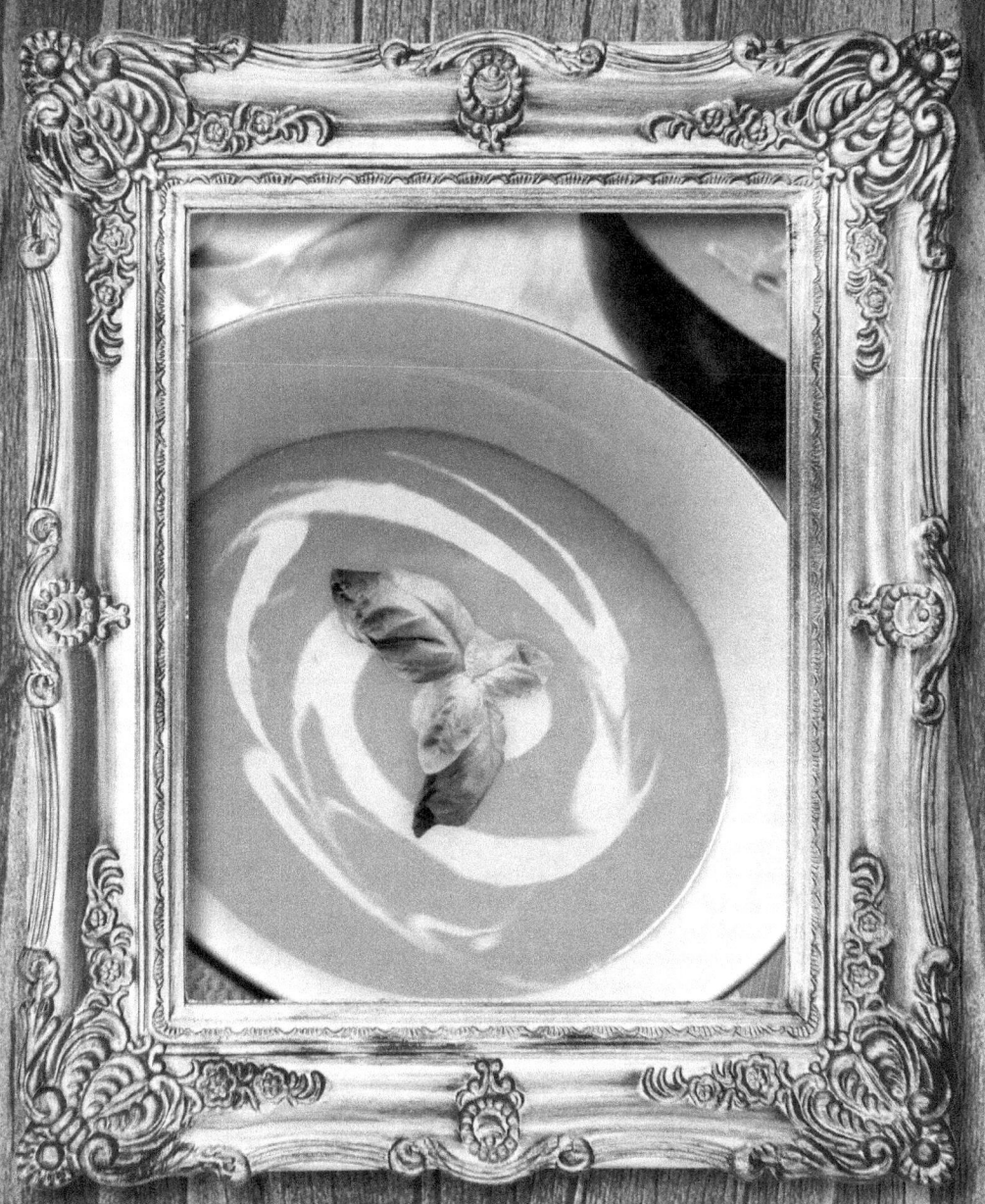

Soups

Vegetable Stock

Making a vegetable stock as a base for soups isn't quite the chore you might think and will always be better than using a stock cube. All you have to do is to prepare the vegetables, chop them into large chunks, fry gently with a few herbs, add some water and then you can leave it to simmer away for a couple of hours. I use root vegetables, particularly carrots, with onions and celery.

Makes around 1 litre

INGREDIENTS

2 Turnips (300 g)
2 Carrots (80 g)
1 large Onion (265 g)
1 stick Celery (40 g)
1 tablespoon (15 g) Macadamia oil or Rapeseed oil
1 Bay leaf (0.3 g)
1 sprig fresh Thyme (10 g) or ½ teaspoon (5 g) dried Thyme
1.4 litres/2½ pints water
1 Garlic bulb (60 g), peeled and chopped finely

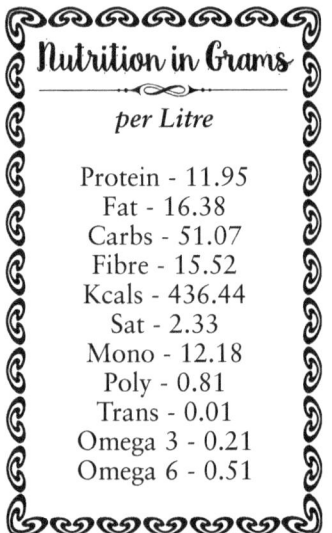

Nutrition in Grams
per Litre

Protein - 11.95
Fat - 16.38
Carbs - 51.07
Fibre - 15.52
Kcals - 436.44
Sat - 2.33
Mono - 12.18
Poly - 0.81
Trans - 0.01
Omega 3 - 0.21
Omega 6 - 0.51

Scrub all the vegetables and skin the onion, and then chop them all into large pieces. Fry the vegetable very gently in the oil and add the herbs. Next add the water and garlic, bring to the boil and allow to simmer for 1-2 hours in a covered pan. Then strain and reserve the liquid for stock. The stock will keep for 3-4 days in the fridge or it can be frozen. The remaining vegetables can be pureed and used for a thick soup or as the basis for a sauce (see below).

Vegetable Soup

This uses the left-over vegetables from making the vegetable stock in the previous recipe and makes a rich soup, high in flavour.

Serves 2

INGREDIENTS

Left-over vegetables from making the Vegetable stock
A little Parsley to garnish

Just liquidise the pulped vegetables and garnish with a little fresh parsley.

Nutrition in Grams
per Serving

Protein - 5.97
Fat - 8.19
Carbs - 25.53
Fibre - 7.76
Kcals - 218.22
Sat - 1.16
Mono - 6.09
Poly - 0.40
Trans - 0.01
Omega 3 - 0.10
Omega 6 - 0.25

Broccoli & Stilton Soup with Crispy Croutons

This is a smoothly blended vegetable soup with the distinct flavour of blue cheese. It makes a great lunch or as a starter for a main meal.

Serves 8

INGREDIENTS
Soup

1 tablespoon (15 g) Macadamia oil or Rapeseed Oil
1 large Onion (265 g), finely chopped
1 stick celery (40 g), sliced
1 leek (100 g), sliced
2 teaspoons (10 g) dried Thyme
1 teaspoon (10 g) Low fat (light) Spreadable Butter
with rapeseed or olive oil (or both)
1 litre Vegetable Stock (see page 80) or use 2 vegetable stock cubes
700 g Broccoli, chopped
100 g Stilton, crumbled

Croutons

2 Slices of Low Carb French stick, 2 cm thick
(for the dough, see the Garlic bread recipe on page 60,
without the Garlic butter)
2 cloves of Garlic (12 g), crushed
2 teaspoon (10 g) Parmesan Cheese
Drizzle of Olive Oil (2 g)
Salt and freshly ground Black Pepper

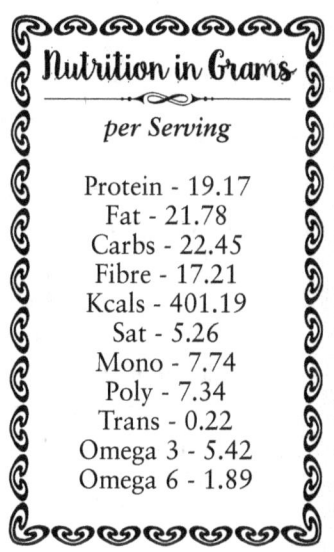

Nutrition in Grams
per Serving

Protein - 19.17
Fat - 21.78
Carbs - 22.45
Fibre - 17.21
Kcals - 401.19
Sat - 5.26
Mono - 7.74
Poly - 7.34
Trans - 0.22
Omega 3 - 5.42
Omega 6 - 1.89

First prepare the Croutons. Heat the oven to gas mark 5 - 175°C (350°F). Prepare the dough as per our bread recipe (first recipe in the Bread & Pizzas chapter). Roll the dough into a large sausage shape about 2 inches in diameter. Grease a baking tray with a little spreadable butter, place the dough onto it and put into the centre of the oven. Bake for about 40-50 minutes, or until it's risen well and is crusty on top. Remove the bread and let it cool on a rack. Cut up the bread into 1 cm squares and place in a bowl. Season with salt and freshly ground black pepper and sprinkle the garlic powder and parmesan cheese over the bread. Drizzle a little Olive Oil over the mixture and with a spoon gently stir together in order to spread the oil evenly over the croutons. Empty the contents onto a baking tray and spread out the croutons so that they are not touching. Place the baking tray into the top half of the oven and cook for 15 minutes or until brown and crispy.

Meanwhile, heat the rapeseed oil in a large saucepan and then add the onions and fry until soft and translucent being careful not to burn them. Add the celery, leek and spreadable butter. Stir until all the spread has melted, cover with a lid and leave for 5 minutes. Remove the lid, and pour in the stock and add the Broccoli and Thyme. Cook for around 15 minutes or until all the vegetables are soft.

Transfer to a blender/food processor and blend until smooth. Stir in the Stilton, allowing a few lumps to remain. Season to taste with salt and freshly ground black pepper. Serve into 4 soup bowls and sprinkle a quarter of the croutons in the centre of each bowl.

Creamy Tomato Soup

This a really easy hearty Tomato Soup made creamy with natural Yoghurt.

Serves 6

INGREDIENTS

2 tablespoons (30 g) Low fat (light) Spreadable Butter with rapeseed or olive oil (or both)

1 large Onion (265 g), finely chopped

2 x 400 g tin of chopped Tomatoes

450 ml Vegetable Stock (see page 80) or use 1 vegetable stock cube

245 ml low fat Natural Yoghurt

2 tablespoons (30 g) fresh parsley, chopped

Salt and pepper to taste

1 tablespoon (15 g) Macadamia oil or Rapeseed Oil for frying

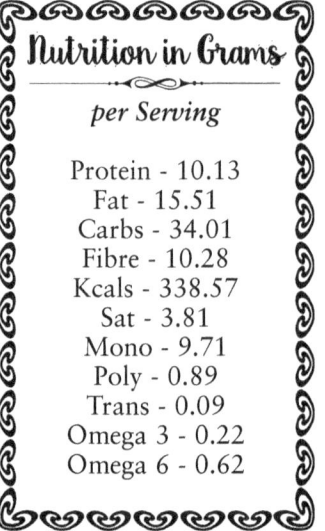

Nutrition in Grams
per Serving

Protein - 10.13
Fat - 15.51
Carbs - 34.01
Fibre - 10.28
Kcals - 338.57
Sat - 3.81
Mono - 9.71
Poly - 0.89
Trans - 0.09
Omega 3 - 0.22
Omega 6 - 0.62

In a large saucepan, fry the onion until translucent. Add the tomatoes, with their liquid, and the stock and bring to a boil. Simmer for 5 minutes. Puree with a blender or food processor until smooth. Stir in the Yoghurt and adjust the seasoning. Sprinkle with the fresh parsley and serve at once.

Cream of Asparagus Soup

Asparagus has a unique flavour unlike any other food and goes well with the crème fraiche in this really easy and quick creamy soup.

Serves 6

Nutrition in Grams
per Serving

Protein - 6.42
Fat - 4.71
Carbs - 16.98
Fibre - 7.13
Kcals - 168.98
Sat - 1.39
Mono - 4.71
Poly - 0.31
Trans - 0.02
Omega 3 - 0.07
Omega 6 - 0.21

INGREDIENTS

900 g Asparagus with the tough ends cut off

1 large Onion (265 g), chopped

1350 ml Vegetable Stock (see page 80) or use 3 vegetable stock cubes

2 tablespoons (30 g) half fat Crème Fraiche

Salt and fresh Pepper, to taste

1 tablespoon (15 g) Macadamia oil or Rapeseed Oil for frying

Heat the oil in a frying pan and cook until soft and translucent. Cut the asparagus in half and add to the pot along with the Vegetable stock and black pepper, to taste. Bring to a boil, cover and cook on a low heat for about 20 minutes or until the Asparagus is very tender. Remove from the heat, add the Crème Fraiche and using a blender or food processor, mix until very smooth. You may have to do this in batches.

Soups

Bortsch Ukraine

Borscht is a sour soup popular in several Eastern European cuisines, including Ukrainian, Russian, Polish, Belarusian, Latvian, Lithuanian, Romanian, and Ashkenazi Jewish cultures. The variety most commonly associated with the name in English is of Ukrainian origin and includes beetroots as one of the main ingredients, which gives the dish a distinctive red colour. The colour and flavour of the soup are superb, and the texture can either be coarse, or smooth if you puree it in a liquidiser.

Serves 4

Nutrition in Grams
per Serving

Protein - 5.47
Fat - 7.71
Carbs - 24.67
Fibre - 7.21
Kcals - 167.26
Sat - 4.1
Mono - 2.49
Poly - 0.41
Trans - 0.11
Omega 3 - 0.07
Omega 6 - 0.33

INGREDIENTS

350 g uncooked Beetroot, peeled

100 g Carrot, scrubbed

100 g Turnip, peeled

1 large Onion (265 g), peeled and finely diced

190 ml Tomato Juice

380 ml Vegetable Stock (see page 80) or use 1 vegetable stock cube

1 teaspoon (5 g) Caraway Seeds

A pinch of Nutmeg (1 g), ground

Salt, freshly ground black pepper

Garnish

150 ml half fat Crème Fraiche

Prepare the vegetables and grate them coarsely. Then put them into a large saucepan with the tomato juice, stock and caraway seeds. Bring them to the boil and season to taste with salt, pepper and a little nutmeg, cover and simmer for 45-50 minutes. Either leave this as a coarse soup or puree it in a liquidiser, blender or food processor. Just before serving garnish with a swirl of Crème Fraiche.

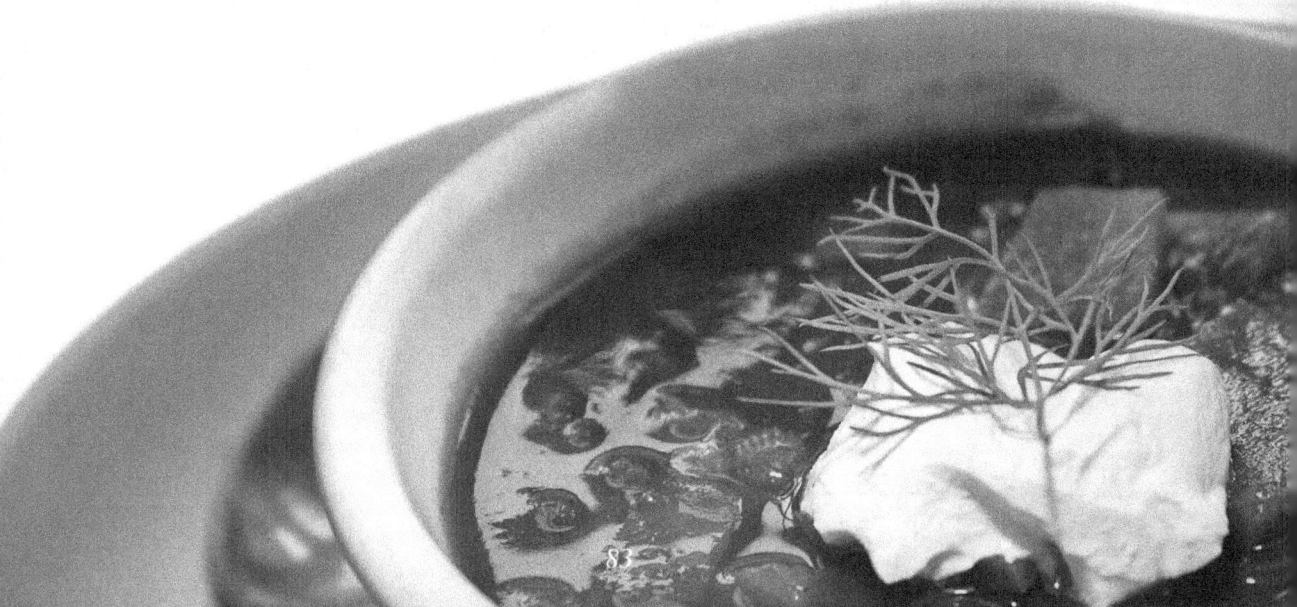

Pennsylvania Chowder

Chowders are thick creamy soups made from a milk or cream sauce base with plenty of vegetables to add flavour and colour. This recipe is simple to make and colourful to look at with its pea and parsley. Milk-based soups should not lie overcooked or the flavour will spoil, so once this soup is hot, serve it straight away.

Serves 4

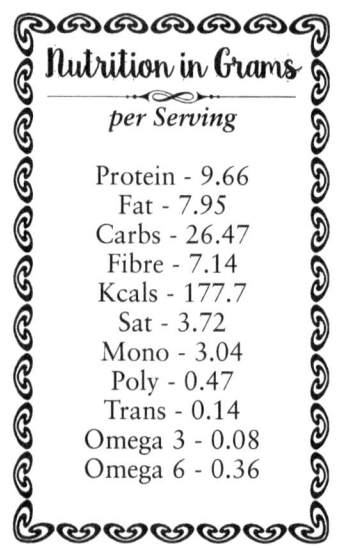

Nutrition in Grams
per Serving

Protein - 9.66
Fat - 7.95
Carbs - 26.47
Fibre - 7.14
Kcals - 177.7
Sat - 3.72
Mono - 3.04
Poly - 0.47
Trans - 0.14
Omega 3 - 0.08
Omega 6 - 0.36

INGREDIENTS

570 ml /1 pint Vegetable Stock (see page 80) or use 1 stock cube

1 large Onion (265 g), peeled and finely chopped

4 sticks Celery (160 g), washed and finely chopped

1 Turnip (300 g), scrubbed and diced

168 g Garden Peas

¼ teaspoon (1¼ g) Paprika

25 g fresh Parsley, finely chopped

570 ml/1 pint semi-skimmed Milk

Salt and freshly ground black pepper

First bring the stock to the boil in a large saucepan and add the Onion, Celery, Carrots and Turnips, then simmer for about 10 minutes. Add the Garden Peas and Paprika and cook for a further 10 minutes on a lower heat. Then stir in the parsley. In a separate pan bring the milk to the boil. Then pour this into the soup. Puree half the mixture in a liquidiser and stir it back into the remaining mixture. Then re-heat the whole soup gently and season generously with salt and pepper. Pour into bowls and garnish with a dusting of Paprika.

Creamed Tomato Soup with Sage

This recipe uses the vegetable stock which is then transformed by a few ingredients into a deliriously rich and creamy soap. Although a lot of garlic us used in the stock, the end result has a mild flavour which gives the overall tomato taste a special quality. It is more subtle than you would expect. I find this soup makes a perfect starter for special meals since it is rich without being heavy.

Serves 6

INGREDIENTS

900 ml Vegetable Stock (see page 80) or use 2 vegetable stock cubes

350 g Tomato Puree

1 teaspoon (5 g) fresh Sage leaves, chopped or ½ teaspoon (2½ g) dried Sage

1 tablespoon (15 ml) Red Wine Vinegar

1 tablespoon (15 ml) Soy Sauce

2 tablespoons (30 ml) Red Wine

275 ml Milk

Salt and freshly ground black pepper

Garnish

4 tablespoons (72 g) Thick Low fat Greek Yoghurt

Fresh sage leaves or sprigs of Parsley

Make up the basic Vegetable stock and include an extra 6 cloves of Garlic. Simmer the stock for 30 minutes, then strain. Dissolve the Tomato Puree in the stock and add the sage, vinegar, soy sauce and red wine. Bring this to the boil and simmer for 10 minutes, stirring occasionally. Let the soup cool slightly, and then pour in the milk. Season well and re-heat gently. Serve hot garnished with a swirl of thick Greek Yoghurt and sprigs of parsley or fresh sage leaves.

Nutrition in Grams per Serving

Protein - 8.60
Fat - 2.55
Carbs - 11.54
Fibre - 0.17
Kcals - 103.05
Sat - 1.13
Mono - 0.74
Poly - 0.16
Trans - 0.01
Omega 3 - 0.04
Omega 6 - 0.12

Mushroom Bisque

Mushrooms have an important role in cookery as they have a good flavour and colour. Also, because they absorb other flavours, they can give richness to many recipes, as well as being delicious in their own right. Flat mushrooms will make the soup dark, and button mushrooms will give it a paler colour.

Serves 6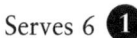

INGREDIENTS

75 g Macadamia oil or Rapeseed oil
1 large onion (265 g), peeled and finely chopped
½ teaspoon (2½ g) Salt
350 g Mushrooms, button or flat
1 teaspoon (5 g) dried Dill
1 teaspoon (5 g) dried Thyme or 1 teaspoon (5 g) fresh Thyme
1 tablespoon (5 g) Paprika
¼ teaspoon (1¼ g) Cayenne Pepper
570 ml Vegetable Stock (see page 80) or use 1 vegetable stock cube
150 ml low fat Natural Yoghurt
Salt and freshly ground black pepper
3 teaspoons (15 g) fresh lemon juice
Garnish: 6 tablespoons (108 g) Yoghurt

Nutrition in Grams per Serving

Protein - 6.74
Fat - 17.13
Carbs - 15.12
Fibre - 4.43
Kcals - 188.72
Sat - 3.19
Mono - 12.41
Poly - 0.56
Trans - 0.04
Omega 3 - 0.09
Omega 6 - 0.45

Gently heat the butter or oil and fry the onion for 10 minutes adding ½ teaspoon of salt while it is frying to bring out the juices. Meanwhile quarter the mushrooms, then add these to the pan with the Dill, Thyme, Paprika and Cayenne pepper. Cook slowly for a further 7-10 minutes on a low heat, covering the mixture with a lid. This extracts a great deal of flavour from both the Onion and the Mushrooms and also draws out juices which improve the final quality of the soup. Pour in the stock and bring to the boil, then reduce the heat and simmer for 3 minutes. Cool slightly and then liquidise. Add salt and pepper and return the soup to a clean pan adding both the natural Yoghurt and the lemon juice. Heat through but do not let it boil otherwise the Yoghurt will curdle. When serving, swirl in a little extra Yoghurt into each bowl.

Soups

French Onion Soup

This rich and flavoursome soup with its large Low Carb croutons has to be my favourite soup for a cold and wintry day.

Serves 8

INGREDIENTS

1 kg Onions (about 4 large), halved and thinly sliced
4 Garlic cloves (24 g), thinly sliced
1 teaspoon (5 g) Cornflour
250 ml dry White Wine
½ teaspoon (2½ g) Stevia
1.3 litres Vegetable Stock (see page 80) or use 3 vegetable stock cubes
4-8 slices Low Carb French bread
(see the Garlic Bread recipe on page 60, without the Garlic butter)
100 g Gruyère, finely grated
1 tablespoon (15 g) Macadamia oil or Rapeseed oil for frying

Nutrition in Grams
per Serving

Protein - 15.77
Fat - 15.53
Carbs - 13.6
Fibre - 10.82
Kcals - 288.25
Sat - 3.77
Mono - 4.68
Poly - 5.9
Trans - 0.16
Omega3 - 4.37
Omega6 - 1.53

Pour some oil into a large saucepan, add the onions and fry with the lid on for 10 minutes until soft. Sprinkle in the Stevia and cook for 20 minutes more, stirring frequently, until caramelised. The onions should be golden and really soft when pricked with a fork. Take care towards the end to ensure that they don't burn.

Add the garlic for the final few minutes of the onions' cooking time, then sprinkle in the cornflour and stir well. Increase the heat and keep stirring as you gradually add the wine, followed by the hot stock. Cover and simmer for 15-20 minutes.

To serve, turn on the grill, and toast the bread. Ladle the soup into heatproof bowls. Put a slice or two of toast on top of the bowls of soup, and pile on the cheese. Grill until melted. Alternatively, you can complete the toasts under the grill, and then serve them on top.

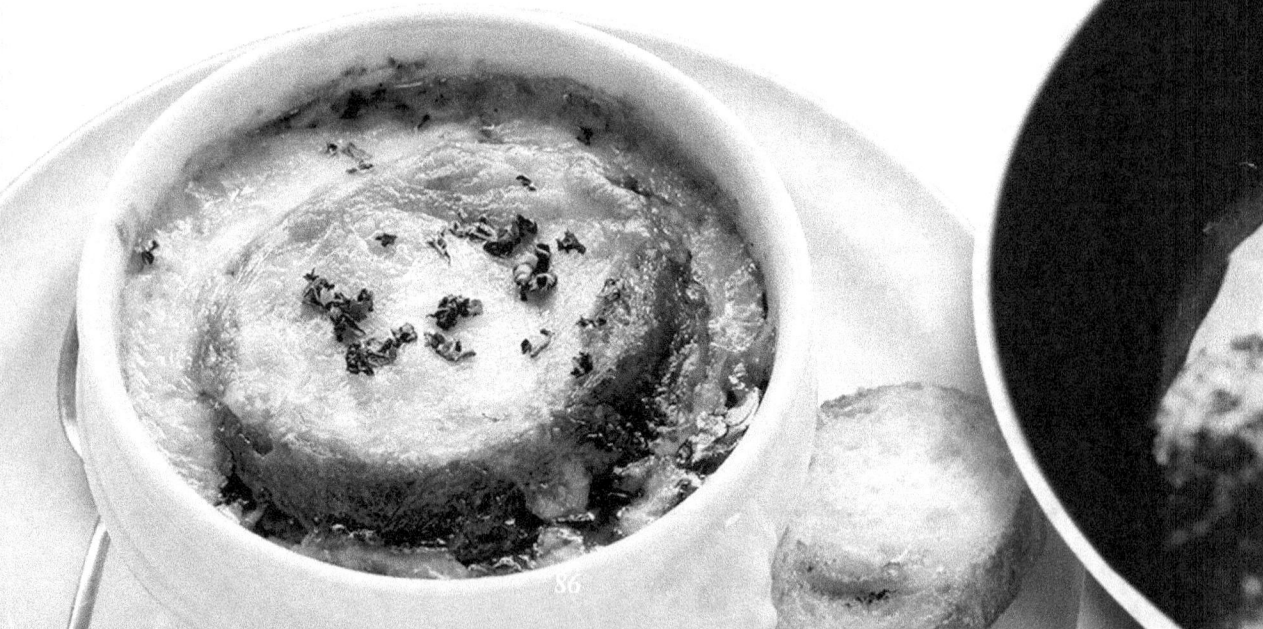

Soups

Broccoli Egg Drop Soup

Serves 4

INGREDIENTS

900 ml Vegetable Stock (see page 80) or use 2 vegetable stock cubes
1 tablespoon (18 ml) Soy sauce
¼ teaspoon (1¼ g) Ginger, ground
40 g Broccoli, chopped
40 g Mushrooms, sliced
2 Large Egg whites (50 g)

In a large saucepan, bring the vegetable stock and soy sauce to the boil and then add the ground ginger. Then, add the broccoli and the mushrooms. Boil for 3-4 minutes or until the broccoli is soft. Lastly, stir in the egg white and remove from the heat. Serve immediately.

Nutrition in Grams
per Serving

Protein - 5.01
Fat - 4.18
Carbs - 14.43
Fibre - 4.28
Kcals - 124.71
Sat - 0.6
Mono - 3.04
Poly - 0.22
Trans - 0
Omega 3 - 0.05
Omega 6 - 0.14

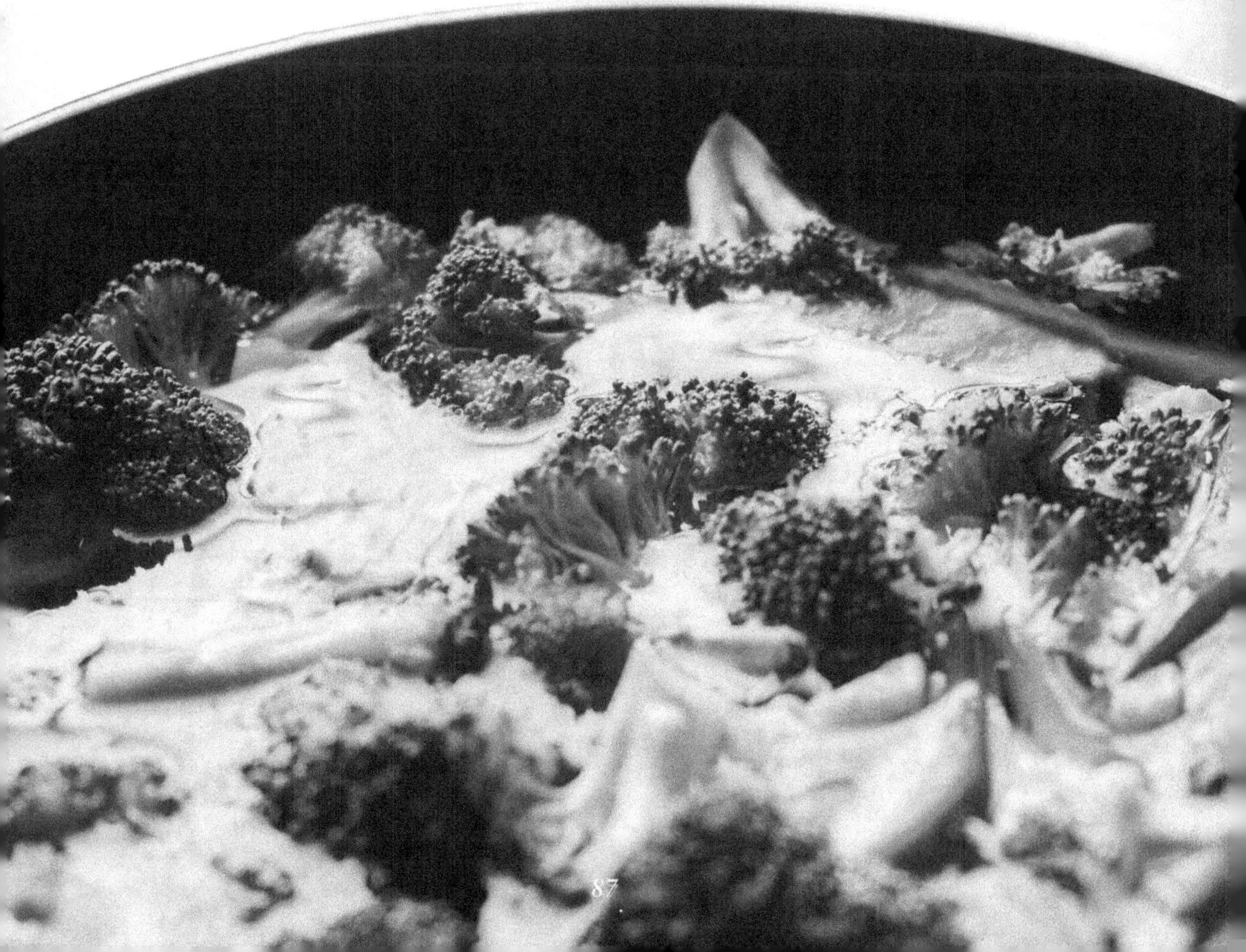

Cream of Pea Soup with Tarragon

This is a light, rich soup that is simple to make, and the combination of milk, cream, peas and tarragon is delicious hot or chilled. If you can't get fresh tarragon, then a good quality dried tarragon would do or you could use fresh mint.

Serves 6

Nutrition in Grams
per Serving

Protein - 8.04
Fat - 9.29
Carbs - 12.44
Fibre - 4.75
Kcals - 180.12
Sat - 5.38
Mono - 2.58
Poly - 0.74
Trans - 0.25
Omega 3 - 0.23
Omega 6 - 0.54

INGREDIENTS

1 bunch Spring Onions (90 g)
30 g Low fat (light) Spreadable Butter with rapeseed or olive oil (or both)
450 g fresh, shelled or frozen Peas
150 ml water
400 ml semi-skimmed milk
170 ml Soured Cream
2 teaspoons (10 g) fresh Tarragon or 1 tablespoon (15 g) dries Tarragon (or fresh Mint)
Salt and freshly ground Black Pepper

First clean the spring onions, then chop the white and green parts finely and reserve some of the green pieces for a garnish. Melt the butter in a medium-sized saucepan on a gentle heat and add the peas, finely chopped spring onions and water. Cook until the peas are tender, which takes about 20-25 minutes. Let this cool slightly and then stir in the milk or cream and fresh tarragon. Season well with salt and pepper.

Put the soup into a liquidiser and liquidise until smooth. Then return it to a clean pan and re heat gently. When serving, garnish each portion with the remaining chopped green spring onion.

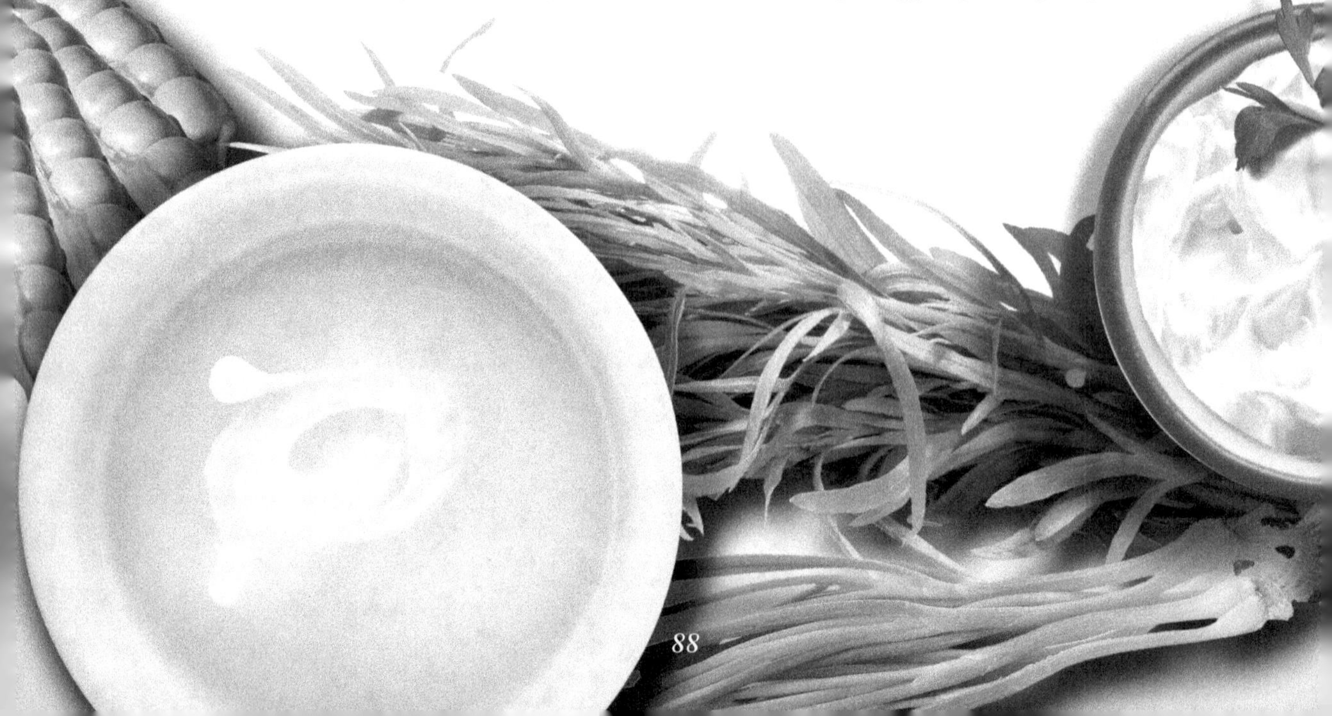

Soups

Mulligatawny Soup

Mulligatawny is an English soup with origins in Indian cuisine. The name originates from the Tamil words millagai / milagu and thanni and can be translated as "pepper-water". The purpose of this particular mulligatawny soup is to get Curcumin into your system to reduce inflammation and therefore insulin resistance.

Curcumin is around 4% of turmeric. It is very badly absorbed by the body with a short half life. But the Bio availability of Curcumin is increased dramatically by Piperine in black pepper (up to 20x), the other chemicals in turmeric (up to 7x), fat and heat (at least 12x).

Serves 2

INGREDIENTS

100 g Celery, grated or very finely chopped
50 g Carrots, grated or very finely cubed
100 g Onion, grated or very finely chopped
20 g of Tomato Puree
10 g medium Curry Powder
5-10 grams Turmeric powder. 5 g for a nice taste,
4 g ground Black Pepper
5 g Bouillon vegetable stock powder
450 g water
60 g whole milk
15 g Rapeseed oil

Nutrition in Grams
per Serving

Protein - 8.33
Fat - 11.05
Carbs - 11.93
Fibre - 3.91
Kcals - 187.27
Sat - 1.97
Mono - 5.45
Poly - 2.6
Trans - 0.03
Omega 3 - 0.78
Omega 6 - 1.82

To make the curry paste, mix the Turmeric, curry powder, milk and the rapeseed oil into a saucepan and mix into a smooth paste and warm gently on a low heat, stirring continually. Put the rest of the ingredients into another saucepan and very gently boil for 15 minutes stirring from time to time. Add the paste from the first saucepan to the soup and simmer but do not boil for a further 15 minutes.

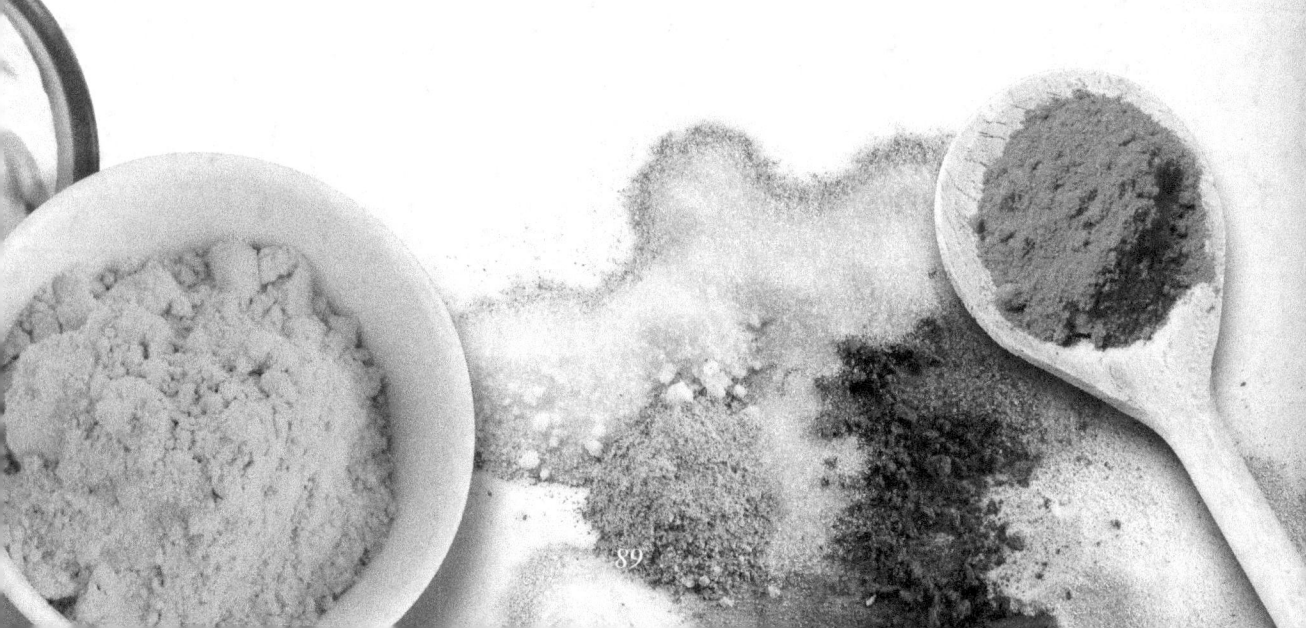

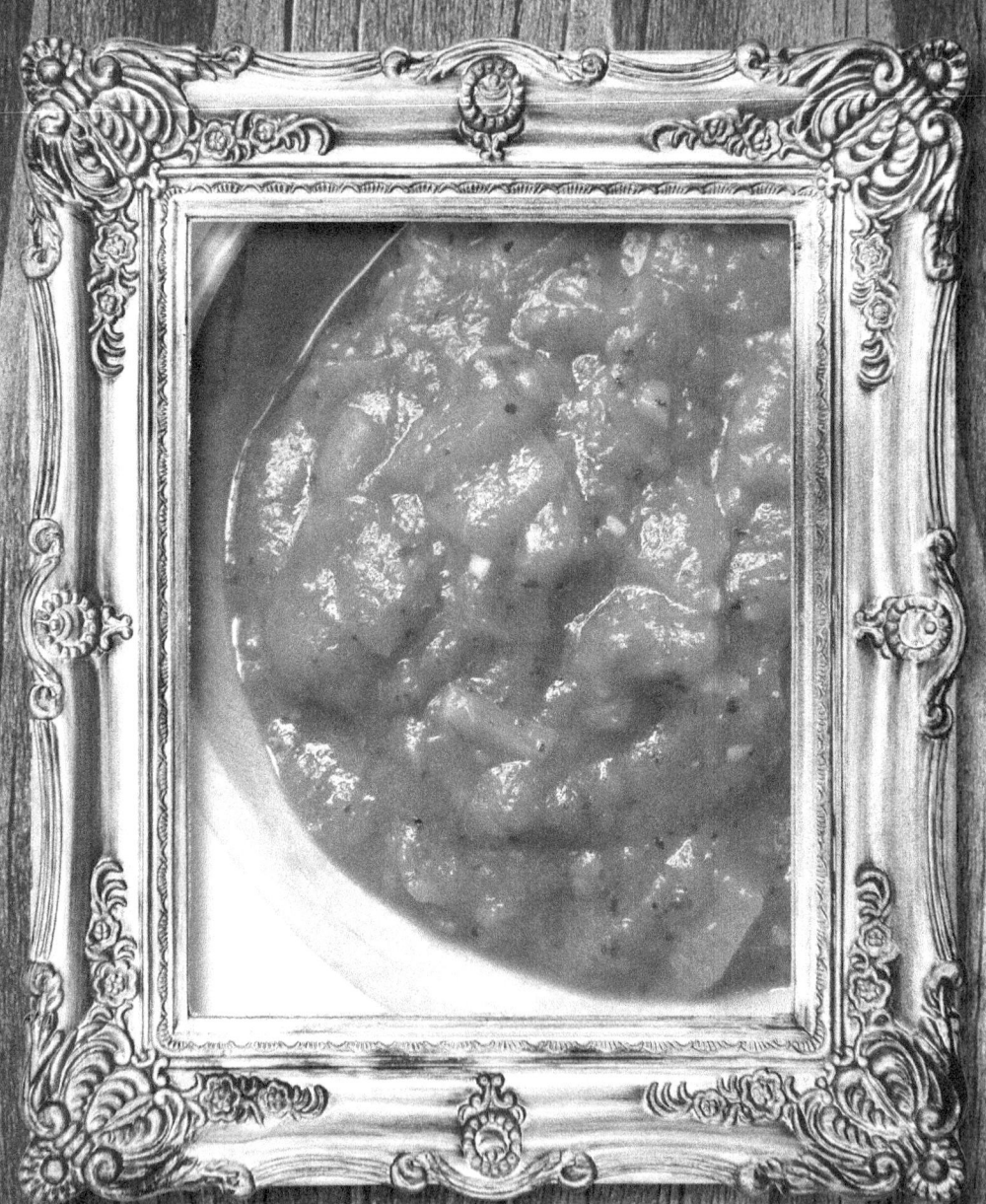

Sauces

Sauces

Savoury Brown Sauce

This rich brown sauce is a great accompaniment for many savoury dishes as a condiment or as an alternative to traditional gravy. The best sauces come from using a good, well flavoured stock, such as our Vegetable stock. The roux should be cooked to a golden colour as this determines the final colour of the sauce, and extra flavouring is added by using yeast extracts or soy sauce. Once you have mastered this, its versatility will become abundantly apparent.

Makes 400 ml/¾ pint sauce - Serves 4

INGREDIENTS

25 g Low fat (light) Spreadable Butter with rapeseed or olive oil

1 large Onion (265 g), peeled and finely chopped

A little salt (1 g)

2 Sticks of celery (80 g), finely chopped

1 teaspoon (5 g) Cornflour

½ teaspoon (2½ g) Mustard powder

670 ml/1 pint Vegetable stock (see page 80) or 2 vegetable stock cubes

1 teaspoon (5 g) dried Thyme or 2 teaspoons (10 g) fresh Thyme

1 Bay leaf (0.3 g)

1 teaspoon (5 g) Yeast extract or 1 teaspoon (5 g) Soy sauce

Salt and freshly ground black pepper

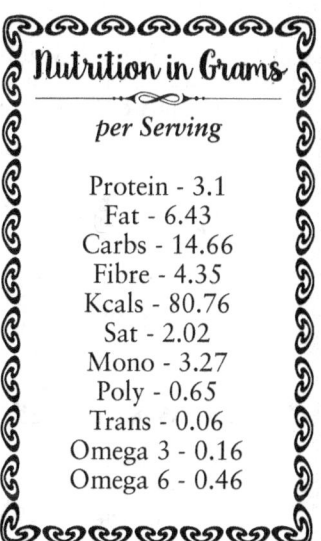

Nutrition in Grams

per Serving

Protein - 3.1
Fat - 6.43
Carbs - 14.66
Fibre - 4.35
Kcals - 80.76
Sat - 2.02
Mono - 3.27
Poly - 0.65
Trans - 0.06
Omega 3 - 0.16
Omega 6 - 0.46

Melt the butter over a gentle heat, and then fry the onion for 5-7 minutes, sprinkling over a little salt so that the juices in the onion are brought out. Then add the celery seed. Sprinkle over the cornflour and mustard powder and allow this roux to cook for 3-5 minutes so that it turns a golden brown colour. Then add the stock gradually, stirring constantly, and bring to the boil adding the thyme, bay leaf and flavourings. Let the sauce cook on a gentle heat for 5-7 minutes, then correct the seasonings and continue cooking for a further 10 minutes in a partially covered pan so that the sauce reduces.

Classic Tomato Sauce

As with the brown sauce, a classic tomato sauce is wonderful on its own as a condiment or as a snack on low carb bread or as an alternative to gravy. This one is very versatile and easy to make; you can also freeze it for later use. Although the sauce is best with fresh tomatoes, a good quality tinned variety is often just as good. This sauce is excellent as a basis for many dishes.

Makes approximately 400 ml/¾ pint sauce - Serves 3

INGREDIENTS

1 tablespoon (15 g) Macadamia oil or Rapeseed oil

1 large Onion (265 g), peeled and finely chopped

1 clove Garlic (6 g), crushed

700 g fresh Tomatoes, skinned and sliced, or 2 x 400 g tins of chopped Tomatoes

2 tablespoons (30 g) Tomato Puree
2 teaspoons (10 g) fresh chopped Basil or 1 teaspoon (5 g) dried Basil
Salt and freshly ground black pepper

Heat the oil in a saucepan and gently fry the chopped onion and garlic for 7-10 minutes until they are soft and translucent, taking care not to colour them. Then add the tomatoes, tomato puree, dried basil (if using), salt and freshly ground black pepper to taste. Lower the heat and cook the sauce for 25-30 minutes in a partially covered pan so that it will reduce slightly. If you are using fresh basil, add it now. Add more seasoning if desired. For a smoother texture the sauce can be liquidised and then re-heated before serving.

Nutrition in Grams
per Serving

Protein - 4.23
Fat - 5.38
Carbs - 14.64
Fibre - 4.40
Kcals - 127.47
Sat - 0.72
Mono - 4.04
Poly - 0.13
Trans - 0.00
Omega 3 - 0.03
Omega 6 - 0.09

Red Wine & Tomato Sauce

Make this special sauce for dinner parties to accompany roasts or as a snack, cold on low carb bread. It is richer than the basic classic tomato sauce as it contains red wine, extra vegetables and herbs.

Makes approximately 1 pint (570 ml) sauce - Serves 4

INGREDIENTS
2 tablespoons (30 g) Macadamia or Rapeseed oil
1 large Onion (265 g), peeled and chopped
1 clove Garlic (6 g), crushed
3 sticks Celery (40 g), chopped
450 g Tomatoes
1.1 litres/2 pints boiling water
2 tablespoons (30 g) Tomato Puree
275 ml/½ pint water
4 tablespoons (60 ml) Red Wine
1 teaspoon (5 g) dried Thyme
1 teaspoon (5 g) dried Basil
½ teaspoon (2½ g) Salt
Freshly ground black pepper

Nutrition in Grams
per Serving

Protein - 2.76
Fat - 7.86
Carbs - 9.9
Fibre - 3.6
Kcals - 136
Sat - 1.11
Mono - 6.08
Poly - 0.17
Trans - 0
Omega 3 - 0.04
Omega 6 - 0.13

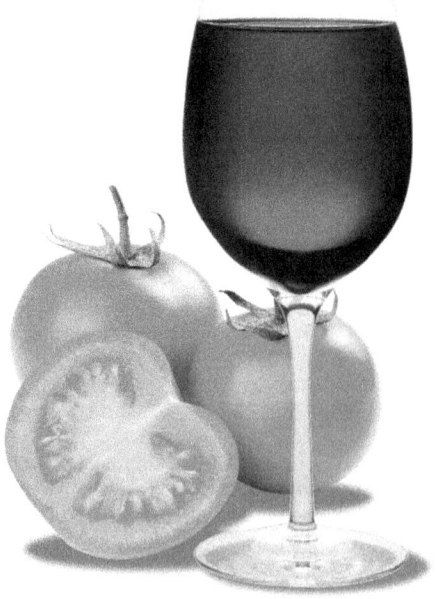

Heat the oil in a saucepan, then add the onion and garlic and cook slowly until softened. Do not let the onion colour. Add the celery and cook for a further 5 minutes. Add the tinned tomatoes or if you are using the fresh tomatoes, put them into a large bowl and pour over the boiling water. Let them stand for a few minutes, then drain, skin and chop. Add these to the pan together with the tomato puree, water, wine and herbs. Season well and simmer uncovered for 30-40 minutes so that the sauce reduces slightly.

Sauces

Green or Red Pesto

Pesto is a sauce originating in Genoa, Italy. Traditionally it consists of crushed garlic, pine nuts, salt, basil leaves, Parmesan cheese and Pecorino Sardo (cheese made from sheep's milk), all blended with olive oil. This alternative cuts down the carbohydrates and fat and is a great addition to Italian dishes or just used as a condiment.

Makes 440 ml, about 20 servings (1 tablespoon per serving)

INGREDIENTS

Green Pesto

150 g garden Peas
2 large stalks of Basil (4 g) (about 15-20 leaves)
½ teaspoon (2½ g) Yeast extract
20 g Parmesan Cheese, grated
20 g Macadamia Nuts, ground
½ teaspoon (2½ g) Salt
Juice of half a Lemon (25 ml)
4 tablespoons (60 ml) Vegetable stock (see page 80)
or use ¼ stock cube
1 clove Garlic (6 g)

For Red Pesto

Replace the peas with 150 g chopped Tomatoes

Green Pesto
Nutrition in Grams
per Serving (1 tbsp)

Protein - 0.9
Fat - 1.1
Carbs - 1.04
Fibre - 0.53
Kcals - 18.93
Sat - 0.29
Mono - 0.67
Poly - 0.05
Trans - 0.01
Omega 3 - 0.01
Omega 6 - 0.04

Combine all the ingredients except for the vegetable stock in a food processor or blender. Slowly add the vegetable stock and continue blending until you achieve your desired consistency. Use it immediately or keep it in an airtight container in the fridge for up to 4 days.

Red Pesto
Nutrition in Grams
per Serving (1 tbsp)

Protein - 0.57
Fat - 1.07
Carbs - 0.57
Fibre - 0.2
Kcals - 13.98
Sat - 0.28
Mono - 0.67
Poly - 0.03
Trans - 0.01
Omega 3 - 0
Omega 6 - 0.03

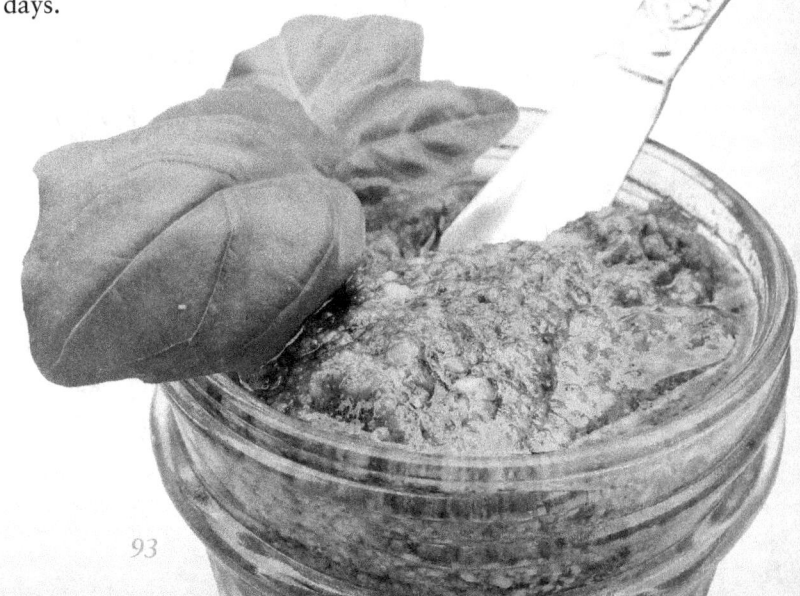

Mayonnaise

Homemade mayonnaise is lighter and creamier in consistency than commercial mayonnaise as well as not having the preservatives. Making mayonnaise also requires the use of eggs that have been 'coddled' or gently cooked in water at just below the boiling point. This process makes the eggs perfectly safe to eat even though they are still a very soft and of a runny consistency. It will keep safely for five to seven days if stored in the fridge.

Makes Approximately 400 ml, about 25 servings (1 tbsp per serving)

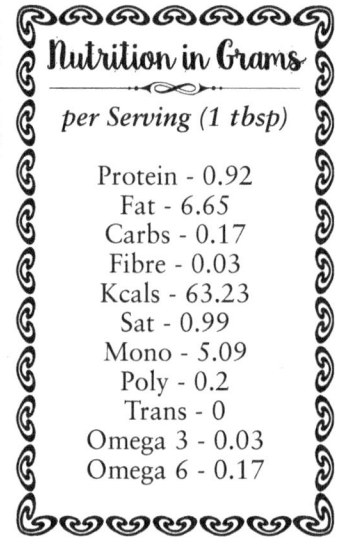

INGREDIENTS

3 coddled large Eggs (175 g)

1 tablespoon (15 g) Mustard, preferably Dijon

1 tablespoon (15 g) apple Cider Vinegar

50 g lemon juice

150 g Macadamia oil

Pinch of salt and freshly ground black pepper

Mayonnaise requires that the egg white still be soft and runny so that it can help make the finished recipe soft and creamy and with the dangers of raw eggs you need to coddle them first. Use eggs that are at room temperature and not straight out of the fridge (this take around half an hour after removal from the fridge). Boil enough water in a saucepan to cover the eggs. While the water is heating up, prepare a bowl full of ice water. When the water has boiled, turn off the heat and immediately place the eggs in the water and leave them for exactly one minute. When the time is up, spoon out the eggs and gently plunge them into the bowl of ice water, being careful not to break the shell. Let them cool for about 2 minutes. Separate 2 coddled yolks and place in food processor, discarding the whites, leaving one whole coddled egg. Add this egg, the mustard, salt, pepper and the lemon juice. Liquidise the mixture for one minute. While still liquidising, slowly add oil by dribbling it in until all the oil has been mixed in. Scrape the sides with a flexible spatula and pour into a jar with a screw top so you can store it if you are not going to be using all at once.

Store any remaining mayonnaise in the fridge for up to 5-7 days. Bring back up to room temperature before serving for the best flavour.

Worcestershire Sauce

Mix together your own Worcestershire sauce to control the ingredients that are being added.

Makes approximately 160 ml about 30 servings (1 teaspoon)

INGREDIENTS

240 ml Apple Cider Vinegar

60 ml Soy Sauce

½ teaspoon (2½ g) Stevia

½ teaspoon (2½ g) ground Ginger
½ teaspoon (2½ g) Mustard powder
½ teaspoon (2½ g) Onion powder
¼ teaspoon (1¼ g) Cinnamon
¼ teaspoon (1¼ g) Chilli powder
¼ teaspoon (1¼ g) ground black pepper
1 clove of Garlic (6 g), crushed

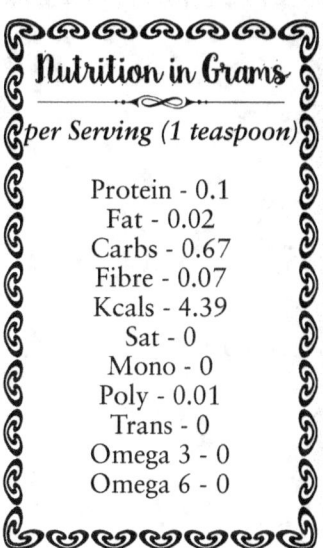

Nutrition in Grams
per Serving (1 teaspoon)

Protein - 0.1
Fat - 0.02
Carbs - 0.67
Fibre - 0.07
Kcals - 4.39
Sat - 0
Mono - 0
Poly - 0.01
Trans - 0
Omega 3 - 0
Omega 6 - 0

Put the apple cider vinegar and soy sauce in a saucepan over a medium heat without a lid. Add the crushed garlic and the dry ingredients, stirring continually. Bring to the boil. When boiling, reduce the heat and simmer for around 20-25 minutes, or until the liquid has reduced by about half. Strain through a sieve and let the sauce cool before using. The sauce can be stored in an airtight container in the fridge for up to 3 months. (It's a good idea to label the container with the date you made the sauce).

Horseradish Sauce

Horseradish sauce made from grated horseradish root and vinegar is a popular condiment in the Britain and Poland. Horseradish is a perennial plant of the vegetable family that includes mustard, wasabi, broccoli, and cabbage. The English word, horseradish, comes from the 16th century. It combines the word horse (used in a symbolic sense to mean strong or coarse) and the word radish. This sauce only takes a few minutes, and the result is demonstrably superior to the supermarket alternative. A great accompaniment to roast meat, particularly beef.

Serves 8 ❷

INGREDIENTS
15 g freshly grated Horseradish, soaked in hot water
1 tablespoon (15 ml) White Wine Vinegar
¼ teaspoon (1.25 g) of Mustard Powder
A pinch of Stevia (1 g)
2 tablespoons (30 g) of chopped fresh Chives
150 ml half fat Crème Fraiche
Salt and Pepper to taste

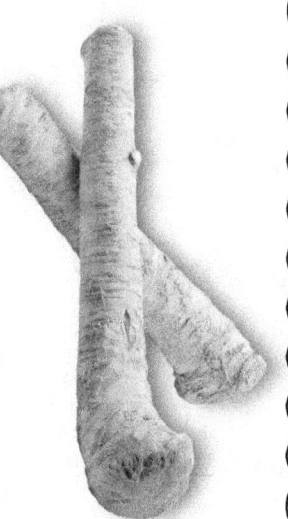

Nutrition in Grams
per Serving

Protein - 0.8
Fat - 2.78
Carbs - 1.52
Fibre - 0.24
Kcals - 34.52
Sat - 1.85
Mono - 0.59
Poly - 0.09
Trans - 0.05
Omega 3 - 0.02
Omega 6 - 0.07

Grate the horseradish on the smallest setting on your grater. But be made aware, onions can make you cry like tear gas does, but horseradish is more like tear gas. Boil some water in a kettle and pour 30 ml into a heatproof bowl. Place the grated horseradish in the water for a couple of minutes and then drain the soaked horseradish. In another bowl, lightly whisk the half fat crème fraiche and stir in the horseradish. Add the other ingredients and mix thoroughly. Kept in a sealed jar it will keep in the fridge for a couple of days.

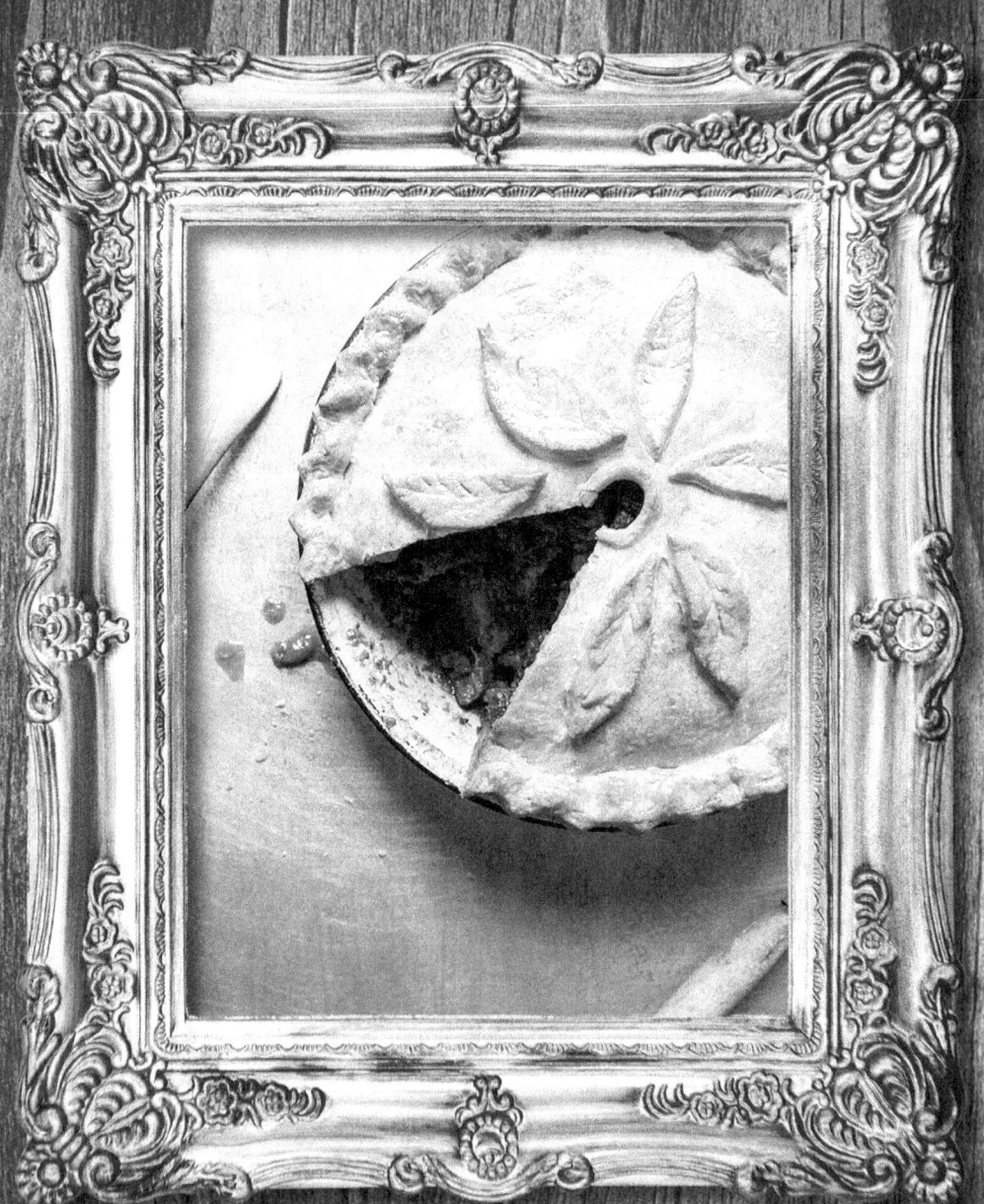

Pastry

Pastry Dishes

Low Carb Flaxseed Pastry

Makes one 23 cm/ 9 inch, 5 cm/ 2 inch deep pie/flan base and sides. Half portion for base only.

INGREDIENTS	Half Portion
150 g Flaxseed, ground	75 g Flaxseed, ground
25 g Low fat (light) Spreadable Butter with rapeseed or olive oil (or both)	12 g Low fat (light) Spreadable Butter with rapeseed or olive oil (or both)
5 g Psyllium Husk	3 g Psyllium Husk
1 medium Egg (65 g)	1 small Egg (45 g)
3 g Baking Powder	1 g Baking Powder
75 ml Water	35 ml Water
1 pinch Salt)	1 pinch Salt

Nutrition in Grams
per whole Portion

Protein - 36.08
Fat - 83.95
Carbs - 3.73
Fibre - 44.3
Kcals - 1025.36
Sat - 16.93
Mono - 16.59
Poly - 44.1
Trans - 0.9
Omega 3 - 34.37
Omega 6 - 9.74

Mix all the dry ingredients together. Beat the egg then add it and the spreadable butter to the mixed powder and mix thoroughly. Slowly add the water, mixing as you go until it becomes dough like (you may not need all the water). Knead until smooth dough is formed. You can then roll it out on a lightly floured hard surface and lightly floured rolling pin (with ground white chia seeds) for your desired shape and thickness.

French Onion Tarts

This is a traditional filling for tarts which is made rich and moist by the succulent onions. When you're cooking the onions, be sure to fry them very slowly so they retain a juicy quality. I like to make small tartlets rather than one large flan as I think there's something especially appetising about an individual serving. These tarts are delicious hot, warm or cold.

Makes 6 Tarts

INGREDIENTS
1 Portion of Short crust Pastry (see page 97)
450 g Onions, peeled and finely chopped
40 g Spreadable butter cut with rapeseed or olive oil or both
½ teaspoon (2½ g) Salt
1 teaspoon (5 g) fresh tarragon
½ teaspoon (2½ g) freshly ground nutmeg
2 medium Eggs (140 g)
50 ml evaporated milk
60 g Extra Mature Cheddar cheese, grated
1 tablespoons (15 g) Low fat (light) Spreadable Butter for greasing the tartlet tins
Salt and freshly ground black pepper

Preheat the oven to gas mark 6 - 200°C (400°F). First prepare the pastry (see page 73) and split the dough into 6 separate and equal amount, making each one into a round ball. Then rest it in the fridge for around 30 minutes. When the dough has rested, roll out the pastry on a lightly floured surface (using extra ground white chia seeds). Grease 6 individual tartlet tins (7 cm diameter) with a little spreadable butter and line them with the individual dough balls and prick well with a fork. Then place in the centre of the oven and bake for 15 minutes until the pastry sets.

Meanwhile fry the onions in the rapeseed oil, taking care not to colour them. During the frying, lightly sprinkle them with salt as this brings out the juices. Then stir in the Tarragon and Nutmeg. Remove from the heat and leave the mixture to cool. In a bowl, beat the eggs thoroughly and mix in the evaporated milk and grated cheese. When the onion filling is cool, season with extra salt and black pepper. Mix it into the cheese and egg mixture and spoon this filling into the pastry cases. Bake for 30 minutes until the pastry shells are cooked and the filling is firm. Serve hot, warm or cold.

Nutrition in Grams
per Serving

Protein - 11.41
Fat - 30.55
Carbs - 8
Fibre - 6.53
Kcals - 367.14
Sat - 7.99
Mono - 7.13
Poly - 13.3
Trans - 0.25
Omega 3 - 9.45
Omega 6 - 3.85

Quiche Gruyère Chanterelle

The use of chanterelle mushrooms dates back to the 16th century although they first gained widespread recognition as a culinary delicacy with the spreading influence of French cuisine in the 18th century, where they began appearing in palace kitchens. Chanterelles are rich in flavour, with a distinctive taste and aroma difficult to characterize. Some species have a fruity odour, others an earthy fragrance, while others can be spicy. The combination of these mushrooms with the Gruyère cheese makes this quiche extremely flavoursome and hearty.

Serves 4 **3**

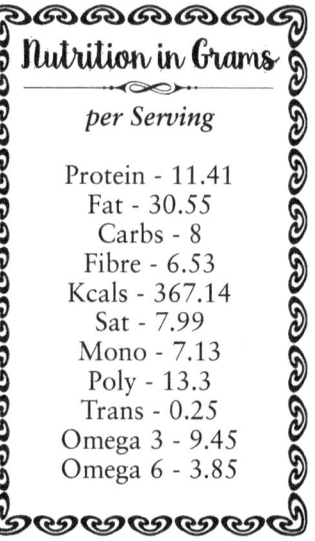

Nutrition in Grams
per Serving

Protein - 25.41
Fat - 45.18
Carbs - 7.79
Fibre - 10.82
Kcals - 562.25
Sat - 11.52
Mono - 11.03
Poly - 19.47
Trans - 0.5
Omega 3 - 14.03
Omega 6 - 5.5

INGREDIENTS
For the pastry
One portion of Low Carb Shortcrust Pastry (see page 97)

For the filling
100 g Gruyère cheese, coarsely grated
4 tomatoes (320 g), thinly sliced
2 Leeks (200 g), sliced
150 g Chanterelle Mushrooms, sliced
3 medium Eggs (195 g), beaten
200 ml semi-skimmed Milk
1 tablespoon half fat cream cheese (30 ml)
Salt to taste freshly ground black pepper
2 sprigs (1 g) of fresh Thyme
1 teaspoon (5 g) Low fat (light) Spreadable Butter with

Pastry Dishes

rapeseed or olive oil (or both) for greasing the flan dish
½ tablespoon (7.5 ml) Rapeseed oil or Macadamia oil for frying

First prepare the pastry (see page 97) Then rest it in the fridge for around 30 minutes. When the dough has rested, roll out the pastry on a lightly floured surface (using extra ground white chia seeds) and line a deep (at least 5 cm/2 inches) 23 cm/9 inch diameter lightly greased flan dish, trimming any excess off. Chill again for 10 minutes.

While the pastry is chilling, heat the Rapeseed oil or Macadamia oil and cook the leeks for 10 minutes, stirring occasionally, until they soften. Then turn up the heat and add the mushrooms. Cook for 5 minutes more, and then turn off the heat. Preheat the oven to gas mark 5 - 190°C (375°F). Remove the flan dish from the fridge and place in the centre of the oven and bake for 15 minutes. Place on a baking tray and bake blind for 20 minutes. Reduce the temperature of the oven to gas mark 3 - 160°C (325°F).

Mix the eggs with the milk, cream cheese and half the Gruyère cheese in a bowl and season well. Pour the leek and mushroom mixture into the bowl and mix. Line the bottom of the pastry case with a layer of half the sliced tomatoes. Pour this into the pastry case and add the remaining sliced tomatoes over the top and sprinkle the remaining cheese and the fresh thyme over the entire flan. Bake in the centre of the oven for 30-40 minutes or until set. Remove from the oven and leave to cool and set further. Serve hot or cold.

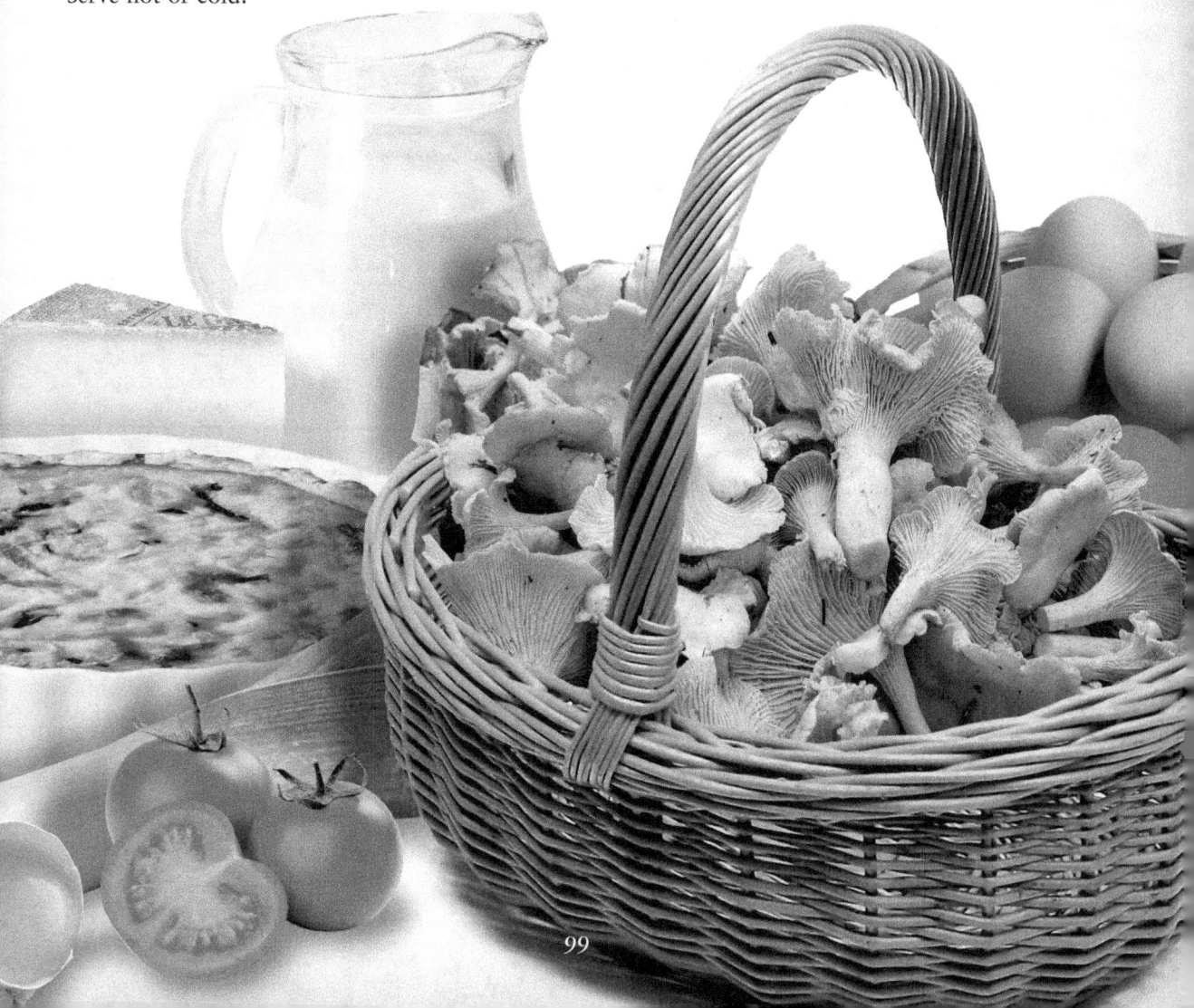

Pastry Dishes

Chicken & Mozzarella Pie

This is a hearty chicken pie that is best served lukewarm. Serve with carrots and broccoli and Tomato Sauce for a rich winter warmer. You can also replace the chicken with lean minced Beef or minced lamb for an alternative choice.

Serves 4

INGREDIENTS

For the pastry

One portion of Low Carb Shortcrust Pastry (see page 97)

400 g Chicken breasts
1 large Onion (265 g), finely chopped
1 Garlic clove (6 g), crushed
1 tablespoon (15 g) of dried Oregano
4 tablespoons (60 g) Tomato Puree
150 ml Chicken Stock using one chicken stock cube
1 tablespoon (15 ml) Rapeseed oil or Macadamia oil for frying
Salt to taste freshly ground black pepper

Topping

80 g Mozzarella cheese, reduced fat
2 large Tomatoes (200 g)

Nutrition in Grams

per Serving

Protein - 41.1
Fat - 38.57
Carbs - 10.45
Fibre - 11.01
Kcals - 575.3
Sat - 7.66
Mono - 9.57
Poly - 18.76
Trans - 0.2
Omega 3 - 13.89
Omega 6 - 4.88

Put some rapeseed oil in a large saucepan and place the Chicken breasts into it on a medium heat and fry until cooked through and golden brown on the outside. When cooked, remove the chicken breasts from the pan and put onto a plate. When the chicken breasts have cooled down a bit, cut them roughly into about 2½ cm/1 inch cubes. In the same frying pan, fry the onion and garlic (adding a little more rapeseed oil if needed) on a medium heat for a few minutes, until the onion is soft and translucent. Add the chicken chunks and keep frying for a couple of minutes, turning the chicken to the cut side to lightly brown them. Add seasoning and the oregano.

Alternatively, if you are going to used either lean minced Lamb or Beef, add the mince after frying the onions and garlic and keep stirring until the meat is consistently browned all over, around 10 minutes will be enough.

Add the Tomato puree and chicken stock. Bring to the boil slowly, lower the heat and let it simmer for about 20 more minutes while you're making the pastry.

Preheat the oven to gas mark 4 - 175°C (350°F). When you have finished the pastry dough, roll it out to about 3 - 4 mm thick. Put a little spreadable butter into a round 23 cm/9 inch diameter by 5 cm/2 inch deep ovenproof pie dish and spread all over the dish with your fingers. Place the rolled pastry into the dish and fit it into the dish, again best done with your fingers. Trim the excess pastry with a knife. Bake the pasty in the centre of the oven for 15 minutes, this pre-cooking is known as blind baking and it makes sure that the inside of the pie crust is cooked before you put the contents in.

When it's cooked, take it out of the oven and place the meat mixture into the pastry crust, using a fork to pat it down. Sprinkle the Mozzarella over the top evenly. Thinly slice the Tomatoes and spread them evenly over the Mozzarella and brush the tomatoes with a little rapeseed oil. Place the pie back in the centre of the oven and bake for 30-40 minutes or until the pie has turned a nice golden brown colour.

Pastry Dishes

Spinach & Goat's Cheese Pie

Spinach is a vegetable rich in flavour and nutrition and is perfectly complemented by the eggs and goat's cheese.

Serves 4

INGREDIENTS

1 portion of shortcrust pastry (see page 97)

2 teaspoon (5 g) Low fat (light) Spreadable Butter with rapeseed or olive oil (or both) for greasing the flan dish

Egg Topping

5 medium Eggs (325 g)

100 ml half fat Crème Fraiche

100 g Goat's cheese, sliced or crumbled

Salt and pepper

Filling

450 g fresh Spinach

1 Garlic clove, crushed (6 g)

1 pinch ground nutmeg (1 g)

Salt and pepper

Nutrition in Grams
per Serving

Protein - 25.74
Fat - 44.95
Carbs - 3.69
Fibre - 12.36
Kcals - 540.89
Sat - 12.05
Mono - 9.42
Poly - 19.57
Trans - 0.26
Omega 3 - 13.93
Omega 6 - 5.65

Preheat the oven to gas mark 4 - 175°C (350°F). First prepare your pastry and line a deep (at least 5 cm/2 inches) 23 cm/9 inch slightly greased flan dish. Bake blind for 15 minutes. Whisk together the eggs and crème fraiche. Add salt, pepper and ground nutmeg and stir together. Chop up the spinach. Fry the garlic in rapeseed oil in a frying pan on a very low heat for about 1 minute, being careful not to brown them. Add the chopped spinach, mix well and fry for a further couple of minutes. Season to taste. Layer the base of the pastry with the chopped spinach mixture. Then pour the egg mixture over the spinach. Crumble or slice (depending on its texture) the goat's cheese all over the top. Bake in the top half of the oven for 30 minutes until nicely browned.

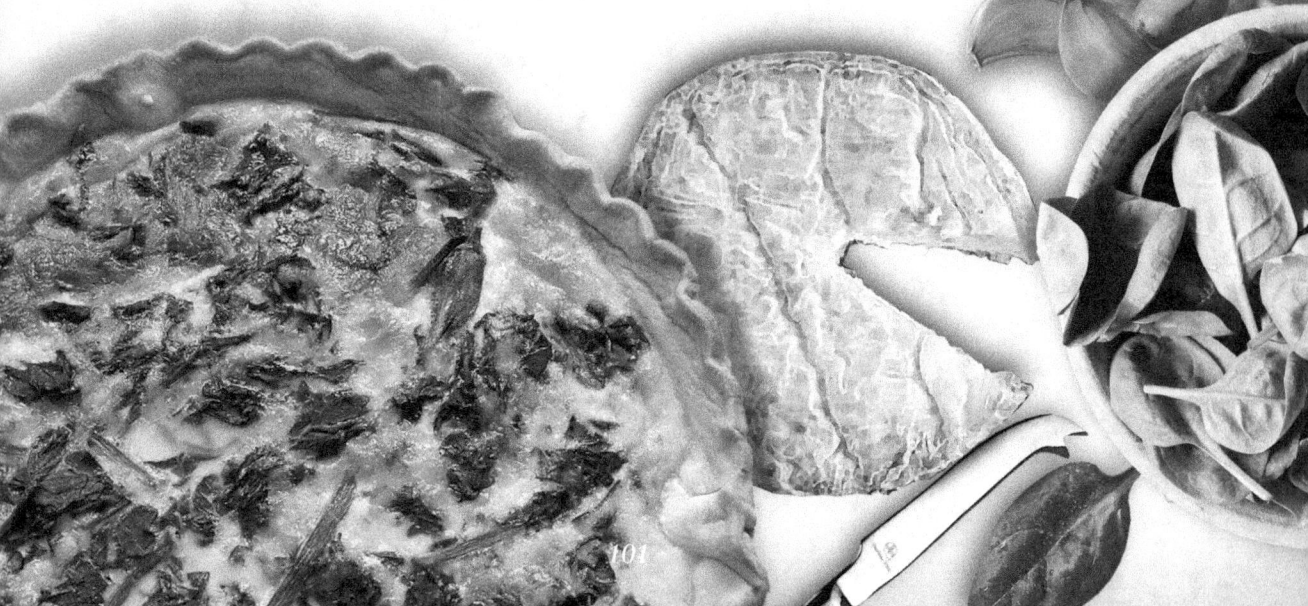

=== Pastry Dishes ===

Mushroom Flan

Serves 4

INGREDIENTS

1 quantity of Shortcrust Pastry (see page 97)
350 g button Mushrooms, wiped and left whole
3 medium Eggs (195 g)
150 ml semi-skimmed Milk
20 g Low fat (light) Spreadable Butter with rapeseed or olive oil (or both)
2 tablespoons (30 g) half fat Crème Fraiche
Salt and freshly ground black pepper
½ teaspoon Paprika (2.5 g)

Nutrition in Grams
per Serving

Protein - 17.13
Fat - 38.33
Carbs - 5.01
Fibre - 8.75
Kcals - 449.23
Sat - 8.76
Mono - 7.41
Poly - 19.16
Trans - 0.32
Omega 3 - 13.87
Omega 6 - 5.3

Preheat the oven to gas mark 6 - 200°C (400°F). Roll out the pastry to fit a 23 cm (9 inch) flan dish. Press the pastry into the case well, prick all over with a fork and bake for 15 minutes. Then allow the case to cool slightly.

Meanwhile prepare the filling. Melt the butter very gently in a frying-pan and fry the whole button mushrooms for 6 minutes over a very gentle heat. In a medium-sized mixing bowl beat the eggs thoroughly, add the milk and crème fraiche and beat thoroughly again.

When the mushrooms are just soft, remove the pan from the heat and allow to cool slightly. Then add them to the egg and milk mixture. Season well and pour this filling into the flan dish. Dust the top with a little paprika then bake in the middle of the oven for 35 minutes or until the centre feels firm to the touch. Serve hot or cold.

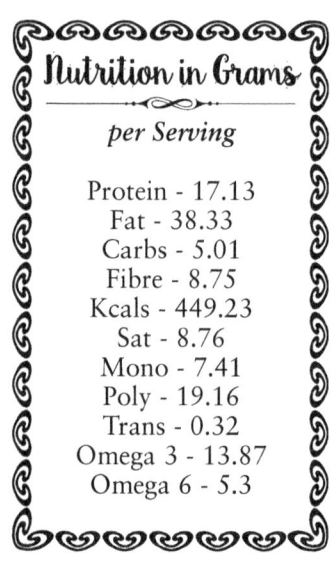

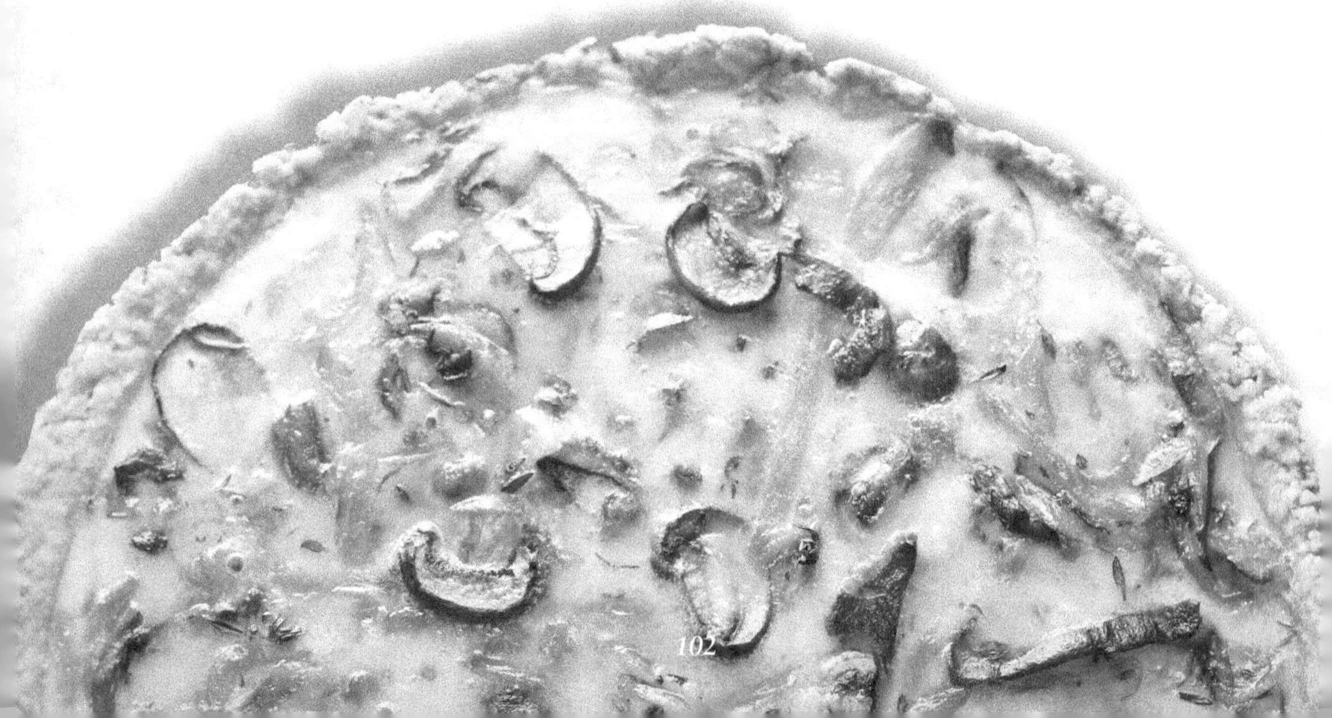

Pastry Dishes

Winter Vegetable Pie

There are all sorts of different combinations of vegetables you can use to make rich and colourful pies, but it is important to achieve the right mix between soft and fibrous vegetables so that you get a good texture. This pie is good served with Savoury Brown Sauce (see page 91) or Tomato Sauce (see page 91), Roast Paprika Turnips (see page 127) and green vegetables.

Serves 6

INGREDIENTS

Double quantity of Shortcrust Pastry (see page 97)
1 large Onion (265 g), peeled and chopped
2 Carrots (160 g), scrubbed and finely chopped
450 g Courgettes, washed and diced
110 g mushrooms, wiped and sliced
2 large (200 g) Tomatoes, washed and chopped
1 teaspoon (2 g) fresh Thyme or ½ teaspoon (2½ g) dried Thyme
1 teaspoon (2 g) fresh Marjoram or ½ teaspoon (2½ g) dried Marjoram
2 tablespoons (15 g) fresh Parsley, finely chopped
2 tablespoons (30 g) Tomato Puree
1 tablespoon (15 g) Soy sauce
1 tablespoon (15 g) Macadamia oil or Rapeseed oil for frying
Beaten small Egg (55 g) and salt for glazing
A little Low fat (light) Spreadable Butter with rapeseed or olive oil (or both) for greasing the flan dish
Salt and freshly ground black pepper

Nutrition in Grams
per Serving

Protein - 13.08
Fat - 41.31
Carbs - 10.41
Fibre - 13.46
Kcals - 494.47
Sat - 5.87
Mono - 8.57
Poly - 24.52
Trans - 0.1
Omega 3 - 18.46
Omega 6 - 6.07

Pre-heat the oven to gas mark 5 - 190°C (375°F). Heat the oil in a large saucepan and gently fry the onions. Then prepare the carrots, courgettes, mushrooms and tomatoes and add them to the pan with the thyme and marjoram. Mix everything together well, cover the pan and cook gently until the vegetables are just soft. This takes about 10-15 minutes. Add the tomato puree, soy sauce and season to taste. Let the mixture cool.

Meanwhile line a 9 inch (23 cm) flan dish with the pastry and bake blind for 15 minutes. Turn the oven temperature up to gas mark 6 - 200°C (400°F). Fill the pastry case with the mixture, packing it down fairly firmly and sprinkle the fresh parsley over it. Cover with a pastry lid and brush with the egg glaze. Cut the pastry lid with a knife with 2 cuts in the centre of the pie about 1 cm in length, so that the steam can escape. Bake the pie in the centre of the oven for 35 or 40 minutes or until the pastry is crisp. Serve hot or warm.

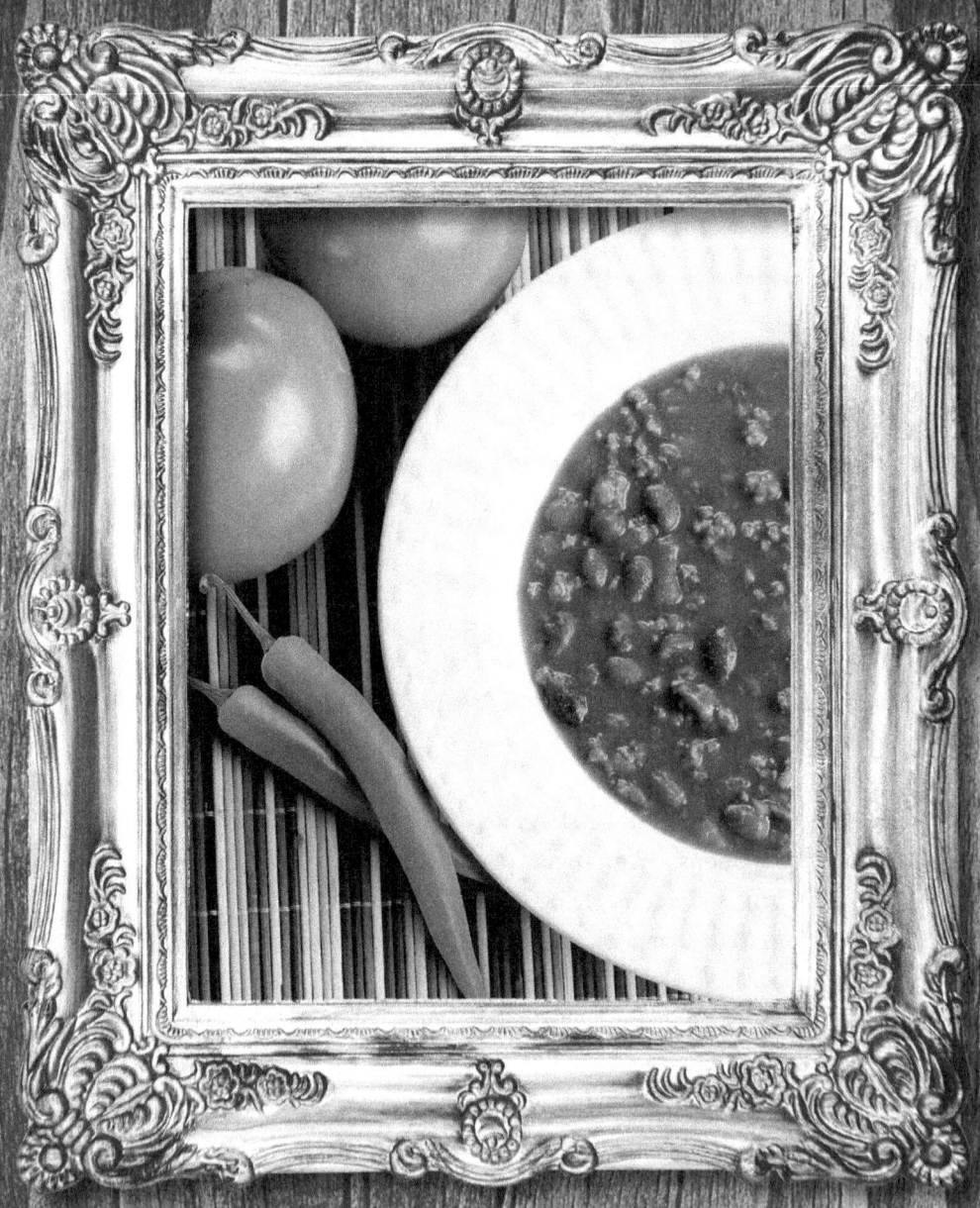

Miscellaneous Main Dishes

Miscellaneous Main Dishes

Chilli Con Carne

Chilli con carne is commonly known in English as simply 'chilli', and comes from the Spanish, literally meaning 'chilli pepper with meat' and is a spicy stew containing chilli peppers, beef, tomatoes and beans.

Serves 5

INGREDIENTS

500 g lean minced Beef (5% fat)
1 large Onions (265 g), chopped
3 Garlic cloves (18 g), peeled and finely chopped
1 teaspoon (5 g) hot Chilli powder (depending on taste) or 1 medium or hot Red Chilli Pepper (finely sliced)
150 ml Red Wine
150 ml Beef stock, made with 1 Beef stock cube
400 g tin of chopped Tomatoes
200 g of tinned Kidney beans, drained and rinsed
3 tablespoons (45 g) Tomato purée
1 teaspoon (5 ml) Cider Vinegar
1 Bay leaf (0.3 g)
1 tablespoon (15 ml) Lemon Juice
Salt and pepper to taste

Garnish:
250 g low fat Natural Yoghurt

Nutrition in Grams
per Serving

Protein - 34.84
Fat - 6.24
Carbs - 17.68
Fibre - 6.04
Kcals - 298.08
Sat - 2.40
Mono - 2.25
Poly - 0.63
Trans - 0.16
Omega 3 - 0.18
Omega 6 - 0.44

Place a large non-stick saucepan over a medium heat and fry the onions and garlic until soft. Add the minced beef and cook for 5 minutes, stirring continuously to break up the mince and brown the meat all over. Add 1-2 teaspoons of chilli powder, depending on how hot you like your chilli or 1 finely chopped red chilli pepper (you can get mild, medium or hot). Fry together for 2 minutes more. Stir well.

Slowly add the wine and then the stock, stirring constantly. Add the cider vinegar and lemon juice. Tip the tomatoes and kidney beans into the pan and stir in the tomato purée and bay leaf. Season with a pinch of salt and plenty of freshly ground black pepper. Bring to boil and simmer, then cover with a lid. Reduce the heat and leave to simmer gently for 45 minutes, stirring occasionally until the mince is tender and the sauce is thick. Adjust the seasoning to taste and serve.

Serve with a swirl of natural yoghurt and either Spiced Cauliflower or Broccoli Rice (see page 160)

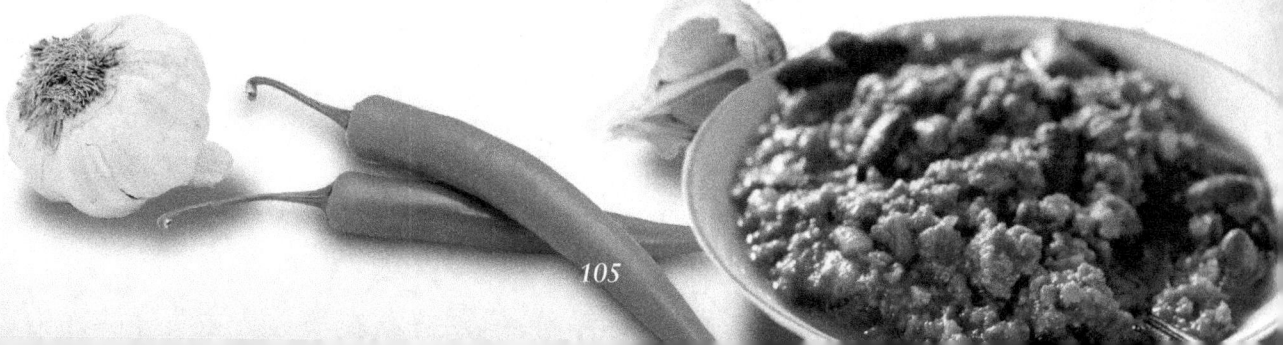

Miscellaneous Main Dishes

Cheese Aubergine Bake

This is one of my favourite dishes; it is rich and colourful yet simple to make and very satisfying to eat. Some people find that aubergines are bitter. To remove the bitterness, slice the aubergines, which need not be peeled, and sprinkle them with salt. Leave them to stand, then wash and dry before frying.

Serves 4

INGREDIENTS

50 ml Macadamia oil or Rapeseed oil
1 large Onion (265 g), peeled and finely chopped
2 cloves Garlic (12 g), crushed
2 x 400 g tin of Tomatoes, drained
2 tablespoons (30 g) Tomato puree
2 teaspoons (10 g) fresh chopped Basil or 1 teaspoon (5 g) dried Basil
Salt and freshly ground black pepper
550 g Aubergines, unpeeled
100 g Mozzarella Cheese, grated
1 tablespoon (15 g) Parmesan Cheese

Nutrition in Grams

per Serving

Protein - 10.36
Fat - 19.50
Carbs - 17.04
Fibre - 7.56
Kcals - 294.91
Sat - 5.77
Mono - 11.63
Poly - 0.47
Trans - 0.24
Omega 3 - 0.09
Omega 6 - 0.38

Pre-heat the oven to gas mark 4 - 180°C (350°F). Heat 1 tablespoon of the Rapeseed oil or Macadamia oil in a saucepan and gently fry the finely chopped onion and crushed garlic for 5 to 7 minutes until they are soft. Then add the tomatoes, tomato puree, basil, salt and pepper, cover the pan and let this mixture simmer on a very low heat for 30 minutes, stirring occasionally. Wash the aubergines and cut them into slices about ¼ inch (½ cm) thick. Put them on a large plate, lightly salt them and then leave them for 20 minutes so that any bitter juices are drawn out. After this, rinse and pat dry. Heat some more Rapeseed oil or Macadamia oil in a deep frying-pan and fry the slices a few at a time so that they become soft and are lightly browned. Drain them on kitchen paper.

Next lightly oil a 3 pint (1.75 litre) ovenproof dish and pour in a little of the tomato sauce. Then make a layer of one-third of the aubergine slices followed by a layer of grated Mozzarella cheese and then some more sauce, repeat these layers ending with a topping of sauce, and cover that with the Parmesan cheese. Cover the dish with foil or a matching lid and bake it for 20 minutes in the centre of the oven. Then uncover it and bake for a further 10 minutes so that the cheese browns nicely on top and serve straight away.

Stuffed Aubergines

Cheese and mushrooms make a delicious filling for aubergines which when baked turn a rich brown colour. This dish goes well with the Classic Tomato Sauce (see page 91) a bright green vegetable such as Spiced Cauliflower or Broccoli Rice (see page 160)

Serves 4

Miscellaneous Main Dishes

INGREDIENTS

4 medium sized (1.2 kg) Aubergines
1 small Onion (150 g), peeled and finely chopped
175 g Mushrooms, wiped and finely chopped
100 g Extra Mature Cheddar cheese, grated
2 teaspoons (8 g) finely chopped fresh Marjoram or 1 teaspoon (5 g) dried Marjoram
¼ teaspoon (1¼ g) Cayenne Pepper
2 medium Eggs (130 g)
Salt and freshly ground black pepper
Olive oil for brushing filling (10 ml)
1 quantity of Savoury Brown Sauce (see page 91)

Nutrition in Grams
per Serving

Protein - 18.18
Fat - 20.64
Carbs - 27.23
Fibre - 13.21
Kcals - 334.69
Sat - 7.9
Mono - 8.59
Poly - 1.76
Trans - 0.29
Omega 3 - 0.31
Omega 6 - 1.4

Pre-heat the oven to gas mark 4 - 180°C (350°F). Cut the aubergine in half lengthways and scoop out the flesh with a teaspoon, taking care not to split the skins and leaving a shell ½ cm/¼ inch thick. Place the shells in boiling water for 5 minutes to blanch. Now prepare the onions, mushrooms and cheese and mix them all together in a large bowl. Mix in the chopped aubergine flesh, marjoram and cayenne pepper. Beat the eggs and add to the aubergine filling, mixing them in thoroughly. Then season to taste. Pile some filling into each of the aubergine shells and lay them in a lightly oiled ovenproof dish. Pour in the Savoury Brown Sauce around the aubergines and brush the filling with some extra oil. Cover the dish with foil or a matching lid and bake for 40 minutes or until the shells are tender and the topping dark brown. Serve immediately.

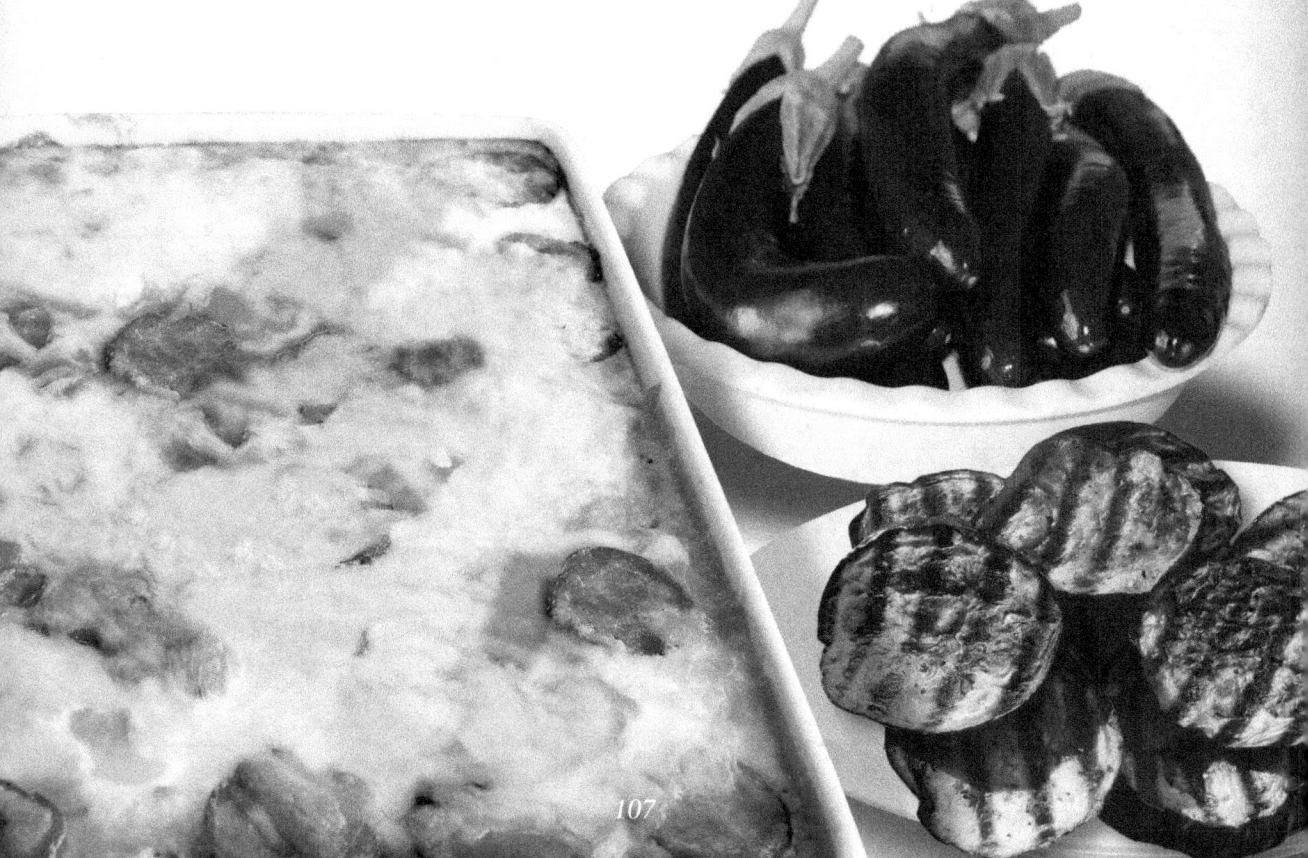

Miscellaneous Main Dishes

Fried Chicken in the Hole

This recipe uses chicken pieces instead of sausages, as sausages are cured and detrimental to diabetics. You could replace the chicken with roast pork pieces or a beef steak, cut up.

Serves 2

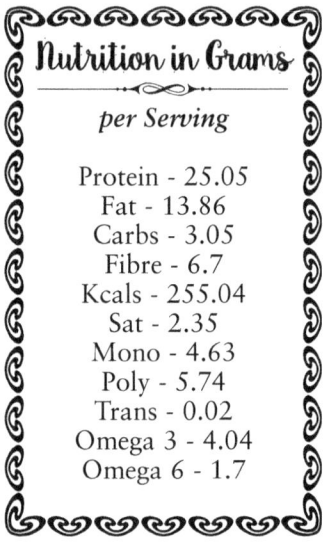

Nutrition in Grams

per Serving

Protein - 25.05
Fat - 13.86
Carbs - 3.05
Fibre - 6.7
Kcals - 255.04
Sat - 2.35
Mono - 4.63
Poly - 5.74
Trans - 0.02
Omega 3 - 4.04
Omega 6 - 1.7

INGREDIENTS

150 g Chicken meat (breast)
½ teaspoon Mixed Herbs

Batter
25 g Flax Seed
12.5 g White Chia Seeds
2 g Psyllium Husk
1 g Baking Powder
80 ml Semi-skimmed Milk
160 ml Water
1 small Egg (55 g)
1 teaspoon (5 ml) Macadamia oil for greasing the baking tray
Pinch of Salt & Pepper

Pre-heat the oven to Gas Mark 7 - 220°C (420°F). In a little Macadamia oil or Rapeseed oil fry the chicken breast, turning regularly until it is browned and flesh is white. Put aside and leave to cool. Then cut the chicken into small chunks (about 2 cm/1 inches by 1 cm/½ inches). For the batter, mix the flaxseed, chia seeds, psyllium husk and baking powder together and finely grind them in a nut mill, blender or food processor, and empty into a bowl. Make a small indent in the middle of the mixture and crack the egg into it. Slowly mix the egg into the mixture, making sure you mix all the dry ingredients with the egg. Mix the milk and water in a jug and add a little to the mixture and mix thoroughly. Gradually add more, continually mixing until you have added all the liquid. Season to taste and add the mixed herbs. Keep stirring until the batter is as smooth as possible and put into the fridge to rest. Meanwhile, in an indented baking tray with 4 indents 10 cm/4 inches in diameter and roughly 1 cm/ ½ inch in depth, pour a little oil into each and spread the oil all over the indent with a brush or your fingers. Place the tray into the top of the oven and leave for 15 minutes.

The secret with all batters is for the oil to be very hot. Once done, remove the batter from the fridge and take the tray out of the oven. Pour a little of the batter mix into each indent, just enough to cover the bottom and place 4 pieces of the sausages into each indent. Pour the rest of the batter on top of the sausages, making sure you cover them. Place the tray back into the top of the oven. Cook for 45 minutes or until the batter has risen and is a dark brown colour. Do not check them for at least 30 minutes as they will quickly deflate. Serve immediately.

Turnip Topped Cumberland Pie

A Shepherd's Pie is traditionally made from minced Lamb (the clue is in the title) while a Cottage Pie is made from minced Beef, a traditional Cumberland Pie can, however, be made from either meat and differs from the others inasmuch as it has an extra layer on top of the mash of breadcrumbs and cheese.

Serves 5

INGREDIENTS

2 Celery sticks (80 g), sliced into 1 cm/½ inch pieces
2 large Leeks (200 g)
1 large Onion (265 g), finely chopped
2 large Carrots (160 g), sliced
5 Bay leaves (1.5 g)
3 Thyme sprigs (1½ g) or 1 teaspoon of dried Thyme
2 tablespoon (30 g) Rapeseed oil or Macadamia oil
2 teaspoon (10 g) plain Flour
2 tablespoon (30 g) Tomato Purée
1 tablespoon (15 g) Yeast Extract/Marmite (don't worry if you hate it, it complements the flavour rather than taking it over)
2 Beef stock cubes (10 g)
400 g 5% fat lean minced Beef or minced lamb
850 g Turnips, cut into 1 cm thick slices
2 x 1 cm slice of the Low carb Bread, crumbled into breadcrumbs (see page 58)
25 g Grated Extra Mature Cheddar Cheese
25 g Grated Parmesan Cheese

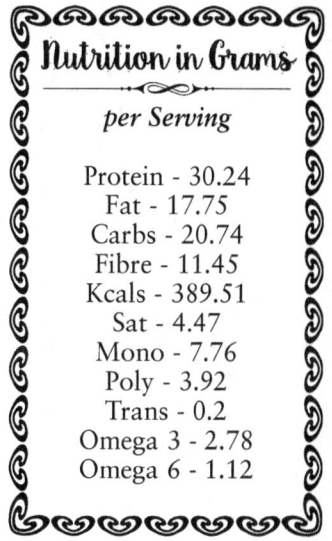

Nutrition in Grams
per Serving

Protein - 30.24
Fat - 17.75
Carbs - 20.74
Fibre - 11.45
Kcals - 389.51
Sat - 4.47
Mono - 7.76
Poly - 3.92
Trans - 0.2
Omega 3 - 2.78
Omega 6 - 1.12

Pre-heat the oven to gas mark 4 - 180°C (350°F). Heat half the Rapeseed oil or Macadamia oil in a large frying pan and add the chopped onions and fry until translucent on a low heat. Add the celery, carrots, leeks, bay leaves and 1 sprig of thyme/dried thyme and cook for around 10 minutes or until soft. Stir in the flour and add the tomato purée, yeast extract and crumble in the Beef stock cubes.

Heat up 200 ml of water (not quite boiling) and gradually stir it into the mixture, add the minced beef and turn the heat up until the sauce is bubbling slightly, stirring occasionally. Turn down the heat and simmer for 20 minutes. Meanwhile, cook the sliced turnips in a pan of boiling water until they're not done but about three quarters of the way there, about 7 minutes. Drain thoroughly (ideally using a colander) and add the remaining thyme and season to taste. Put the grated parmesan and cheddar in a bowl and add the low carb breadcrumbs. Layer all the sliced turnips over the meat followed by a layer of the cheese mixture. Brush a little Rapeseed oil or Macadamia oil over the top. Pop the dish in the top half of the oven and bake for 30 minutes until golden and crispy, and the sauce is bubbling.

Classic Shepherd's Pie

A classic shepherd's pie made with minced lamb and topped with mashed swede and turnips.

Serves 6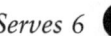

INGREDIENTS

1 tablespoon (5 g) Macadamia oil or Rapeseed oil
1 large Onion (265 g), finely chopped
2 large Carrots (160 g), chopped
500 g pack lean Lamb Mince
2 tablespoon (30 g) Tomato Purée
1 tablespoon (15 ml) Worcestershire Sauce (see page 94) or use bought version

Miscellaneous Main Dishes

500 ml Beef Stock made with 2 Beef stock cubes (10 g)
450 g Swede, cut into small chunks
450 g Turnips, cut into small chunks
30 g Low fat (light) Spreadable Butter with rapeseed or olive oil
3 tablespoons (45 ml) semi-skimmed Milk
50 g Extra Mature Cheddar, grated
2 large Tomatoes (160 g) sliced thinly (for the topping) - optional

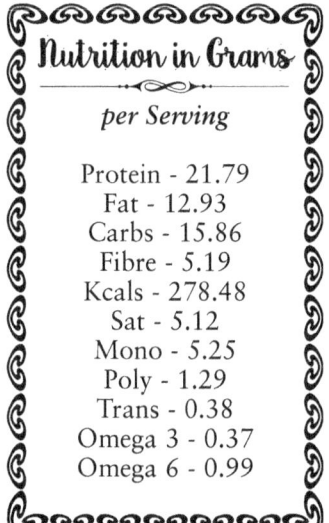

Nutrition in Grams
per Serving

Protein - 21.79
Fat - 12.93
Carbs - 15.86
Fibre - 5.19
Kcals - 278.48
Sat - 5.12
Mono - 5.25
Poly - 1.29
Trans - 0.38
Omega 3 - 0.37
Omega 6 - 0.99

Boil the Swede and Turnips in salted water. The Swede takes longer (around 25 minutes) until it is nice and soft (it needs to be very soft otherwise it becomes difficult to mash), the turnips take about 15 minutes.

Meanwhile, heat the oil in a large frying pan for a minute or two, then add the chopped onions and fry until translucent. Keep moving them around in the pan and try not to burn them as they can become a little bitter if you do. Add the chopped carrots and cook for a few minutes until they are soft. Add the lamb mince and cook until lightly brown, tipping off any excess fat. Add the Tomato Purée and Worcestershire Sauce and fry for a few minutes. Pour the stock in, put the lid on, and turn the heat up until it starts to bubble, then turn the heat down and simmer for 40 minutes. Remove the lid after 20 minutes if there is too much liquid.

Pre heat the oven to gas mark 4 - 180°C (350°F). Then drain the Swede and Turnips and add together in a saucepan, add the spreadable Butter and milk and mash thoroughly until smooth. Boil the potatoes in salted water for 10-15 minutes until tender. Drain, then mash with the butter and milk.

Put the mince into an ovenproof dish, top with the mash and smooth evenly with a fork. I then like to scrape the fork all over the surface to give a pleasant ruffled look. Sprinkle the cheese evenly over the top and add the sliced tomatoes spreading them evenly over the top and then brush them lightly with Macadamia oil or Rapeseed oil. Put into the centre of the oven and bake for 20-25 minutes until the top is starting to colour and the mince is bubbling at the edges.

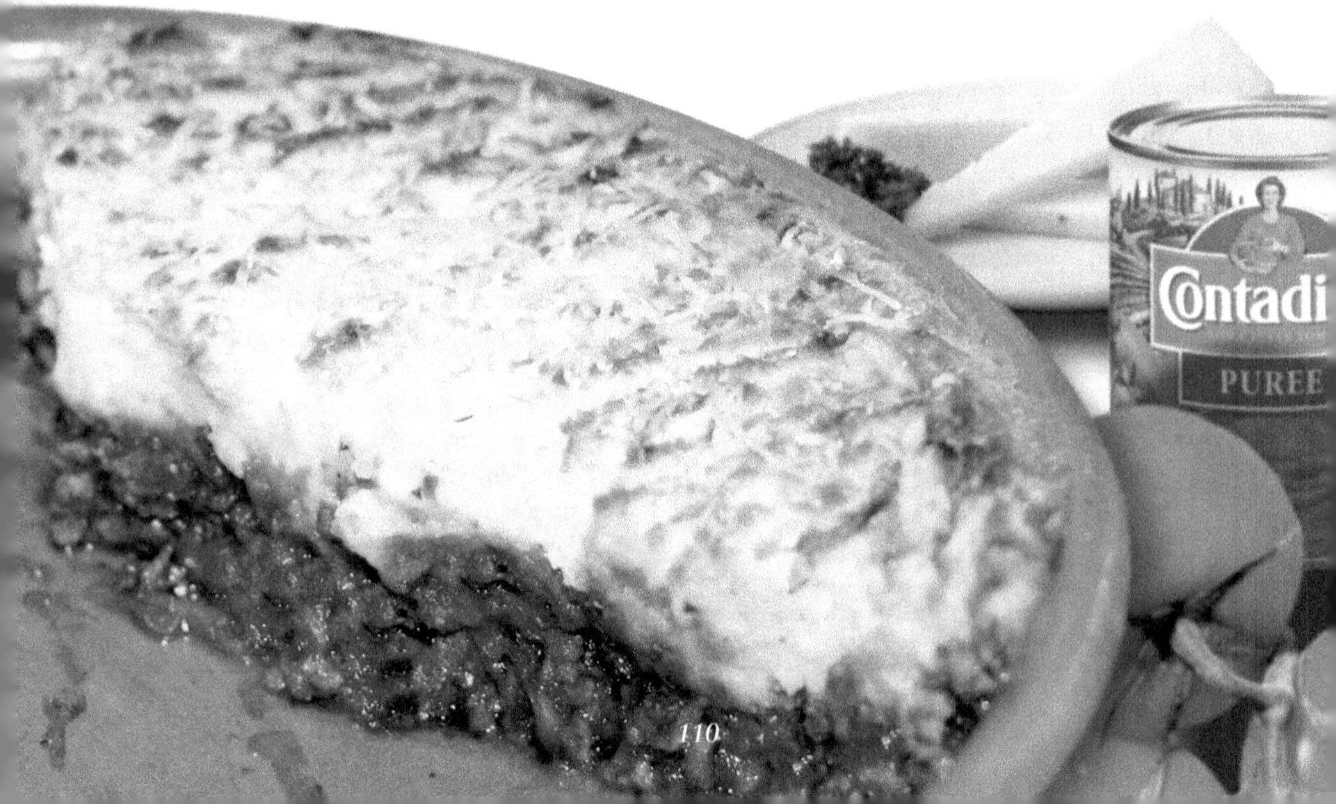

Miscellaneous Main Dishes

White Tuscan Pie

This makes a good supper dish. It is like shepherd's pie but is made with a rich bean and vegetable mixture topped with mashed Swede and Turnip. Cannellini Beans are white kidney beans, also known as 'Italian white kidney beans' or 'fasolia beans.' They are medium sized - about 1 cm/½ inch long and kidney shaped, with a tough seed coat, and are the least carby of all beans along with kidney beans. This specific variety is very popular in Italian cuisine. Serve this pie with green vegetables and a tomato or mushroom sauce.

Serves 6

Nutrition in Grams
per Serving

Protein - 3.62
Fat - 6.40
Carbs - 15.17
Fibre - 5.67
Kcals - 142.63
Sat - 2.68
Mono - 2.84
Poly - 0.29
Trans - 0.08
Omega 3 - 0.10
Omega 6 - 0.20

INGREDIENTS

120 g Cannellini Beans
100 g Cauliflower rice
1 tablespoon (15 g) Macadamia oil or Rapeseed oil
1 large Onion (265 g), peeled and finely chopped
225 g Carrots, scrubbed and diced
2 tablespoons (30 ml) Soy sauce
2 tablespoons (30 g) Tomato puree
¼ teaspoon (1¼ g) dried Oregano
¼ teaspoon (1¼ g) Basil
¼ teaspoon (1¼ g) Thyme
¼ teaspoon (1¼ g) Rosemary
275 ml Vegetable stock (see page 80) or use 1 stock cube
Salt and freshly ground black pepper

Mashed Topping
200 g Swede, peeled
200 g Turnips, peeled
100 g Carrots, scrubbed
25 g Spreadable butter (cut with Rapeseed oil or olive oil or both)

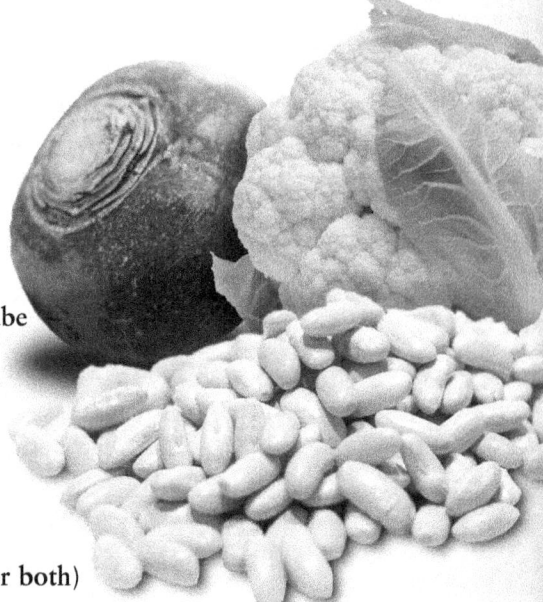

Pre heat the oven to gas mark 4 - 180°C (350°F). Wash the Cannellini beans and soak them overnight, or steep them in boiling water for 1 hour. Drain and rinse, then bring them to the boil in fresh water and cook for 30 minutes.

Heat the oil in a saucepan and fry the onion for 5 minutes. Add the carrots and cook for 2-3 minutes. Then add the cooked beans. Mix the soy sauce, tomato puree and herbs with the stock. Pour this over the bean and vegetable mixture. Bring to the boil and simmer for 20-30 minutes, so that the flavours are well blended. Season to taste. Add a little more liquid if necessary so that the final mixture is moist. Transfer into a greased 3 pint (10 litre) casserole.

Boil the Carrots, Swede and Turnips until soft and mash them with butter. Season well. Spread the mash over the beans and vegetables. Bake for 35-40 minutes until the mash is crisp and brown.

Miscellaneous Main Dishes

Spiced Turnip Mini Shepherd's Pies

This is a spicy twist on the traditional Shepherd's Pie, that look beautiful when presented individually although you can also put it all in a large ovenproof dish. You can add more Chilli powder, if you like your spices hot. I'd suggest using the fresh Coriander as it has a unique flavour that is slightly lost in the ground version.

Serves 6

Nutrition in Grams
per Serving

Protein - 22.82
Fat - 10.12
Carbs - 12.17
Fibre - 6.38
Kcals - 237.28
Sat - 3.25
Mono - 4.95
Poly - 0.88
Trans - 0.16
Omega 3 - 0.21
Omega 6 - 0.68

INGREDIENTS
For the Sauce
- 1 large Onion (265 g), finely chopped
- 2 Garlic cloves (12 g), crushed
- 1 inch of fresh Ginger (7½ g), peeled and granted
- 1 teaspoon Cumin (5 g), ground
- 1 teaspoon (5 g) Coriander, ground
- 1 teaspoon (5 g) Turmeric ground
- 1 teaspoon (5 g) Chilli powder
- 500 g minced lean Beef (5 % fat) or Lamb
- 400 g can of chopped Tomatoes
- 100 g Spinach
- 1 tablespoon (15 g) Macadamia oil or Rapeseed oil

For the Mash
- 600 g Turnips, peeled and chopped into large chunks
- 1 green Chilli (45 g), deseeded and chopped
- Large bunch of fresh Coriander (100 g), finely chopped or 2 teaspoons (10 g) ground Coriander
- 2 teaspoons (10 g) Turmeric
- The juice of 1 lemon (50 ml)
- 30 g Low fat (light) Spreadable Butter with rapeseed or olive oil (or both)

Pre-heat the oven to gas mark 6 - 200°C (400°F). For the sauce, heat the oil in a pan and add the onion. Cook until soft, then add the garlic, ginger, cumin, coriander, turmeric and chilli powder and cook until aromatic. Turn up the heat, add the mince, fry until browned, then add the tomatoes and simmer for 20 minutes until thickened. A few minutes before the end, add the spinach.

Meanwhile, in a saucepan of water, bring the turnips to the boil and cook for 10 minutes. Drain, season and mash with the butter, green chilli, fresh coriander, turmeric and lemon juice. Assemble the pies in 6 individual ovenproof dishes or small casserole dishes by placing some meat sauce on the bottom and top with the mash, alternatively you can used a large ovenproof dish or casserole and make one large pie. Score the tops with a fork, and then bake for 20 minutes until golden and bubbling.

Miscellaneous Main Dishes

Lancashire Hotpot

This famous lamb stew topped with sliced Swede is a great winter warmer and is enough on its own for a hearty main meal.

Serves 4

INGREDIENTS

30 g Macadamia oil or Rapeseed oil

400 g diced Lamb

3 Lamb Kidneys (120 g), sliced with the fat removed

1 large Onion (265 g), finely chopped

4 Carrots (320 g), peeled and finely chopped

1 teaspoon (5 g) plain Flour

2 teaspoons (10 g) Worcestershire Sauce (see page 94) or use a bought version

500 ml Lamb or Chicken stock (use 1 stock cube - 5 g)

2 Bay leaves (0.6 g)

900 g Swede, peeled and sliced

Nutrition in Grams per Serving

Protein - 28.44
Fat - 16.80
Carbs - 26.47
Fibre - 9.48
Kcals - 389.77
Sat - 4.78
Mono - 9.28
Poly - 0.85
Trans - 0.62
Omega 3 - 0.48
Omega 6 - 0.58

Prepare the stock by mixing two stock cubes into a jug containing 500 ml of boiling water. Pre-heat the oven to gas mark 3 - 140°C (280°F). Heat some Rapeseed oil or Macadamia oil in a large frying pan, and fry the diced lamb until the pieces are brown all over, turning frequently. Remove and put on a plate. Then do the same with the lamb kidneys. Add a little more Rapeseed oil or Macadamia oil and fry the onions and carrots until they have begun to soften while mixing continuously. Sprinkle over the flour and cook for a couple of minutes. Add in the Worcestershire sauce and the stock, and then bring to the boil. Add the diced lamb and kidneys and the bay leaves, then remove from the heat. Pour the mixture into an ovenproof dish or casserole and spread evenly over the bottom. Arrange the sliced swede on top of the meat and brush with a little Rapeseed oil or Macadamia oil. Cover with baking foil, then place in the top half of the oven for 1½ hrs or until the swede is soft when pricked with a fork. Remove the foil, brush the top with a little more oil, and then grill for 7 minutes until golden brown.

No Pasta Lasagne

Pasta is a no-no when on a low carb diet but this recipe has a viable alternative in this traditional Italian dish.

Serves 6

INGREDIENTS

Sauce

1 tablespoon (15 ml) Macadamia oil or Rapeseed oil

450 g lean minced Beef (5% Fat)

Miscellaneous Main Dishes

1 large Onion (265 g)
1 Garlic clove (6 g), crushed
75 g Tomato puree
400 g tinned Tomatoes
½ tablespoon (2½ g) dried Basil
1 teaspoon Salt (5 g)
½ teaspoon (2½ g) black Pepper

Pasta
6 medium Eggs (390 g)
150 g half fat Cream Cheese
1 teaspoon Salt (5 g)
30 g ground Psyllium Husk powder

Cheese layer
200 g Low fat Natural Yoghurt
50 g reduced fat Mozzarella Cheese, grated
1 tablespoon (15 g) grated Parmesan Cheese
½ teaspoon Salt (2½ g)
¼ teaspoon (1¼ g) black Pepper
2 g fresh Parsley, finely chopped

Nutrition in Grams
per Serving

Protein - 35.48
Fat - 14.80
Carbs - 13.05
Fibre - 5.59
Kcals - 332.97
Sat - 5.43
Mono - 6.33
Poly - 1.25
Trans - 0.29
Omega 3 - 0.16
Omega 6 - 1.08

Fry the finely chopped onion and garlic in Rapeseed oil or Macadamia oil until soft. Add the minced beef and fry on a low heat until brown, stirring continuously so as not to burn it. Add the tinned tomatoes, tomato puree and dried basil. Season to taste. Turn the heat up until the sauce is lightly bubbling, then lower the heat and let the sauce simmer for about 15 minutes.

For the lasagna, preheat the oven to 150°C (300°F). Whisk together the eggs, cream cheese and salt into a smooth paste. Continue to whisk while stirring in the psyllium husk, adding a little at a time. Leave to stand for a few minutes. Spread the mixture on a baking tray covered with baking paper using a spatula. Place another sheet of baking paper on top and flatten with a rolling pin until the mixture is roughly 33 x 45 cm (13 x 18 inches) in size. Leaving the baking paper in place, bake for about 10-12 minutes in the centre of the oven. Remove from the oven and let it cool before removing the paper. Cut into slices to fit your baking dish.

Turn the oven up to 200°C (400°F). Mix the grated Mozzarella cheese with the crème fraiche. Season to taste and stir in the parsley. Place a layer of the sauce in the bottom of an ovenproof dish, using about half the mixture. Place your lasagne sheets over the sauce, covering the sauce completely, but not overlapping them. Then spread a layer of the cheese mixture over the pasta, covering it all. Repeat, ending with a layer of the cheese mixture and finally sprinkle the Parmesan cheese over the top. Bake in the oven for about 30 minutes. Serve with a tomato salad and Vinaigrette dressing (see page 177).

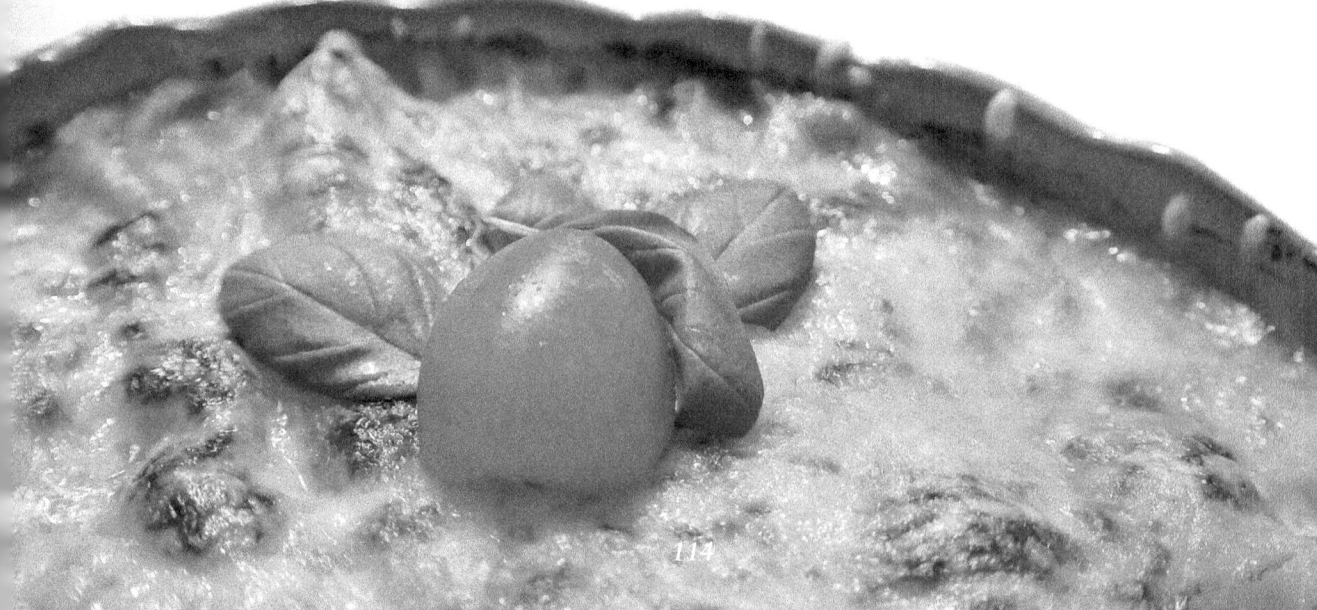

Miscellaneous Main Dishes

Broccoli & Cauliflower Chicken Gratin

This is an easy to cook one dish meal in itself.

Serves 4

INGREDIENTS

450 g Chicken breasts
1 Leek (100 g), cut into 1 cm
1 large Onion (265 g), finely chopped
450 g Broccoli, cut into individual florets
225 g Cauliflower, cut into individual florets
2 tablespoons (30 g) mustard, preferably Dijon
225 g low fat Natural Yoghurt
100 g reduced fat Mozzarella cheese, grated
100 g of low carb breadcrumbs
1 tablespoons (15 ml) Macadamia oil or Rapeseed oil
1 teaspoon fresh thyme (1 g) or ½ teaspoon (2½ g) dried Thyme
Salt and pepper, to taste

Nutrition in Grams
per Serving

Protein - 29.22
Fat - 11.87
Carbs - 11.21
Fibre - 7.26
Kcals - 287.65
Sat - 3.76
Mono - 4.1
Poly - 2.73
Trans - 0.15
Omega 3 - 1.83
Omega 6 - 0.92

Finely chop the onion and put about 2 tablespoons of Rapeseed oil or Macadamia oil into a large frying pan. Fry the Onions until they are soft and translucent. Add in all the chopped vegetables and fry for about 10 minutes, continually turning, until they start to soften (this may take longer, just keep checking by sticking a fork into them) and season to taste. When done, put onto a plate to cool and remove any excess oil with a kitchen towel. Meanwhile, on a medium heat, fry the chicken breast, turning occasionally, until brown on the outside and the flesh is white, about 15 minutes. Preheat the oven to 225°C (450°F).

Once the vegetables have begun to soften slightly, place them into an ovenproof casserole dish. In a bowl thoroughly mix the mustard with the yoghurt and pour all over the vegetables. Cut the fried chicken in to small pieces and layer the pieces evenly over the vegetables and sprinkle the thyme over them. Mix the mozzarella cheese and the breadcrumbs together in a bowl (this is what makes it a gratin) and sprinkle the mixture all over the surface and place the casserole dish in the top half of the oven and bake for 15 minutes.

Burgers with Tomato Relish

Serves 4

INGREDIENTS

Burger
400 g 5% Fat lean minced Beef
1 large Egg, (75 g)
5 ml Mustard, preferably Dijon
5 ml Worcestershire sauce (see page 94) or use bought version
1 small Onion (150 g), finely grated

Miscellaneous Main Dishes

1 clove Garlic (6 g), crushed
Salt and freshly ground black Pepper

Tomato Relish
1 tablespoon (15 ml) Macadamia oil or Rapeseed oil
1 small Onion (150 g), finely chopped
2 Garlic cloves (12 g), crushed
1 small fresh red Chilli (45 g), halved, deseeded, finely chopped
500 g ripe vine-ripened Tomatoes, coarsely chopped
2 tablespoons (30 ml) Red Wine Vinegar

4 low carb Buns (see page 59)

Nutrition in Grams
per Serving inc. Bun

Protein - 47.51
Fat - 24.39
Carbs - 15.15
Fibre - 18.18
Kcals - 511.77
Sat - 4.16
Mono - 7.58
Poly - 10.75
Trans - 0.15
Omega 3 - 8.02
Omega 6 - 2.72

For the relish, heat the oil in a medium saucepan over medium-low heat. Add the onion and garlic and cook, stirring often, for 5 minutes or until soft. Add the chilli, and cook for 2 minutes. Add the tomato to the onion mixture and cook, stirring occasionally, for 5 minutes or until the tomato breaks down. Add the red wine vinegar, and cook for 10 minutes or until the mixture thickens. Set aside to cool.

For the burgers, whisk egg in a bowl with the mustard, Worcestershire sauce, finely chopped onion and crushed garlic. Season to taste. Then, crumble in the minced beef using a fork, and gently mix together. Using your hands, shape the mixture into 4 round burgers about 2 cm/¾ inch thick. Don't press down too firmly. Using your thumb, make a small depression in the centre of each side of each burger to prevent them puffing up during cooking.

With a little Rapeseed oil or Macadamia oil in a frying pan, fry the burgers for about 6 – 8 minutes, turn over gently with a spatula and repeat on the other side. With a fork, check that they aren't pink in the centre. Leave for longer if they are. Serve the burgers in 4 lightly buttered low carb buns with a healthy dollop of relish. Serve with Turnip Chips (see page 161) and a tomato salad (see page 173).

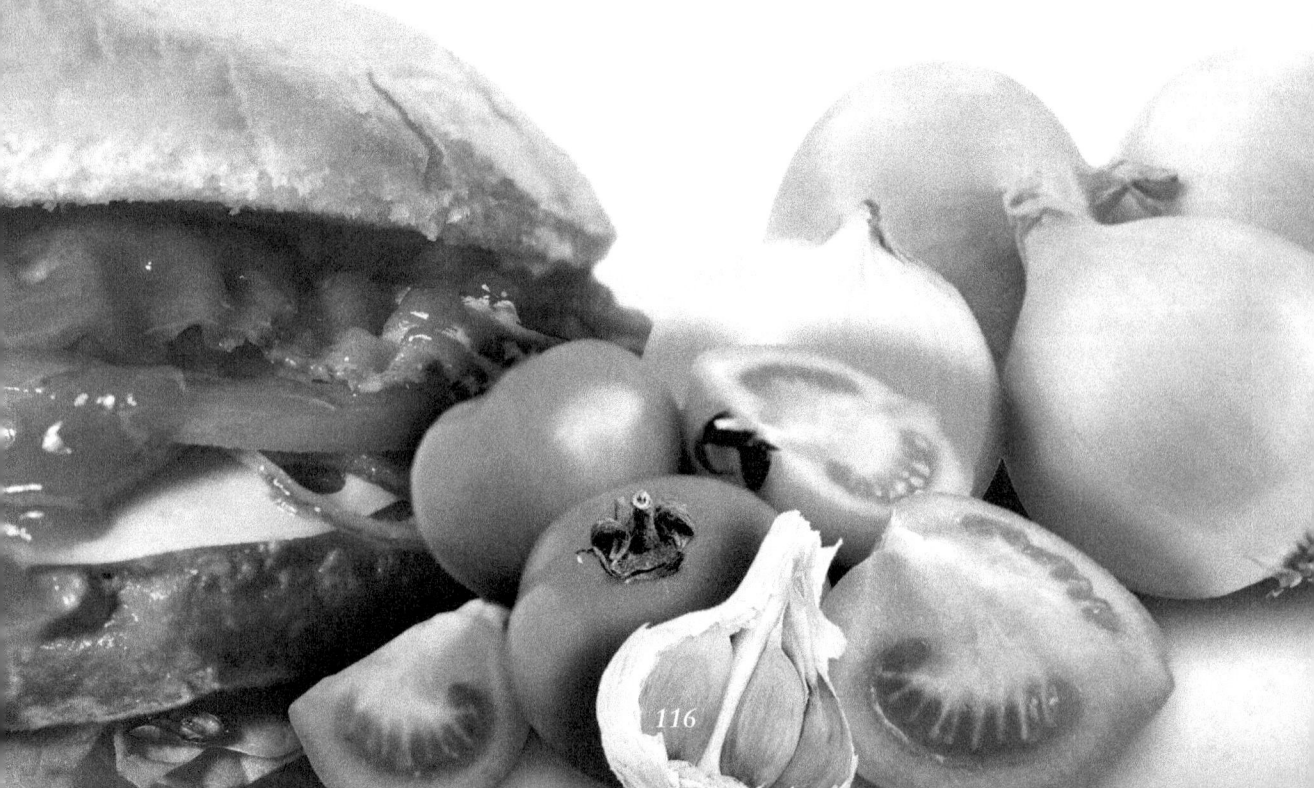

Miscellaneous Main Dishes

Green Cabbage Casserole

An easy recipe that makes a great evening meal.

Serves 6

INGREDIENTS

680 g Green Cabbage
20 g Low fat (light) Spreadable Butter with rapeseed or olive oil (or both)
450 g lean minced Beef (5% fat)
1 teaspoon Salt (5 g)
1 small Onion (150 g)
2 Garlic cloves (12 g), crushed
¼ teaspoon (1¼ g) ground black Pepper
1 tablespoon (15 ml) White Wine Vinegar
100 g Extra Mature Cheddar cheese, grated
1 teaspoon (5 ml) Rapeseed oil or Macadamia oil for frying
2 tablespoons TexMex Seasoning (see below)

Nutrition in Grams
per Serving

Protein - 23.45
Fat - 13.94
Carbs - 8.17
Fibre - 4.11
Kcals - 259.97
Sat - 5.79
Mono - 5.87
Poly - 0.90
Trans - 0.29
Omega 3 - 0.15
Omega 6 - 0.74

TexMex Seasoning

3 tablespoons (45 g) Chilli powder
2 tablespoons (30 g) Cumin
1 tablespoon (15 g) ground black Pepper
1 teaspoon (5 g) Salt
1 tablespoon (10 g) Garlic powder
1½ teaspoons (7½ g) crushed Red Peppers

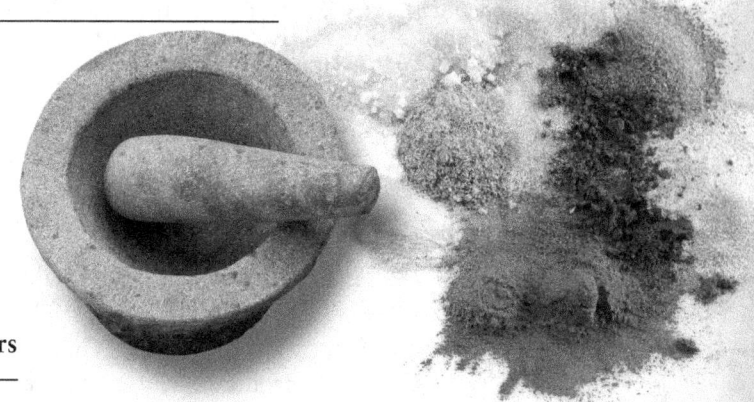

Shred the cabbage by hand or in a food processor, as finely as possible. Fry the cabbage in the spreadable butter in a large frying pan on a medium heat until soft, stirring continually so as not to let the cabbage go brown. It takes a little while for the cabbage to turn soft.

For the TexMex seasoning, mix the spices and crushed red pepper (you can then store the rest for future use) and add 2 tablespoons of the seasoning to the cabbage. Place the remainder in an airtight container for future use, it will last indefinitely. Add the white wine vinegar, stir thoroughly and continue to fry for a couple of minutes. Transfer to a bowl to use later.

Preheat the oven to 200°C (400°F). Finely chop the onion and put a little Rapeseed oil or Macadamia oil into a large frying pan. Fry the onion and garlic until they are soft and translucent. Add the minced beef and fry on a medium heat until browned all over, stirring continuously so as not to burn the onions. Stir in the cabbage mixture and fry on a low heat for a minute. Season to taste. Add two thirds of the cheese to the cabbage mixture and stir in and place in a ovenproof dish. Sprinkle the rest of the cheese on top and bake for 15–20 minutes or until the cheese has turned brown on top.

Miscellaneous Main Dishes

Garlic Chicken with Mash

This is a really easy and quick but delicious baked chicken with loads of garlic.

Serves 4

INGREDIENTS

900 g Chicken thighs

1 tablespoon (15 ml) Macadamia oil or Rapeseed oil

7 Garlic cloves (42 g), crushed

The juice of 1 Lemon (50 ml)

15 g fresh Parsley, finely chopped

4 portions of the Ultimate Mash (see page 168)

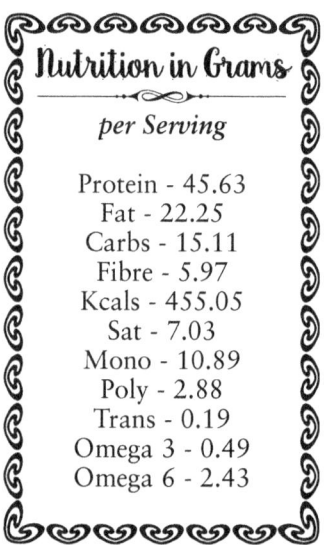

Nutrition in Grams

per Serving

Protein - 45.63
Fat - 22.25
Carbs - 15.11
Fibre - 5.97
Kcals - 455.05
Sat - 7.03
Mono - 10.89
Poly - 2.88
Trans - 0.19
Omega 3 - 0.49
Omega 6 - 2.43

Preheat the oven to gas mark 7 - 225°C (450°F). Place the chicken pieces in an ovenproof dish lightly greased with Rapeseed oil or Macadamia oil. Salt and pepper generously. Sprinkle the garlic and parsley over the chicken pieces, and drizzle the lemon juice and Rapeseed oil or Macadamia oil on top. Bake the chicken until golden and the garlic slices have turned brown and roasted, which will take around 35 minutes. Just keep checking the chicken by sticking a fork in the fleshy parts of the thighs and see if the flesh is white not pink, which indicates that the chicken is done. Lower the temperature to gas mark 2 - 150°C (300°F) for the last 10 minutes. Serve with our ultimate mash (see page 168).

Brussel Sprouts & Hamburger Gratin

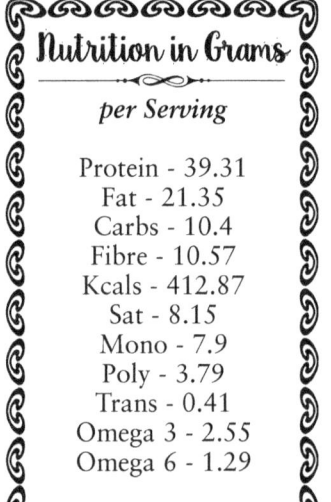

Nutrition in Grams

per Serving

Protein - 39.31
Fat - 21.35
Carbs - 10.4
Fibre - 10.57
Kcals - 412.87
Sat - 8.15
Mono - 7.9
Poly - 3.79
Trans - 0.41
Omega 3 - 2.55
Omega 6 - 1.29

In cooking, the word gratin refers to a recipe that is prepared in the au gratin style, which means that it's topped with seasoned breadcrumbs and cheese and then baked. Brussel Sprouts have a kind of bad reputation, in the UK anyway. Like the yeast extract, Marmite, people either love them or hate them, but I think their slightly nutty and peppery flavour gives them a unique taste. This is a great combination of sprouts and cheese covered with minced beef, finished au gratin style.

Serves 4

INGREDIENTS

450 g lean minced Beef (5% fat)

225 g Turnips, sliced

450 g Brussel Sprouts, cut in halves

2 tablespoons (30 g) half fat Crème Fraiche

15 g Low fat (light) Spreadable Butter with rapeseed or olive oil

½ teaspoon (2½ g) Rosemary, dried

1 teaspoon (5 g) dried Basil

Miscellaneous Main Dishes

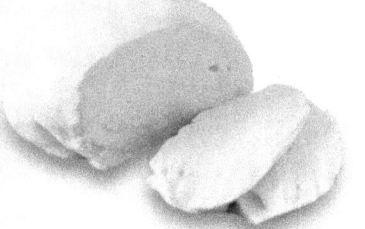
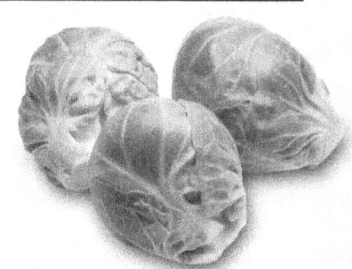

1 teaspoon (5 g) dried Marjoram
100 g Mozzarella cheese, grated
100 g of low carb breadcrumbs (see page 68)
½ teaspoon (2½ g) Paprika
Salt and pepper to taste
1 tablespoon (15 ml) Rapeseed oil or Macadamia oil for frying

In a large frying pan and fry the halved Brussel sprouts in the spreadable butter, on a low heat for 5 minutes, constantly stirring. Then add the crème fraiche and mix thoroughly. Season to taste and then empty into a medium sized ovenproof dish. Slice the turnips into thin slices and put in a saucepan of water and bring to the boil and cook for 10 minutes or until soft.

Pre-heat the oven to 220°C (425°F). Meanwhile, fry the minced beef in a little Rapeseed oil or Macadamia oil, until you have browned the meat all over, stirring continuously. Season with salt and pepper and add the herbs, mix together and then pour on top of the Brussels sprouts. Then layer the sliced, cooked turnips over the whole surface of the minced beef. In small bowl, mix the mozzarella cheese and the bread crumbs and sprinkle over turnips. Sprinkle with the paprika. Place in the middle of the oven for 15 minutes or until the cheese and breadcrumbs have browned. Serve with a fresh salad and some homemade mayonnaise (see page 94).

Tortilla with Minced Beef & Salsa

Treat yourself to this delicious beef and cheese filled tortilla. With your own low carb tortilla and spice mix this is a quintessential Mexican favourite.

Serves 4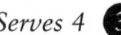

INGREDIENTS

4 low carb Tortilla breads (see page 59)
400 g lean minced Beef (5% fat)
1 tablespoon (15 ml) Macadamia oil or Rapeseed oil
1 teaspoon Salt (5 g)

Salsa

4 large Tomatoes (400 g), peeled and finely chopped
1 fresh green Chilli (45 g), deseeded and finely chopped
1 small Red Onion (150 g), very finely chopped
1 Garlic clove (6 g), crushed
1 teaspoon (5 ml) Red Wine Vinegar
Juice of 1 lime (50 ml)
Handful of fresh Coriander, roughly chopped (80 g)
Salt and pepper to taste

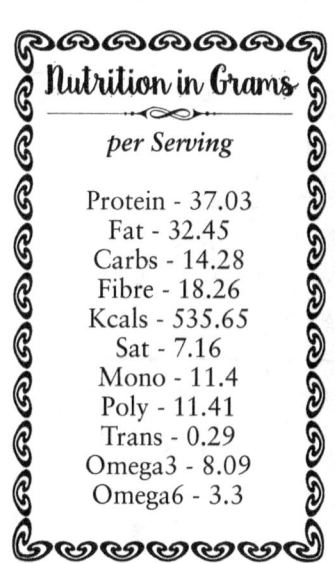

Nutrition in Grams

per Serving

Protein - 37.03
Fat - 32.45
Carbs - 14.28
Fibre - 18.26
Kcals - 535.65
Sat - 7.16
Mono - 11.4
Poly - 11.41
Trans - 0.29
Omega3 - 8.09
Omega6 - 3.3

Miscellaneous Main Dishes

Mexican Seasoning

2 teaspoons (10 g) Chilli powder
2 teaspoons (10 g) Paprika powder
1 teaspoon (5 g) ground Cumin
2 teaspoons (10 g) Garlic powder
1 pinch Cayenne Pepper (1 g)
Pinch of Salt (1 g)

Topping
60 g Extra Mature Cheese, grated
Handful of baby Spinach (50 g), chopped
1 large leaf of Swiss Chard (20 g), chopped

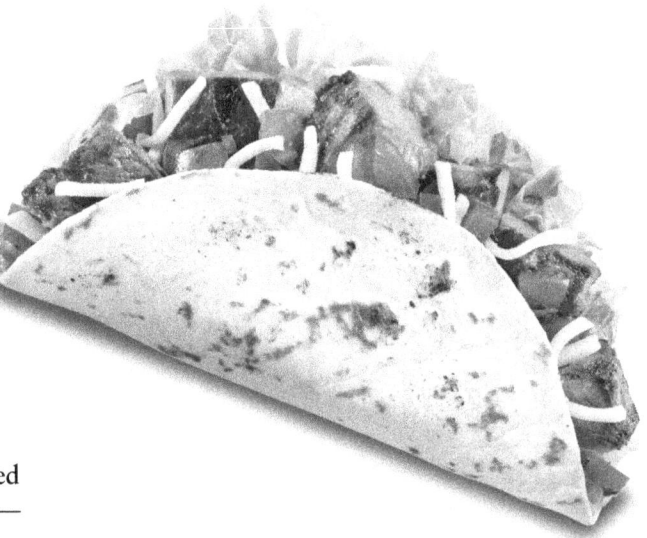

Start by making two portions of the low carb tortilla bread (see page 59) Then, place a little Rapeseed oil or Macadamia oil in a large frying pan and add the minced beef on a low heat. Fry for about 10 minutes, stirring continuously, so as to brown the meat all over without burning it. Then add the Mexican seasoning with about 100 ml of water and mix well. Turn the heat up and bring to the boil before reducing the heat and simmering the mixture, stirring occasionally, until most of the water has evaporated. Add the spices for the Mexican seasoning and stir.

Meanwhile, make the salsa. With a little Rapeseed or Macadamia oil and on a low heat, fry the onions and garlic until they are soft and translucent, stirring constantly. Add the chopped tomatoes, finely chopped green chilli, red wine vinegar, lime juice and fresh coriander. Season to taste. Lay out the 4 tortillas flat. Place the minced beef equally into the 4 tortillas on the centre half of the tortillas, and pour the tomato mix equally on top. Finally top with the baby spinach, Swiss chard and grated cheddar. Fold the tortillas from both sides over the mixture and serve with a green salad.

Aubergine & Mushroom Parmigiana

Parmigiana is an Italian dish made with a shallow sliced aubergine filling, layered with cheese and tomato sauce, then baked.

Serves 4 ❷

INGREDIENTS

2 large Aubergines, diced (600 g)
6 large flat Mushrooms, chopped (45 g)
2 large Onions, finely chopped (330 g)
3 Garlic cloves, crushed (18 g)
100 g Mozzarella cheese, grated
2 x 400 g tins of chopped Tomatoes
140 g Tomato puree

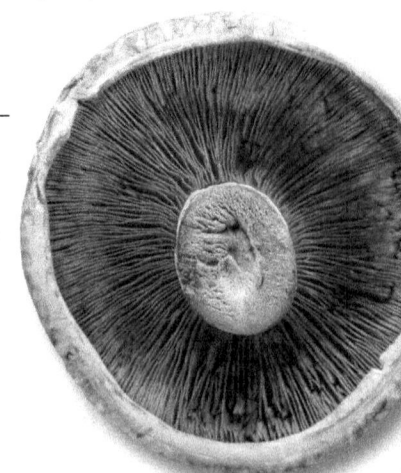

3 teaspoons (15 g) Basil, dried

1 teaspoon (5 g) Vegetable Bouillon

Preheat the oven to gas mark 2 - 150°C (300°F). Take the stalks off the aubergines then dice them into 1 cm slices, cut in half. Chop the mushrooms up and place them and the aubergines in the bottom of a greased (with Rapeseed oil or Macadamia oil) ovenproof dish. Spread evenly. Place in the centre of the oven and bake for 20 minutes.

Finely chop up the onions and fry them with the crushed garlic until they are soft and translucent. Add the chopped tomatoes, the puree, the bouillon and the basil to the onions and fry for another 10 minutes on a low heat, stirring occasionally. Remove the aubergines and mushrooms from the oven and pour the tomato mixture over them, spreading the sauce out evenly. Sprinkle the grated Mozzarella all over the top. Turn the oven up to gas mark 4 - 180°C (350°F). Place back in the centre of the oven and bake for around 30 minutes or until the top is golden brown and the dish is bubbling. Serve with a tomato salad (see page 173).

Nutrition in Grams
per Serving

Protein - 11.84
Fat - 5.99
Carbs - 23.20
Fibre - 9.02
Kcals - 208.62
Sat - 3.58
Mono - 1.32
Poly - 0.48
Trans - 0.20
Omega 3 - 0.06
Omega 6 - 0.41

Spanish Cauliflower

Serves 4

INGREDIENTS

450 g minced Beef, or minced Turkey

350 g Cauliflower, riced

180 g Red Peppers

1 x 400 g tin of chopped Tomatoes

130 g Fresh salsa (see page 119)

2 Garlic cloves, crushed (12 g)

1 tablespoon (15 ml) Macadamia oil or Rapeseed oil for frying

Salt and freshly ground black Pepper, to taste

Nutrition in Grams
per Serving

Protein - 31.10
Fat - 9.20
Carbs - 15.74
Fibre - 7.93
Kcals - 278.66
Sat - 2.67
Mono - 4.98
Poly - 0.45
Trans - 0.15
Omega 3 - 0.12
Omega 6 - 0.37

First, prepare the salsa. Then, the fiddly bit, unless you're using a food processor. Holding the stalk end of the Cauliflower or Broccoli floret (I advise wearing some gloves to protect from grating your fingers) grate the heads of the florets on the smallest setting on your grater. If you have no protection stop grating when you reach the top of the stalk, you really only want the flowery heads of the florets anyway. Pour the oil into a large frying pan. Add the garlic and red peppers and fry for 2-3 minutes over medium heat. Add the cauliflower rice and cook on a low for around 10 minutes or until the cauliflower has softened. Add the minced beef/turkey and over medium heat brown the meat, stirring continuously until all the meat has been browned. Pour and mix in the tinned tomatoes and salsa. Turn the heat up until the sauce is slightly bubble, stirring thoroughly. Once bubbling, turn the heat down and cover with a lid and simmer for 5 minutes.

Miscellaneous Main Dishes

Watercress Soufflé

Chopped watercress gives this soufflé a pleasant and subtle peppery flavour.

Serves 4

INGREDIENTS

20 g Low fat (light) Spreadable Butter with rapeseed or olive oil (or both)

20 g plain Flour

275 ml warm semi-skimmed Milk

50 g Extra Mature Cheddar cheese, grated

½ teaspoon (2½ g) Mustard, preferably Dijon

1 bunch Watercress (160 g), very finely chopped

4 large Egg whites (75 g)

4 large Egg yolks (150 g)

Salt and freshly ground black pepper

Nutrition in Grams
per Serving

Protein - 13.79
Fat - 12.77
Carbs - 8.16
Fibre - 0.23
Kcals - 199.94
Sat - 5.39
Mono - 4.45
Poly - 1.27
Trans - 0.17
Omega 3 - 0.20
Omega 6 - 1.05

Preheat the oven to gas mark 6 - 200°C (400°F). Melt the butter in a small saucepan, stir in the flour and cook the roux gently for 2 or 3 minutes. Pour in the warmed milk and bring the sauce to the boil, stirring constantly. When the mixture comes to the boil, let it simmer over a very gentle heat, for 3-5 minutes, stirring occasionally. Then remove the pan from the heat and add the grated cheese and mustard. When the sauce has cooled a little, beat in the egg yolks and then season to taste. Add the chopped watercress to the sauce. In a mixing bowl beat the egg whites, with a whisk, until they are stiff enough to stay in shape when you move it.

Then, stir a spoonful of beaten egg white into the cooked sauce. Fold in the remaining egg. Put this mixture immediately into a greased 900 ml (1½ pint) soufflé dish and bake for 25 minutes or until it is well risen and firm to the touch in the centre. Serve the soufflé straight away.

Chinese-Style Vegetables

This combination of vegetables is flavoured with soy sauce, ginger and white wine, and uses the quick stir-fry method of cooking to preserve all the freshness in colour and texture of the crisp peppers and crunchy bean sprouts. Serve with Spiced Cauliflower Rice (see page 160) without the spices.

Serves 4

INGREDIENTS

525 ml boiling water

1 tablespoon (15 ml) Macadamia oil or Rapeseed oil

1 teaspoon (7½ g) fresh root ginger, grated

Miscellaneous Main Dishes

1 large Onion (265 g), peeled and chopped
1 large Red Pepper (180 g), de-seeded and cut into strips
225 g Mushrooms, wiped and sliced
225 g Bean Sprouts, rinsed
2 tablespoons (30 ml) Soy sauce
2 tablespoons (30 ml) White Wine
1 teaspoon Cornflour (5 g) dissolved in 1 tablespoon water
Salt and freshly ground black Pepper

Nutrition in Grams
per Serving

Protein - 4.84
Fat - 4.17
Carbs - 11.88
Fibre - 3.47
Kcals - 112.30
Sat - 0.61
Mono - 3.03
Poly - 0.21
Trans - 0.00
Omega 3 - 0.06
Omega 6 - 0.19

First prepare the Cauliflower rice, if using. Meanwhile, heat the oil in a Wok or large frying pan and fry the ginger and onions for 5 minutes. Then add the pepper and mushrooms and fry for a further 3-5 minutes. Add the bean sprouts and stir, then add the soy sauce, white wine and dissolved cornflour. Cook over a high heat for about 3 minutes, stirring constantly. When the rice is done, turn it onto a warm serving dish, pile the cooked vegetables over the top and serve straight away.

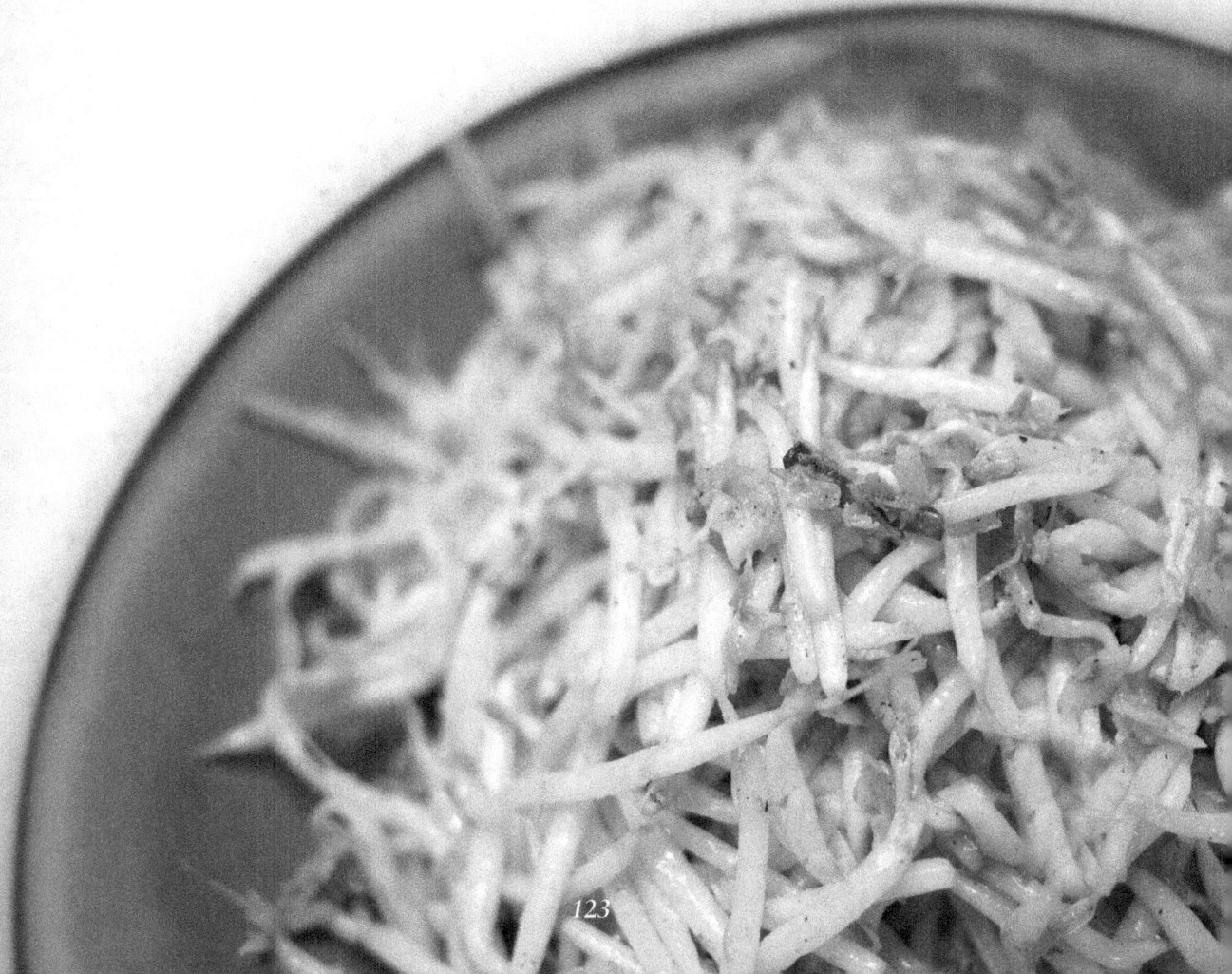

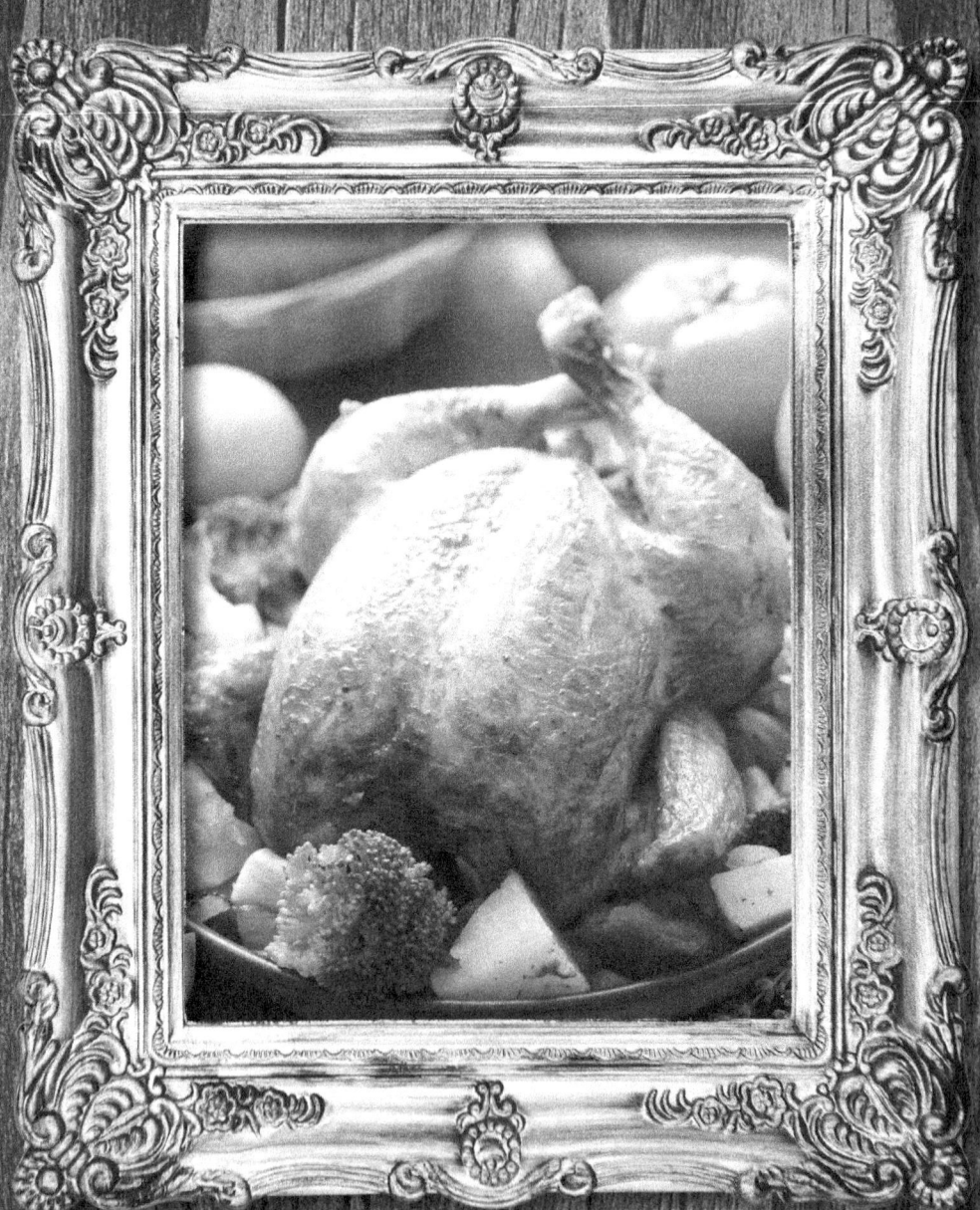

Roasts

Roast Paprika Chicken

The paprika in this recipe, which is rubbed into the skin, gives the skin a lovely flavour while the onion moistens the chicken and gives it a subtle underlying taste, as well as being great to add to the gravy.

Serves 6

INGREDIENTS

2 kg Chicken

1 small Onion (150 g)

2 tablespoons (30 g) smoked Paprika or plain Paprika

1 tablespoon (15 ml) Macadamia oil or Rapeseed oil

Gravy

Juices from the chicken

Chicken stock cubes, gravy granules or gravy browning powder such as Bisto

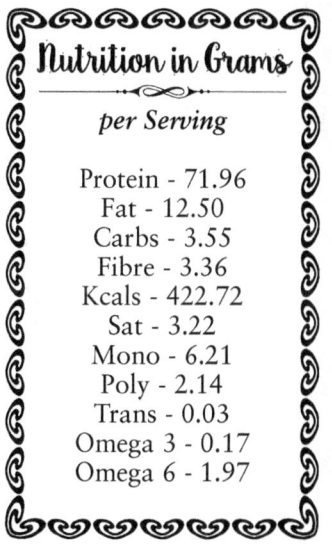

Nutrition in Grams
per Serving

Protein - 71.96
Fat - 12.50
Carbs - 3.55
Fibre - 3.36
Kcals - 422.72
Sat - 3.22
Mono - 6.21
Poly - 2.14
Trans - 0.03
Omega 3 - 0.17
Omega 6 - 1.97

Preheat the oven to gas mark 5 - 190°C (375°F). As with all raw chicken, it is paramount that you don't taint utensils and your hands without cleaning with hot water and an antibacterial gel. If you are worried about this it would advisable to wear some disposable latex gloves. Pour a little Rapeseed oil or Macadamia oil into a large ovenproof dish or roasting tin. Remove the chicken from the packaging and place in the dish or tin. Drizzle a little of the oil over the chicken's back and rub the oil all over the skin. Wash your hands thoroughly. Sprinkle the paprika all over the skin and then rub this into the skin so that you have an even covering. Wash hands. Peel the onion and make a cut halfway through the onion and place it deep into the cavity where you put the stuffing. You can then stuff the chicken with the homemade Sage and Onion Stuffing (see page 153) Place in the centre of the oven. Check the packaging for cooking times, but the rough guide is 20 minutes per 450 g plus 20 minutes. So for a 2 kg bird it would be around 1 hr 50 minutes although the best way to check that it is properly cooked is to cut the skin at the point the legs connect with the body and see that the flesh is white and the juices are clear. If it is pink after the allotted time, keep checking every 10 minutes until it satisfies these criteria. Although the onion helps with keeping the chicken moist, it is best to baste the breasts every half hour as this is the part of the chicken that can become dry (just use a spoon to pour the juices from the bottom of the dish all over the top of the chicken). Alternatively, you cook the chicken upside down for the first 40 minutes so that the juices seep into the breasts and turn over for the remainder of the time (in this situation, I rub the paprika into the skin when the chicken is turned).

When cooked, remove the chicken from the oven and using two forks take it out of the roasting tin/dish and drain as much of the juices into the tin/dish. Place a plate, remove the stuffing and using a fork, fish the onion out of the cavity and let it cool. This can now be finely chopped for use in the gravy or used as a side dish to your roast (because it is cooked the strong flavour has gone and it makes a great addition as an accompanying vegetable). Now pour the juices into a glass measuring jug and left until you can clearly see the separation of fat/oil from the juices with the fat at the top. Pour as much of the fat layer away so that you a reducing the amount of fat you will intake and that can make the gravy a little greasy. Use water that you have used for boiling vegetables to top up the juices to your required amount of gravy and pour into a saucepan. You can now add the onions (if using) and the gravy granules, chicken stock cubes or gravy granules (Note: if you are using stock cubes the gravy can be a little thin, so you may need to add a little thickener such as cornflour).

Serve with roast paprika turnips or swede (see page 127) cauliflower mash, spiced shredded green cabbage (see page 136), lemon broccoli (see page 158) and spiced cider carrots (see page 156).

Roast Lamb with Garlic & Rosemary

Serves 6

INGREDIENTS
2 kg leg of Lamb
3 cloves of Garlic (18 g)
A handful of fresh Rosemary (30 g)
The zest of a Lemon (15 g)
1 large Onion (265 g)
2 tablespoons (30 ml) Macadamia oil or Rapeseed oil

Mint Sauce
A handful of fresh mint (30 g)
1 teaspoon (5 g) Stevia
3 tablespoons (45 ml) White Wine Vinegar

Nutrition in Grams
per Serving

Protein - 70.73
Fat - 15.98
Carbs - 1.39
Fibre - 1.03
Kcals - 436.39
Sat - 4.29
Mono - 8.75
Poly - 1.33
Trans - 0.44
Omega 3 - 0.30
Omega 6 - 1.03

Preheat the oven to gas mark 6 - 200°C (400°F). Break the garlic bulb up into cloves, then peel and crush 3, leaving the rest whole. Roughly chop half the rosemary leaves, keeping the rest as separate sprigs. Put the garlic into a bowl and add the chopped rosemary. Finely grate the lemon zest and add to the mixture. Pour in the oil and mix together. Season the lamb with salt and black pepper, then drizzle with the oil mixture over the lamb and rub all over the meat. With a sharp knife make small incisions in the skin and place the sprigs of the remaining rosemary into each incision, so that the look like they've been planted in the skin. Place in the centre of the oven.

Meanwhile, you can make the mint sauce if you are going to use it. Pick and finely chop the mint leaves, then place in a small bowl. Mix in the Stevia, a good pinch of salt, 1 tablespoon of hot water and the white wine vinegar.

Nutrition in Grams
Mint Sauce per Serving

Protein - 0.16
Fat - 0.06
Carbs - 1.49
Fibre - 0.36
Kcals - 3.43
Sat - 0.01
Mono - 0
Poly - 0.03
Trans - 0
Omega 3 - 0.03
Omega 6 - 0

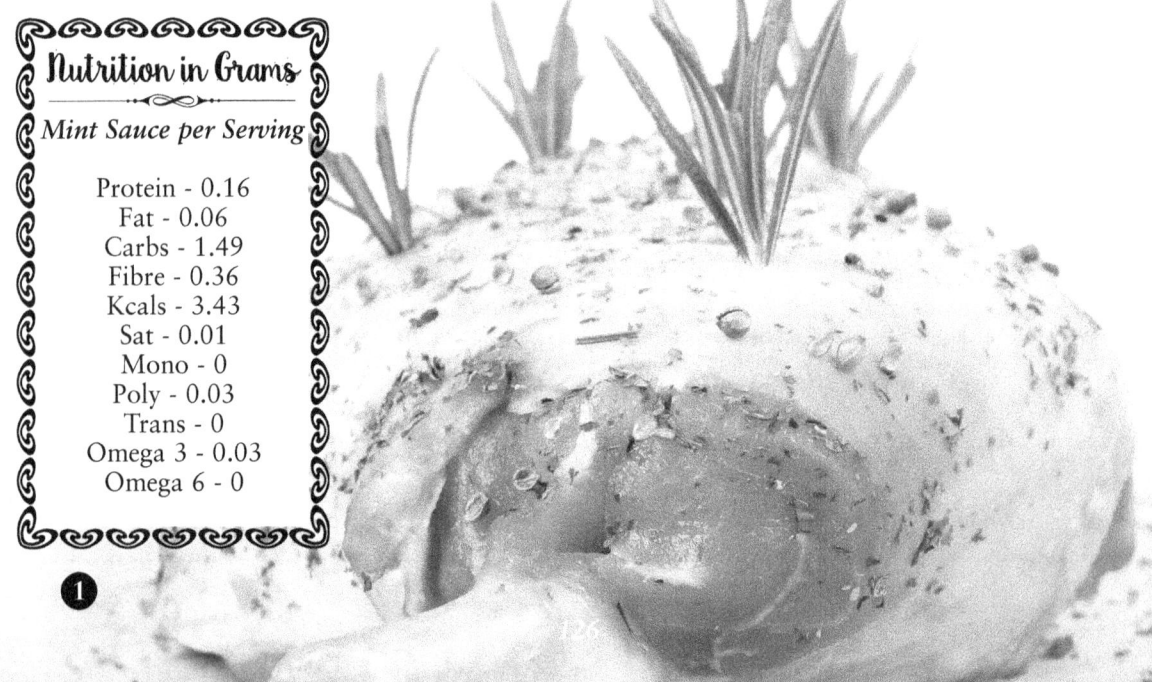

Roast Pork with Garlic & Rosemary

Serves 8

INGREDIENTS

2 kg loin of Pork on the bone, rind removed
3 cloves garlic (18 g)
2 tablespoons fresh rosemary (30 g)
2 tablespoons (30 ml) Macadamia oil or Rapeseed oil
100 ml White WineSalt and freshly ground black pepper

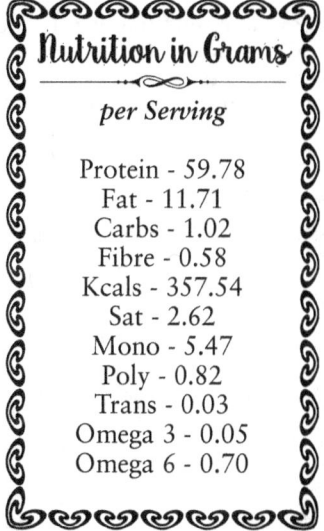

Nutrition in Grams

per Serving

Protein - 59.78
Fat - 11.71
Carbs - 1.02
Fibre - 0.58
Kcals - 357.54
Sat - 2.62
Mono - 5.47
Poly - 0.82
Trans - 0.03
Omega 3 - 0.05
Omega 6 - 0.70

Preheat oven to gas mark 4 - 180°C (350°F). Crush the garlic cloves and mix into a paste with the fresh rosemary and salt and pepper. Place the joint into a large roasting tin and stick a sharp knife into the surface of the pork in several places and insert the garlic paste into the holes. Mix any leftover paste with the oil and rub all over the loin.

Place the pan into the preheated oven and cook for 2 hours, turning regularly and spooning any juices over the joint. After 2 hours remove roast to a large plate and leave to rest for 10 minutes. Meanwhile remove as much fat and oil from the roasting tin, leaving the juices. Pour the wine into the tin and stir to with any browned bits leftover in the tin. Transfer to a saucepan and heat up. Pour the mixture over the joint and serve. Any leftover slices of pork can be refrigerated and used as part of a full English Breakfast (see page 166).

Nutrition in Grams

Turnips per Serving

Protein - 1.28
Fat - 4.10
Carbs - 5.57
Fibre - 2.68
Kcals - 69.92
Sat - 0.56
Mono - 3.07
Poly - 0.26
Trans - 0.00
Omega 3 - 0.06
Omega 6 - 0.20

Roast Paprika Turnips or Swede

These are a great alternative to roast Potatoes and actually are quite flavoursome, more so than Potatoes. Once you have these for a while, you won't miss Potatoes. I've suggested Smoked Paprika because its smell and flavour are simply divine, but you can just as easily use unsmoked.

Serves 4

INGREDIENTS

450 g Turnips or Swede, peeled and sliced into large chunks
1 tablespoon (15 ml) Rapeseed oil or Macadamia oil
½ tablespoon (7½ g) smoked Paprika
Salt and freshly ground black pepper

Pre-heat the oven to gas mark 4 - 180°C (350°F). If you are usingTurnips then all you have to do is peel them and chop them into roastie sized chunks into a saucepan. If using Swede, peel and chop up and put into a saucepan and cover with water. Boil them for about 15 minutes and drain. While in the saucepan, drizzle the oil over your chosen vegetable and shake the pan so that all their surfaces are slightly covered. Drain any excess oil, to keep the amount of oil used to a minimum. Sprinkle the Paprika and seasoning over them and again shake the pan to work the Paprika all over. Empty into a roasting tin (if you cooking a roast dinner with meat, don't roast them in the same dish as the meat as they will soak up the unwanted Oil from the meat) and spread out evenly. Cook for 45 minutes.

Yorkshire Pudding

Yorkshire pudding was first devised in England and is made from a batter consisting of eggs, flour, and milk or water. Often served with beef and gravy it has become an integral part of a traditional British Sunday roast. When wheat flour began to be widely used in the making of cakes and puddings, chefs the county of Yorkshire, in the north of England, devised a means of making use of the fat that dripped from roasting meat to cook a batter pudding. During 1737, a recipe for a 'dripping pudding' was published in the book 'The Whole Duty of a Woman,' and was later renamed as a Yorkshire pudding, in honour of its original invention.

Nutrition in Grams
per Serving

Protein - 8.21
Fat - 12.57
Carbs - 2.71
Fibre - 6.23
Kcals - 172.84
Sat - 1.94
Mono - 4.13
Poly - 5.5
Trans - 0.01
Omega 3 - 4.01
Omega 6 - 1.5

Serves 2 ❸

INGREDIENTS

25 g Flax Seed
12.5 g White Chia Seeds
2 g Psyllium Husk
1 g Baking Powder
80 ml Semi-skimmed Milk
160 ml Water
1 small Egg (55 g)
1 teaspoon (5 ml) Macadamia oil or Rapeseed oil for greasing the baking tray
Pinch of Salt & Pepper

Pre-heat the oven to gas mark 2 - 150°C (300°F). Mix all the dry ingredients together and finely grind them in a nut mill, blender or food processor, and empty into a bowl. Make a small indent in the middle of the mixture and crack the egg into it. Slowly mix the egg into the mixture, making sure you mix all the dry ingredients with the egg. Mix the milk and water in a jug and add a little to the mixture and mix thoroughly. Gradually add more, continually mixing until you have added all the liquid. Keep stirring until the batter is as smooth as possible and put into the fridge to rest. Meanwhile, in an indented baking tray with 4 indents 10 cm/4 inches in diameter and roughly 1 cm/½ inch in depth, pour a little oil into each and spread the oil all over the indent with a brush or your fingers. Place the tray into the top of the oven and leave for 15 minutes. The secret with all batters is for the oil to be very hot. Once done, remove the batter from the fridge and take the tray out of the oven. Pour the batter into each indent, filling them to about three quarters of their depth and place the tray back into the top of the oven. Cook for 40 minutes or until the batter has risen and is a dark brown colour. Do not check them for at least 30 minutes as they will quickly deflate. Serve immediately.

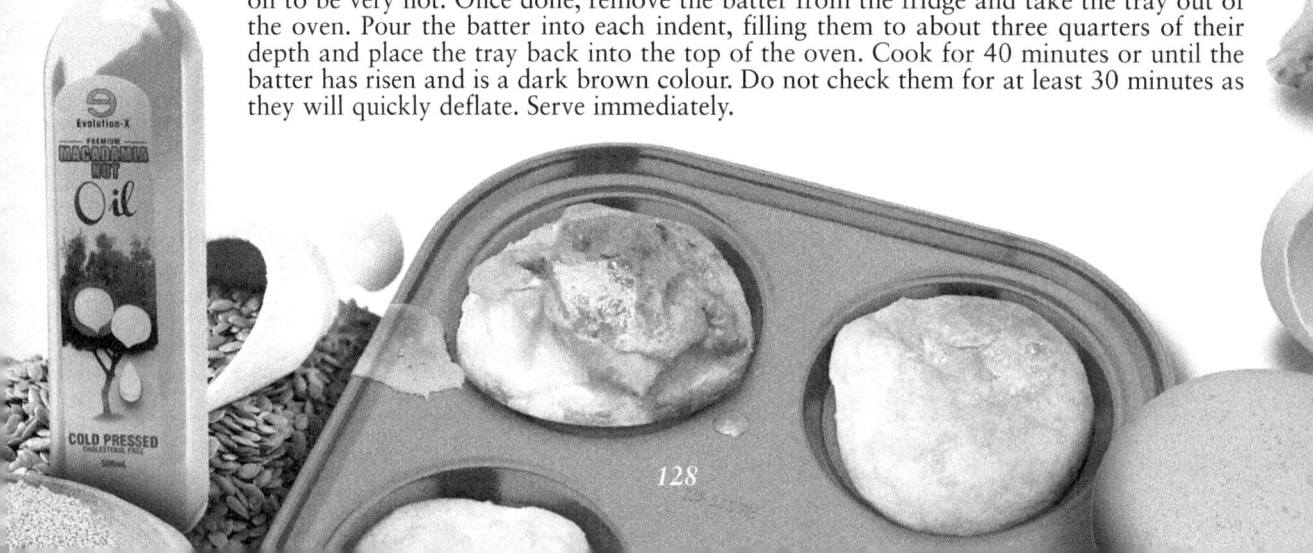

Roasts

Sage & Onion Stuffing

A lovely, easy to make, fresh alternative to the packaged dry ingredients of readymade stuffing that are high in carbohydrates.

Serves 4

INGREDIENTS
3 large Onions (795 g)
8 Sage leaves (3.5 g)
100 g of low carb Breadcrumbs
1 medium Egg yolk (43 g)
30 g Low fat (light) Spreadable Butter with rapeseed or olive oil (or both)
Salt and Pepper to taste

Nutrition in Grams
per Serving

Protein - 3.73
Fat - 4.79
Carbs - 8.17
Fibre - 3.78
Kcals - 100.04
Sat - 1.34
Mono - 1.35
Poly - 1.73
Trans - 0.04
Omega 3 - 1.17
Omega 6 - 0.58

Bring a pan of water to boiling, peel the Onions and put them into the boiling water. Simmer for around 10 minutes adding the Sage leaves for the final couple of minutes. Remove the Onions and Sage and finely chop them both. Put into a bowl and add the bread, seasoning (plenty of salt and pepper) and spreadable butter, mix together thoroughly. Add the yolk of an egg and stir in thoroughly. The stuffing is now ready to use.

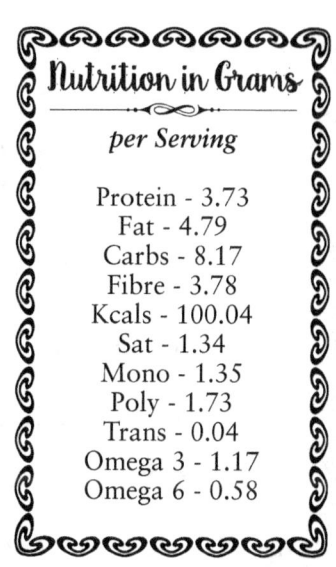

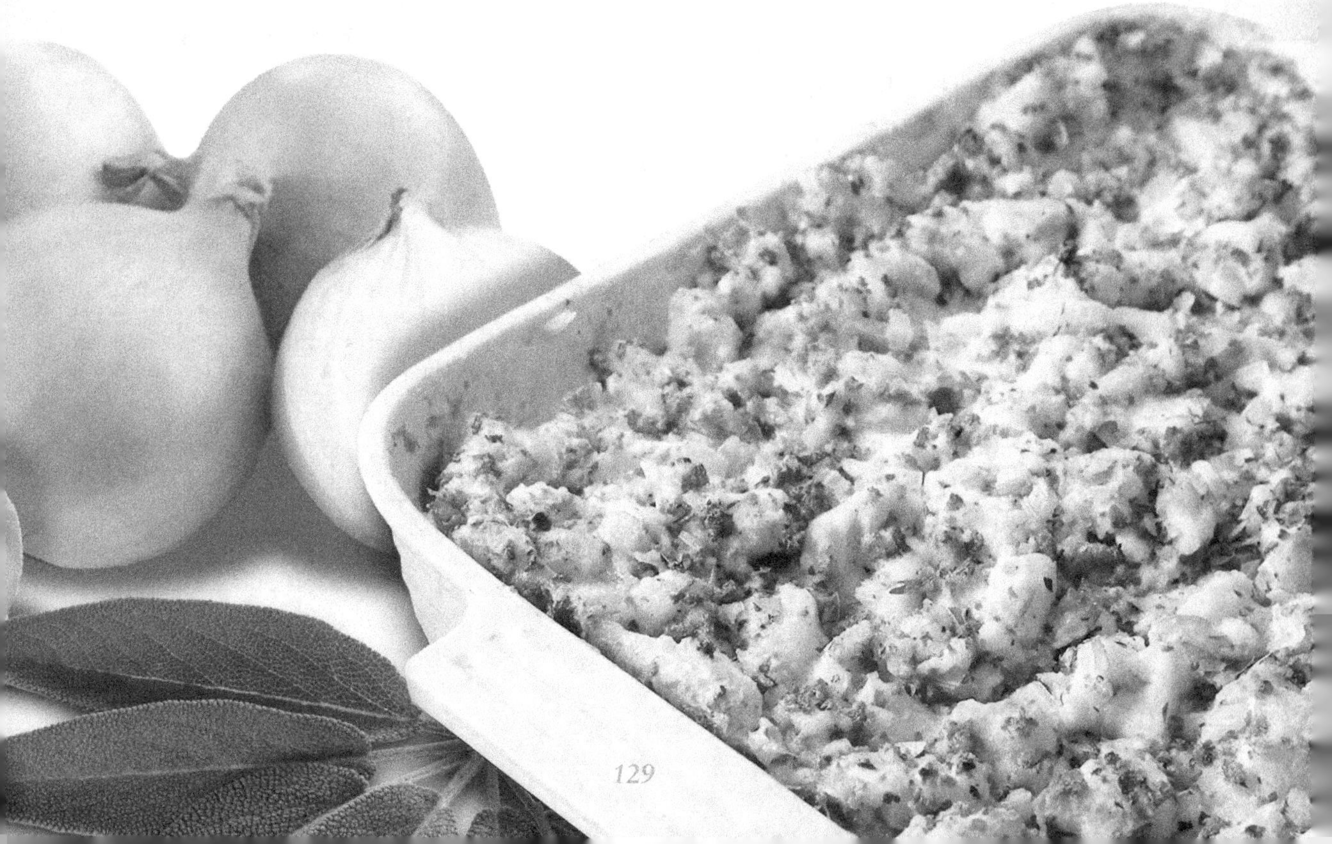

Macadamia & Mushroom Roast

Nut loaves and roasts have had a bit of a bad reputation when vegetarian cooking became popular. They were considered bland and tasteless but are in fact a great alternative to roast meat and this recipe contains loads of taste. Layering the contents makes for a visually aesthetically pleasing result.

This recipe is delicious hot served with a green vegetable, roasted Turnips (see page 127) and a rich Tomato Sauce (see page 91). Alternatively, you can serve it cold with a mixed green salad (see page 172).

Serves 6

INGREDIENTS

1 small Onion (150 g), finely chopped
2 cloves of Garlic (12 g), crushed
225 g Macadamia Nuts, finely chopped
150 g fresh low carb Breadcrumbs
3 medium Turnips (750 g)
1 tablespoon (15 g) Low fat (light) Spreadable Butter with rapeseed or olive oil (or both)
1 teaspoon (7 g) fresh Rosemary or ½ teaspoon (3 g) dried Rosemary
1 teaspoon fresh Thyme (7 g) or ½ teaspoon (3 g) dried Thyme
1 teaspoon (5 g) of Marmite/Yeast Extract
150 ml Vegetable Stock (use 1 stock cube (5 g) - or make your own - (see page 80)
225 g Mushrooms, chopped
1 tablespoon (15 ml) of Macadamia oil or Rapeseed oil
Salt and freshly ground black pepper

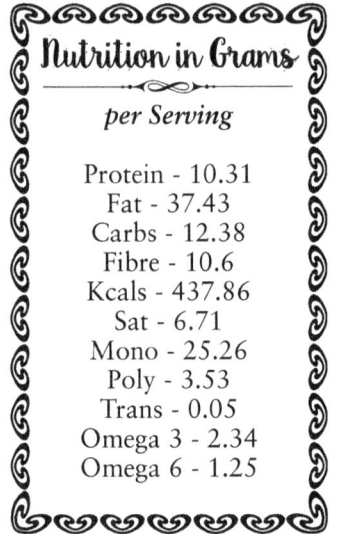

Nutrition in Grams

per Serving

Protein - 10.31
Fat - 37.43
Carbs - 12.38
Fibre - 10.6
Kcals - 437.86
Sat - 6.71
Mono - 25.26
Poly - 3.53
Trans - 0.05
Omega 3 - 2.34
Omega 6 - 1.25

Pre-heat the oven to gas mark 4 - 180°C (360°F). Heat the oil and fry the onion and garlic until soft and the onion is translucent, keep stirring them to prevent them from burning. Grind the Walnuts in a nut mill, blender or food processor, put in a bowl and then mix with the breadcrumbs. Beat the Egg thoroughly and add it to the dry ingredients. Boil the Turnips for 15 minutes until soft, drain and add the spreadable butter and mash until very smooth. Add the herbs to the mash, stir and add to the onion mix. Dissolve the yeast extract in the vegetable stock and add to the other ingredients. Season well.

Put some Macadamia oil or Rapeseed oil in a frying pan and sauté the chopped Mushrooms until soft. Grease a 900 g loaf tin with a little spreadable butter, and then put in half the nut mixture, pushing the mixture firmly down. Cover with a layer of half the chopped mushrooms and put the rest of the nut mixture over the mushrooms, again pushing down firmly. Then cover the top with the remaining chopped mushrooms, cover with foil and bake in the centre of the oven for 1 hour. When cooked, remove the loaf from the oven and leave to stand for 10 minutes before turning it out. It can be eaten either hot or cold.

Roasts

Slow-Cooked Pot Roast with Creamy Gravy

This pot roast takes time but very little effort and can be left to cook overnight or while you're at work.

Serves 6

INGREDIENTS
900 g Pork joint
½ tablespoon (2½ g) Salt
1 Bay leaf (0.3 g)
5 Peppercorns (1 g)
1 teaspoon (5 g) dried Thyme
1 teaspoon (5 g) dried Rosemary
2 Garlic cloves (12 g), crushed
45 g fresh Ginger
1 tablespoon (15 ml) Olive oil
1 tablespoon (5 g) Paprika powder
½ teaspoon (2½ g) ground black Pepper

Creamy Gravy
360 ml low fat Natural Yoghurt
Juices from the roast

Garnish:
Chopped Spring Onions

Nutrition in Grams
per Serving

Protein - 35.24
Fat - 15.27
Carbs - 5.13
Fibre - 1.30
Kcals - 302.80
Sat - 5.41
Mono - 6.90
Poly - 1.59
Trans - 0.04
Omega 3 - 0.21
Omega 6 - 1.53

Preheat the oven to gas mark 1- 100°C (200°F). Place the meat in a deep ovenproof dish and sprinkle the salt over it. Add water to cover 2/3 of the meat and add the bay leaf and peppercorns. Place the baking dish in the oven for 7–8 hours. Remove the meat from the ovenproof dish and put on a large plate and save the juices in a jug for making the gravy. Put the crushed garlic and ginger in a small bowl. Add the olive oil, herbs and pepper and stir together. Then rub the mixture over the pork. Return the meat to the ovenproof dish and turn up the oven to gas mark 8- 220°C (450°F). Roast for about 10–15 minutes.

Meanwhile, sieve the juices to remove any solid bits and put in a saucepan. Boil and reduce to about half the volume. Add the natural yoghurt and heat, stirring continually, being careful not to boil. Cut the meat into thin slices and serve with the creamy gravy. Cauliflower mash (see page 167) and Green Cabbage go great with this dish. Garnish with finely chopped spring onions.

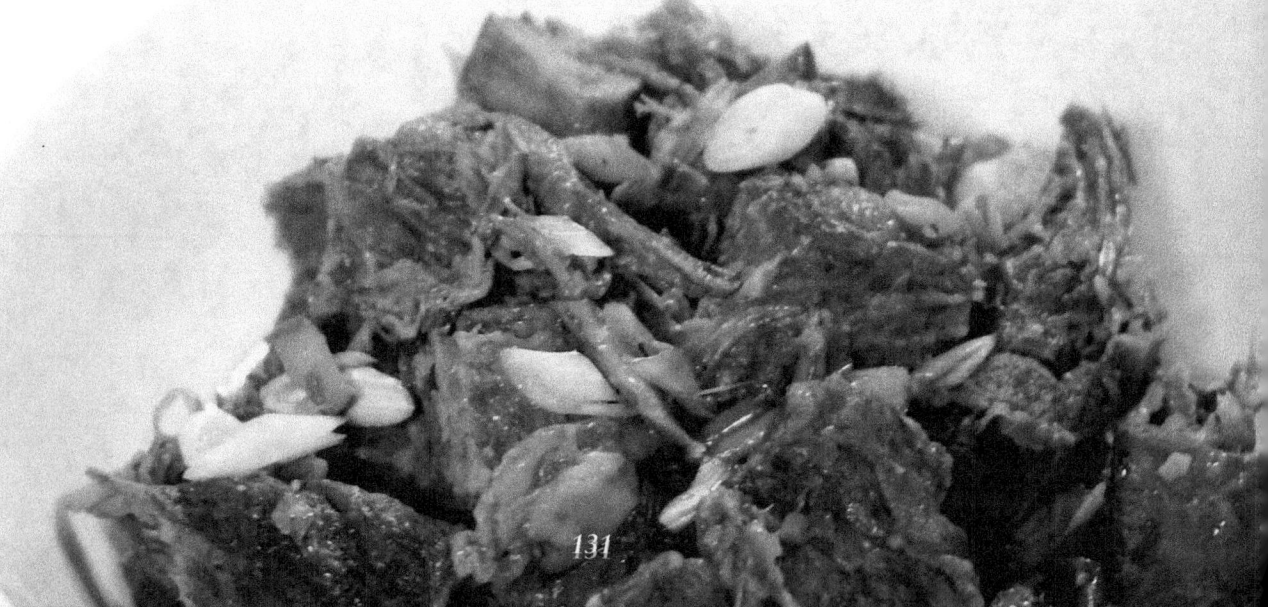

Roasts

Roast Beef with Roasted Vegetables

Serves 6 ❷

INGREDIENTS

1.5 kg topside of beef
2 Onions, cut into small chunks (530 g)
2 Carrots, roughly chopped (200 g)
2 sticks Celery, sliced (100 g)
450 g Turnips, peeled and chopped into chunks
450 g Swedes, peeled and chopped into chunks
1 bulb of Garlic (48 g)
1 tablespoon (15 g) fresh Thyme
1 tablespoon (15 g) fresh Rosemary
1 tablespoon (15 g) fresh Sage
3 Bay Leaves (0.9 g)
2 tablespoons (30 ml) Macadamia or Rapeseed Oil

Nutrition in Grams

per Serving

Protein - 59.55
Fat - 13.16
Carbs - 22.23
Fibre - 7.80
Kcals - 464.41
Sat - 3.58
Mono - 7.02
Poly - 1.21
Trans - 0.28
Omega 3 - 0.39
Omega 6 - 0.90

Remove the beef from the fridge 30 minutes before you want to cook it. Preheat the oven to gas mark 9 - 240°C (475°F). Wash and roughly chop the vegetables. Break the garlic bulb into the individual cloves, peel and chop them in half. Put all the chopped vegetables, garlic and herbs into the a large roasting tray, sprinkle the herbs over them and drizzle with half the oil. Place the beef on top of the vegetables. Drizzle the beef with the remainder of the oil and season well with salt and black pepper, then rub all over the surface of the joint.

Place the tray in the oven, Turn the heat down f the oven to gas mark 6 - 200°C (400°F) and cook for 50 minutes for medium-rare, 1 hour for a medium beef or 1 hour 15 minutes for well done. Baste the beef after 30 minutes if the vegetables are dry just splash a little water on them. When cooked, take the tray out of the oven and transfer the beef to a plate and cover it with tin foil and leave to rest for 15 minutes. Serve with Lemon Broccoli (see page 158), Gravy and Horseradish Sauce (see page 95 for homemade version).

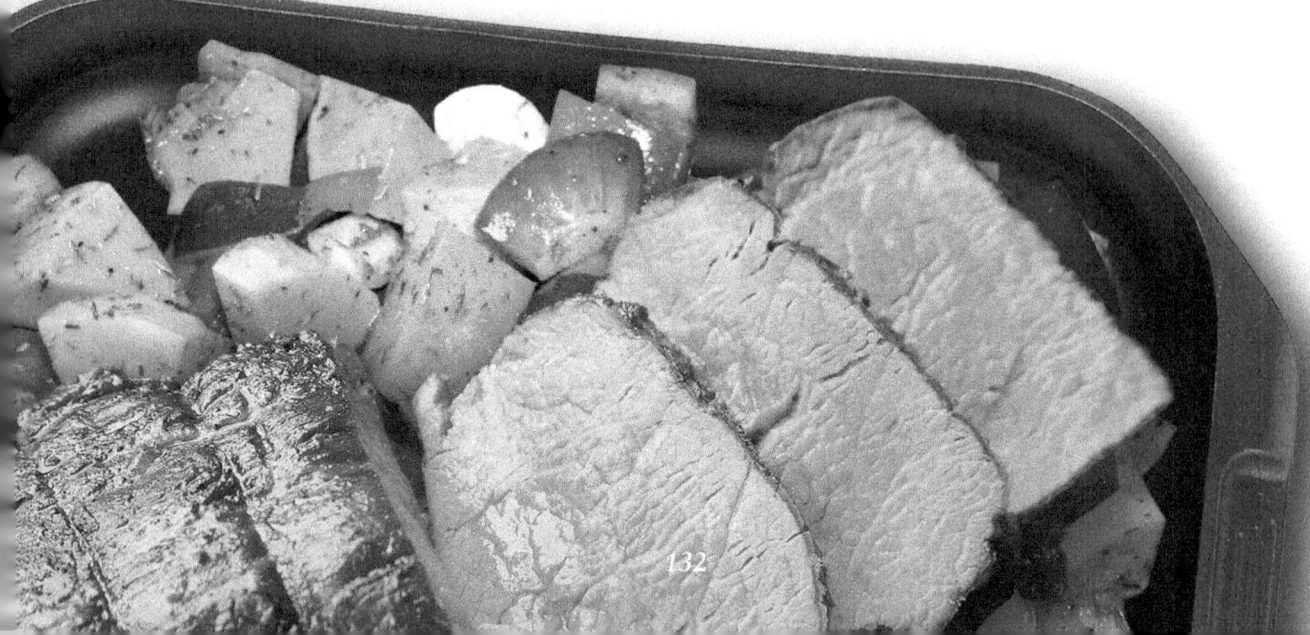

―― Roasts ――

Layered Cheese & Tomato Nut Roast

This nut roast has a deliciously crunchy texture. You can simply mix all the ingredients together but I think it is worth the extra effort to keep them separate and make a layered loaf as this looks much more attractive.

The roast can be eaten hot or cold, but when hot it is fairly crumbly so I tend to serve it straight from the dish. If you do want to turn it out to serve it, you'll find it easier if you line the tin with foil or greaseproof paper. It is delicious with a Barbecue Sauce (see page 63) and could be served with roast turnips (see page 127) and Ratatouille (see page 156).

Serves 4

INGREDIENTS

50 g Extra Mature Cheese, grated

75 g fresh Low Carb Breadcrumbs (see page 58)

2 tablespoons (30 g) Macadamia or Rapeseed oil

1 Onion, (265 g) peeled and finely chopped

2 sticks Celery (100 g), finely chopped

75 g Macadamia Nuts, roughly chopped

50 g ground Almonds

1 teaspoon fresh Marjoram (5 g) or

½ teaspoon dried Marjoram (2½ g)

1 teaspoon fresh Thyme (5 g) or

½ teaspoon dried thyme (2½ g)

Salt and freshly ground Black Pepper

400 g tin of Tomatoes, drained

5 g Low fat (light) Spreadable Butter with rapeseed or olive oil (or both) for greasing the tin

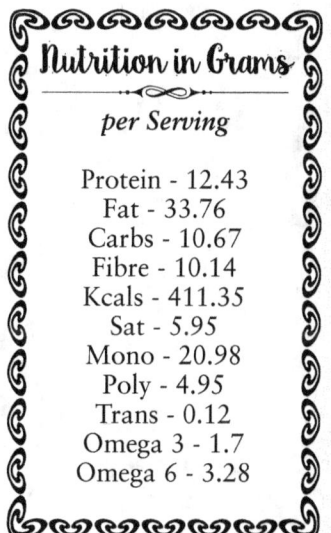

Nutrition in Grams

per Serving

Protein - 12.43
Fat - 33.76
Carbs - 10.67
Fibre - 10.14
Kcals - 411.35
Sat - 5.95
Mono - 20.98
Poly - 4.95
Trans - 0.12
Omega 3 - 1.7
Omega 6 - 3.28

Pre-heat the oven to gas mark 5 - 190°C (375°F). Mix together the grated cheese and breadcrumbs in a large bowl and moisten thorn with 1 tablespoon of oil. Heat the remaining tablespoon of oil in a frying-pan and gently fry the onion and celery until fairly soft. Roughly chop the walnuts and add them to the frying pan along with the ground almonds and herbs. Mix together well and remove the pan from the heat. Season well. Liquidise or sieve the drained tomatoes.

Line and thoroughly grease a 700 g (1½ lb) loaf tin. Press in a layer of the cheese and breadcrumbs, then a Layer of nuts and celery, then a layer of liquidised tomatoes. Repeat these layers, ending with a topping of cheese and breadcrumbs. Press down well. Bake for 1 hour or until firm to the touch. Serve hot or cold. If you want to turn the terrine out while it's hot, be sure to let it stand at least 10 minutes so that it firms up before removing it from the tin.

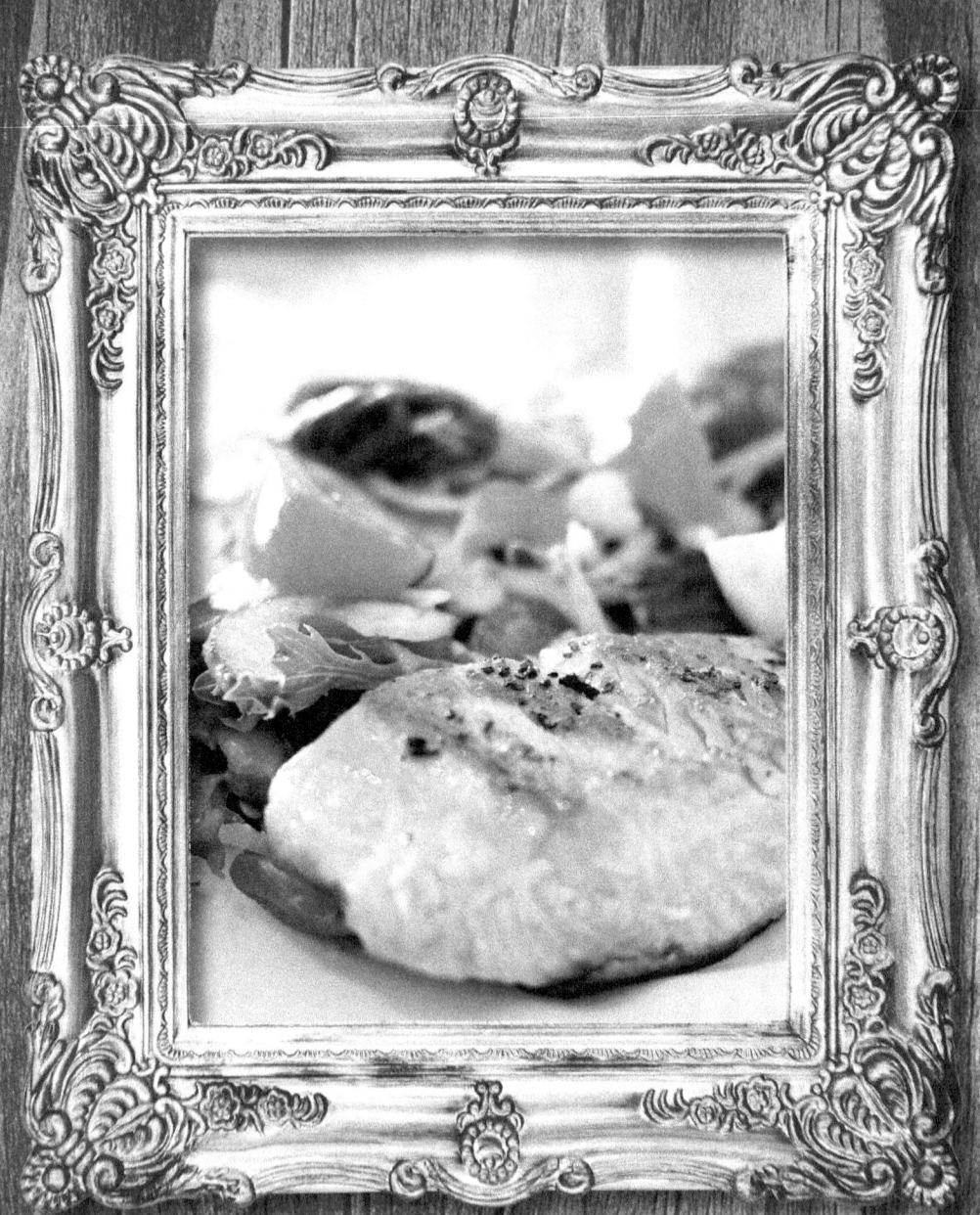

Fish

Fish Pie

This is a very easy and delicious Fish dsh and a good source of marine Omega 3.

Serves 4

INGREDIENTS
400 g Skinless Cod Fillet
400 g Skinless Salmon Fillets
600 ml semi-skimmed Milk
1 small Onion (150 g), quartered
4 Cloves
2 Bay leaves (0.6 g)
4 Large Eggs (300 g)
Small bunch Parsley (80 g), leaves only, chopped
15 g Low fat (light) Spreadable Butter with rapeseed or olive oil (or both)
15 g plain Flour
½ teaspoon (2½ g) of freshly grated Nutmeg
1 kg Swede, peeled and cut into even-sized chunks
50 g Extra Mature Cheddar, grated

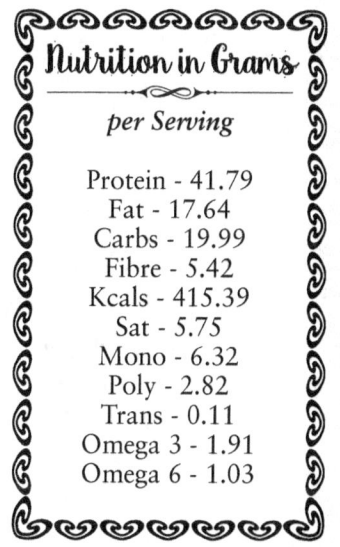

Nutrition in Grams
per Serving

Protein - 41.79
Fat - 17.64
Carbs - 19.99
Fibre - 5.42
Kcals - 415.39
Sat - 5.75
Mono - 6.32
Poly - 2.82
Trans - 0.11
Omega 3 - 1.91
Omega 6 - 1.03

First you need to poach the fish. Put the fish in a medium saucepan and pour over 500 ml of the milk. Push one clove into each of the onion quarters, and add to the milk with the bay leaves. Bring the milk to the boil. Reduce the heat immediately and simmer for 8 minutes. Lift the fish onto a plate and drain off the milk into a jug to let it cool. With a fork, flake the fish into large pieces into an ovenproof dish. Bring a small pan of water to boiling point and very slightly reduce the heat so that is gently boiling. Carefully lower the eggs in with a spoon. Keeping the water gentle boiling, and boil the eggs for 8 minutes. Lift the eggs out and put into a bowl of cold water to cool for 5 minutes. Remove the shell and slice the eggs and arrange on the top of the fish, then sprinkle most of the chopped parsley over the top, retaining a little to sprinkle on the top of the pie when it is cooked.

To make the sauce, melt half the spreadable butter in a small saucepan, stir in the flour to make a roux and cook for 1 minute over a moderate heat, stirring constantly. Remove from the heat; pour in about a quarter of the cold milk you used for poaching the fish and stir until completely blended. Gradually add the milk, mixing continually until you have a smooth sauce. Returning the pan to the heat, bring the sauce to the boil and simmer for 5 minutes, stirring continually until it nicely thickens up. Remove from the heat, season with salt, pepper and nutmeg, and then pour over the fish.

Pre-heat the oven to gas mark 4 - 180°C (350°F). Boil the Swede for 25 minutes until really soft. Drain completely, season to taste with salt and freshly ground black pepper and mash thoroughly with the remaining spreadable butter and milk. Spread the mash over the top of the pie with a fork, making sure to seal the edges with the mash. Fluff the top with a fork then sprinkle the cheese evenly over the top and place in the centre of the oven and cook for 30 minutes. Remove from the oven and sprinkle the remaining Parsley over the pie.

Fish

Dill Weed Salmon Pie

This is a scrumptious, creamy fish pie with the distinctive flavour of Dill. Dill, also known as dill weed, is a green herb with thin, wiry leaves. It has a distinctive taste of a blend of fennel, anise and celery. Salmon is a great source of marine Omega 3.

Serves 4

INGREDIENTS

Pie Crust

1 portion low carb shortcrust pastry (see page 97)

Filling

400 g Salmon
100 ml Thick Low fat Greek Yoghurt
2 medium Eggs (130 g)
2 tablespoons (45 g) fresh Dill, finely chopped
1 large Onion (265 g), finely chopped
80 ml half fat Cream Cheese
80 g Extra Mature Cheddar, grated
3 tablespoons (12 g) fresh parsley for a garnish
Salt and freshly ground black pepper to taste
Small amount of Low fat (light) Spreadable Butter with rapeseed or olive oil (or both) to grease tin

Nutrition in Grams
per Serving

Protein - 40.8
Fat - 48.73
Carbs - 10.4
Fibre - 9.62
Kcals - 665.17
Sat - 9.86
Mono - 12.16
Poly - 22.85
Trans - 0.47
Omega 3 - 16.49
Omega 6 - 6.35

Follow the instructions for Shortcrust Pastry on page 73 Put the dough in the fridge until you are ready to use it. Preheat the oven to gas mark 4 - 175°C (350°F).

Using a small amount of spreadable butter; grease a 23 cm/10 inch diameter, 5 cm/2 inch deep round baking tin, making sure you completely cover both the bottom and the sides. Roll out the pastry dough to about a 4 mm thick round shape and carefully place over the tin and, with slightly greased fingers, ease the pastry into the tin. Trim any excess with a knife, and use these pieces to fill any gaps you may have, smoothing the joins with a little water on your fingers. Place the pastry into the centre of the oven and bake for 15 minutes. When cooked, remove from the oven and let it cool down.

Fry the chopped Onion in a little oil on a low heat until they are soft and translucent. Leave to cool down. In a large bowl, crack open the eggs and mix thoroughly, add the Ricotta, Cheddar and Greek Yoghurt and stir into the eggs. When you have a smooth paste, sprinkle in the Dill and add the onions. Season to taste and mix together.

Pour half the mixture into the cooled Pastry crust and spread evenly. Cut the Salmon into chunks and spread evenly over the pie. Pour in the remaining mixture and spread over the fish. Place in the centre of the oven and cook for 35 minutes. Garnish with a little parsley.

Fish Casserole with Mushrooms & Mustard

This is a hearty and quick low carb fish dish with a creamy French-mustard sauce.

Serves 6 ❷

INGREDIENTS

700 g White Fish
450 g Button Mushrooms, chopped
20 g Low fat (light) Spreadable Butter with rapeseed or olive oil (or both)
2 tablespoons (8 g) fresh Parsley
200 g half fat Crème Fraiche
225 ml semi-skimmed Milk
2 tablespoons (30 g) Mustard, preferably Dijon
100 g Extra Mature Cheddar cheese, grated
Salt and freshly ground black pepper to taste

Nutrition in Grams
per Serving

Protein - 31.68
Fat - 15.86
Carbs - 6.19
Fibre - 1.01
Kcals - 294.52
Sat - 8.61
Mono - 4.24
Poly - 1.23
Trans - 0.34
Omega 3 - 0.44
Omega 6 - 0.79

Preheat the oven to gas mark 4 - 175°C (350°F). Cut the mushrooms into wedges. Fry in the spreadable butter until the mushrooms have turned a nicely brown. Add salt and pepper to taste and add the herbs. Pour in the crème fraiche and mustard and lower the heat. Simmer for 5-10 minutes to reduce the sauce a bit. Season the fish with salt and pepper and place in a greased baking dish. Sprinkle three-quarters of the cheese over the fish and pour the creamed mushrooms on top. Top with the remaining cheese and place in the top half of the oven.

Bake for about 20 minutes, and then check with a knife to see if the fish is cooked. The fish is done if it comes apart easily.

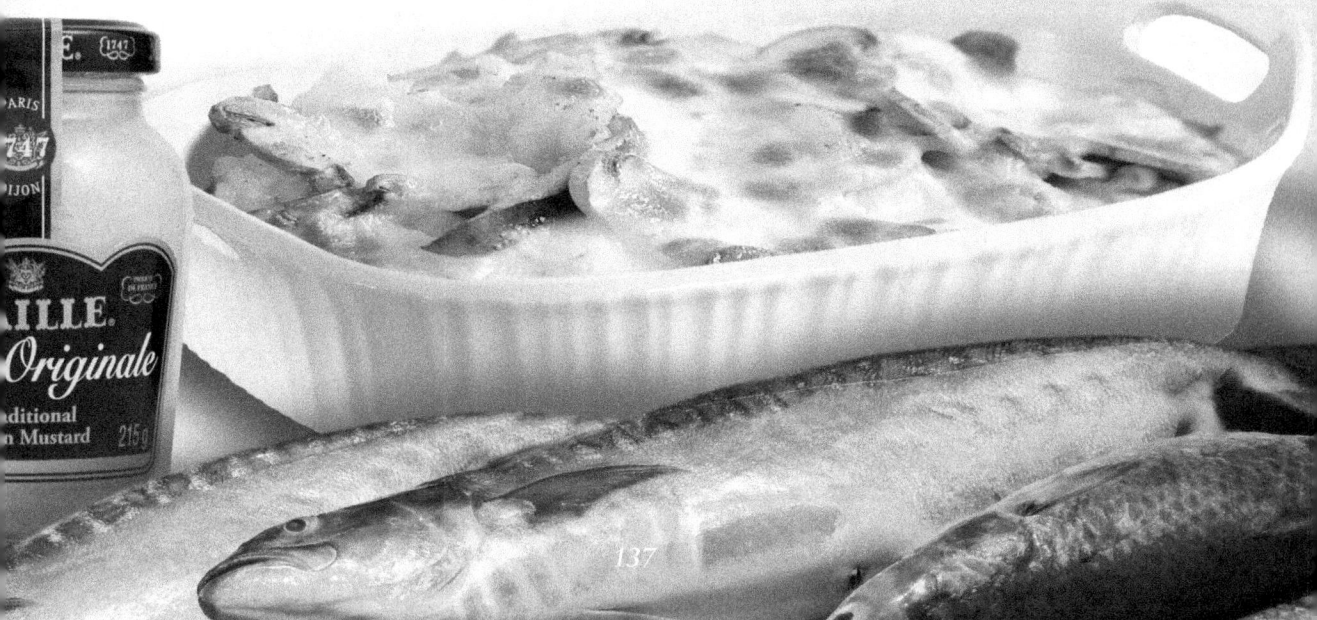

Fish

Salmon with Pesto & Spinach

A simple and delicious salmon dish is so quick and easy and it also has under 3 carbs per portion!

Serves 4

INGREDIENTS

700 g Salmon

4 tablespoons (60 g) homemade Mayonnaise (see page 94)

4 tablespoons (60 g) Green or Red homemade Pesto (see page 93)

25 g grated Parmesan Cheese

450 g fresh Spinach

1 tablespoon (15 ml) Macadamia oil or Rapeseed oil

Salt and pepper

Nutrition in Grams
per Serving

Protein - 44.10
Fat - 33.79
Carbs - 2.86
Fibre - 4.63
Kcals - 491.08
Sat - 6.45
Mono - 15.36
Poly - 8.23
Trans - 0.10
Omega 3 - 4.19
Omega 6 - 3.94

Preheat the oven to gas mark 6 - 200°C (400°F). Salt and pepper the salmon pieces and place them in a greased baking dish, skin down. In a mixing bowl, mix the mayonnaise, pesto and parmesan cheese and then spread over the salmon. Bake for 20 minutes or until the salmon is done, which is when it comes apart easily.

Meanwhile, fry the spinach in a little Rapeseed oil or Macadamia oil until it shrinks. It will only take a couple of minutes. Add salt and pepper to taste. Serve immediately with the oven-baked salmon.

Lemon Baked Salmon

The salmon in this dish is ideally complemented with the flavour of the butter and lemon.

Serves 6

INGREDIENTS

1.2 kg Salmon

1 teaspoon Salt (5 g)

Freshly ground Black Pepper

50 g Low fat (light) Spreadable Butter with rapeseed or olive oil (or both)

1 Lemon, sliced (85 g)

The juice of one lemon (50 ml)

Rapeseed oil or Macadamia oil for greasing baking dish (15 g)

Nutrition in Grams
per Serving

Protein - 45.51
Fat - 32.03
Carbs - 6.16
Fibre - 2.54
Kcals - 494.18
Sat - 8.21
Mono - 13.44
Poly - 6.31
Trans - 0.30
Omega 3 - 4.74
Omega 6 - 1.49

Preheat the oven to gas mark 6 - 200°C (400°F). Place the salmon with the skin down in a greased baking dish. Add salt and pepper generously. Slice the lemon thinly and place on top of the salmon. Cover with half of the butter in thin slices. Bake on middle rack for about 20 minutes. The salmon is done when it comes apart easily. Melt the rest of the butter in a small sauce pan on a low heat. Remove from the heat and put aside to cool a little and carefully add the lemon juice. Serve the fish with the lemon butter and a side dish of your choice.

Cheesy Tuna Casserole

Serves 4 ❷

INGREDIENTS

340 g tinned Tuna in brine, drained
340 g Green Beans
85 g Mushrooms, chopped
1 stalk Celery (40 g), finely chopped
1 large Onion (265 g), finely chopped
120 ml Vegetable Stock (using one stock cube - 5 g)
or make your own (see page 80)
100 g low fat Natural Yoghurt
100 g Extra Mature Cheddar Cheese, grated
1 tablespoon (15 ml) Macadamia oil or Rapeseed oil for frying
Salt and pepper, to taste

Nutrition in Grams

per Serving

Protein - 26.08
Fat - 6.06
Carbs - 9.62
Fibre - 4.05
Kcals - 205.58
Sat - 1.49
Mono - 3.54
Poly - 0.49
Trans - 0.02
Omega 3 - 0.29
Omega 6 - 0.20

Preheat the oven to gas mark 4 - 175°C (350°F). In a large saucepan, cook the green beans until nice and soft, then drain them well and return to the saucepan. Meanwhile, fry the mushrooms, celery and onion in the Rapeseed oil or Macadamia oil until they are very soft and just starting to brown a little. Add the vegetable stock and bring to the boil. Let the liquid reduce by half, and then stir in the yoghurt. Cook on a low heat for a couple of minutes, or until the sauce has reduced a little and thickened, stirring frequently. Add the tuna, stir well and season to taste. Stir the tuna and mushroom mixture into the saucepan with the green beans. Mix in the cheese and pour into a large ovenproof dish. Place in the centre of the oven and bake for 15-20 minutes or until the sauce is bubbling.

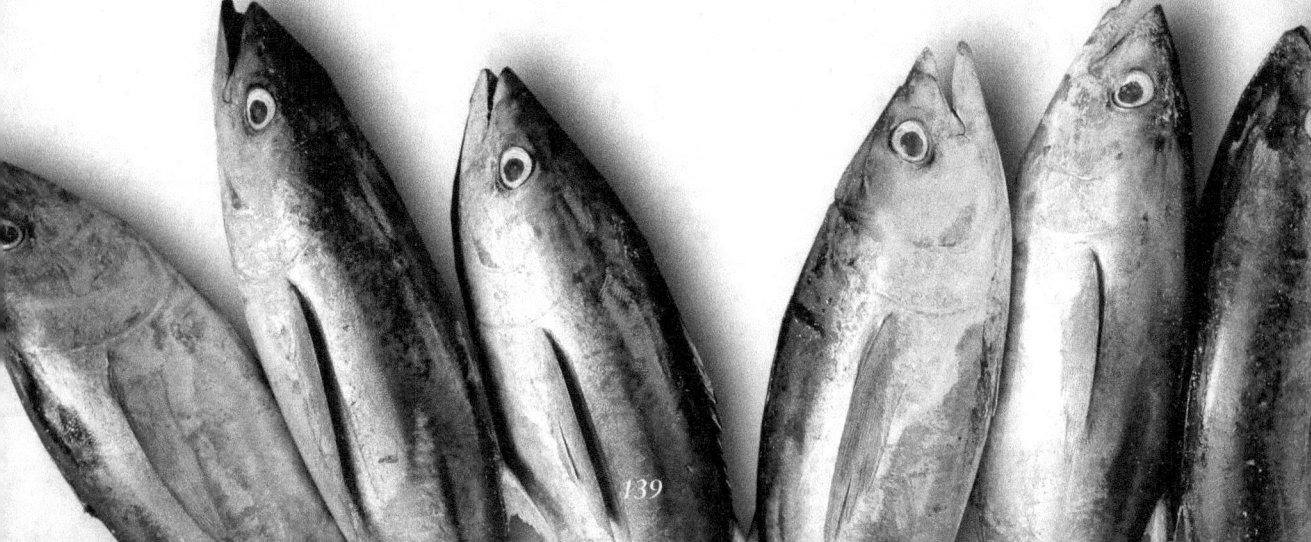

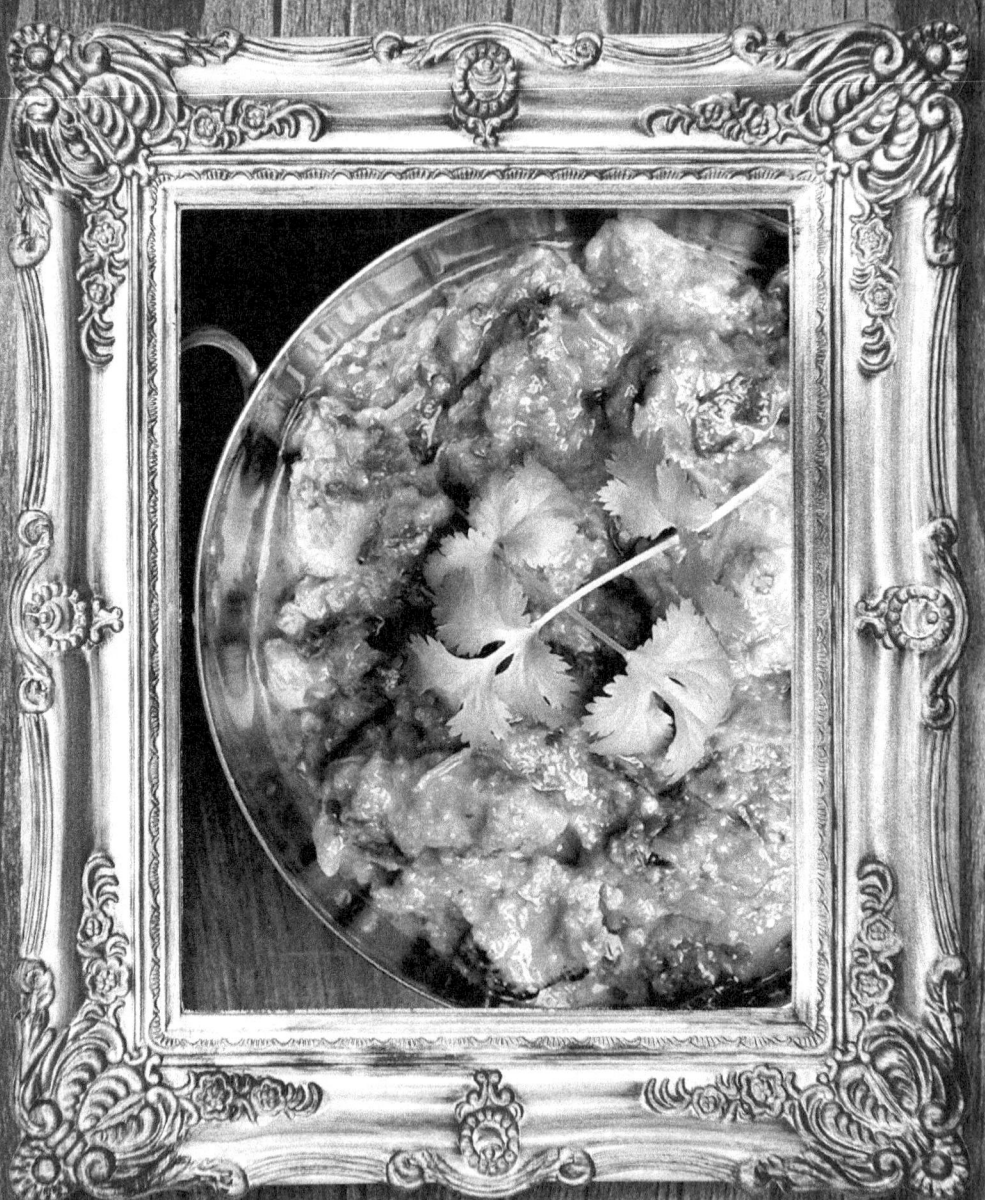

Curries

Garam Masala Chicken

This Chicken Curry is really easy to make and full of flavour. If you don't want to mix up your own Garam Masala, you can buy it premixed from most anywhere. This goes great with Cauliflower or Broccoli Rice.

Serves 4

INGREDIENTS

700 g Chicken breasts
1 Red Pepper (165 g), finely sliced
280 ml thick Low fat Greek Yoghurt
1 tablespoon fresh Parsley (4 g), finely chopped
1 tablespoon (15 ml) Macadamia oil or Rapeseed Oil for frying
Salt and Pepper to taste

Garam Masala

1 teaspoon (5 g) ground Cumin
2 teaspoon (10 g) Coriander seeds, ground or ground Coriander
(grinding the seeds produces a fresher taste)
1 teaspoon (5 g) ground Cardamom
1 teaspoon (5 g) Turmeric, ground
1 teaspoon ground Ginger (5 g) or 7½ g chopped fresh ginger
1 teaspoon (5 g) Paprika powder
½- 1 teaspoon (2½ g - 5 g) chilli powder (dependent on taste)
1 pinch of ground nutmeg (1 g)

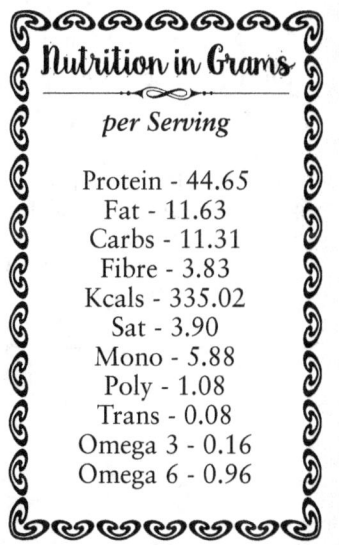

Nutrition in Grams
per Serving

Protein - 44.65
Fat - 11.63
Carbs - 11.31
Fibre - 3.83
Kcals - 335.02
Sat - 3.90
Mono - 5.88
Poly - 1.08
Trans - 0.08
Omega 3 - 0.16
Omega 6 - 0.96

Mix all the Garam Masala ingredients in a bowl. If you are using the Coriander seeds, you need to ground them in a nut mill or a pestle and mortar. Alternatively you can buy a pre-mixed Garam Masala. Preheat the oven to gas mark 6 - 200°C /400°F.

Cut the raw chicken breasts in half along their length. Add the Rapeseed Oil or Macadamia oil in a large frying pan and fry on a medium heat until the meat has turned a nice brown colour (around 15-20 minutes). Sprinkle half the Garam Masala spices and stir thoroughly. Season to taste. Place the chicken fillets, including the juices, in a large ovenproof roasting dish.

Chop up the green Pepper into 1 cm square chunks. Put the Yoghurt in a bowl and stir in the Peppers and the rest of the Garam Masala and mix thoroughly. Spread this mix all over the chicken, making sure you cover the chicken evenly. Bake in the centre of the oven for about 20 minutes. When nicely browned, remove from the oven and sprinkle the parsley over the top.

Thai Fish Curry

A really quick and simple way to cook fish with a lot of flavour.

Serves 4

INGREDIENTS

700 g Salmon or White Fish

2 tablespoons (30 g) Low fat (light) Spreadable Butter with rapeseed or olive oil (or both)

2 tablespoons (30 g) curry paste or rajah curry powder or Fiddes Payne Madras curry powder

400 g Thick Low fat Greek Yoghurt

25 g fresh Coriander, chopped

Salt and freshly ground Black Pepper

A little Rapeseed Oil or Macadamia oil for greasing the baking dish

Nutrition in Grams
per Serving

Protein - 41.94
Fat - 13.2
Carbs - 9.31
Fibre - 4.16
Kcals - 339.84
Sat - 5.86
Mono - 4.57
Poly - 1.58
Trans - 0.2
Omega 3 - 0.64
Omega 6 - 0.94

Preheat the oven to gas mark 6 - 200°C (400°F). Cut the fish into 4 equal portions. Grease a deep ovenproof dish with a little Rapeseed Oil or Macadamia oil. The dish should be just big enough to take the fish. Place the fish pieces in the dish. Salt and pepper to taste and put a little knob of butter on each fish piece. In a bowl, mix the yoghurt, curry powder and chopped coriander and pour evenly over the fish. Place in the top half of the oven and cook for 20 minutes or until the fish is done. Serve with boiled cauliflower or broccoli, cauliflower mash or cauliflower rice.

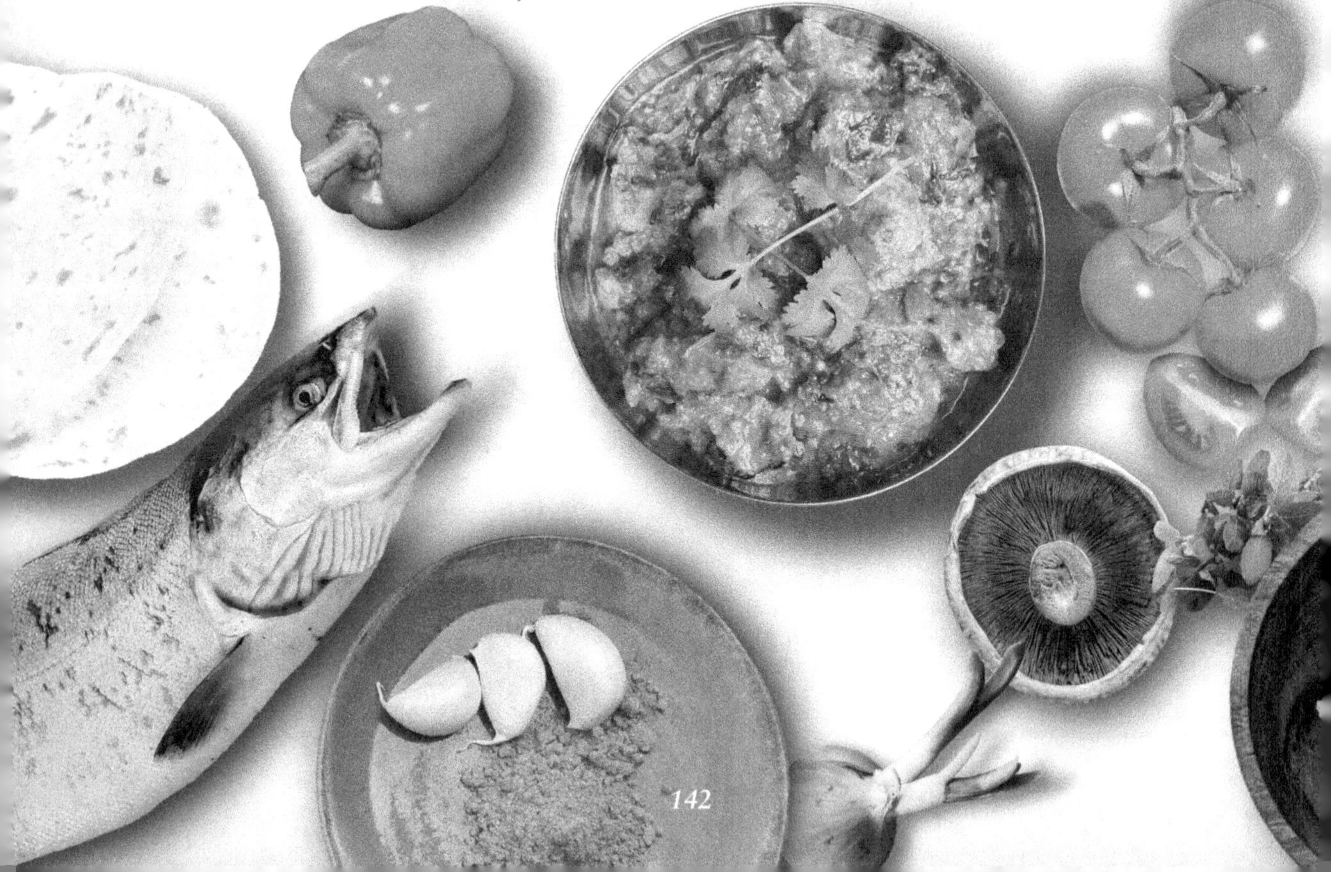

Curry Chicken with Broccoli & Green Beans

A delicious, fast and easy curry with the strong flavour of curry powder, ginger and warming chilli pepper.

Serves 4

INGREDIENTS

450 g Chicken thighs, boneless

225 g Broccoli, chopped into small pieces

115 g fresh Green Beans, cut in half

1 large Onion (265 g), finely chopped

100 ml low fat Natural Yoghurt

2 tablespoons (30 g) curry powder (we recommend Rajah or Fiddes Payne Madras curry powder)

1 Red Chilli Pepper (45 g), finely chopped or grated

1 tablespoon (15 g) grated fresh Ginger

4 cloves of Garlic (24 g), finely sliced

1 tablespoon (15 ml) Macadamia oil or Rapeseed Oil, for frying

Salt and pepper, to taste

Nutrition in Grams
per Serving

Protein - 26.69
Fat - 10.9
Carbs - 12.68
Fibre - 9.16
Kcals - 272.8
Sat - 2.95
Mono - 5.86
Poly - 1.28
Trans - 0.05
Omega 3 - 0.13
Omega 6 - 1.15

Pour a little Rapeseed Oil or Macadamia oil in a frying pan and fry the onion, garlic, ginger and chilli pepper for a couple of minutes. Add the curry powder and chicken thighs and fry the chicken on a medium heat for 10 minutes or until light brown. Add a little more oil if needed. Chop the broccoli and French beans and add to the chicken. Finally add the yoghurt, season to taste, cover with a lid and let simmer for 15 minutes. Serve with cauliflower or broccoli rice.

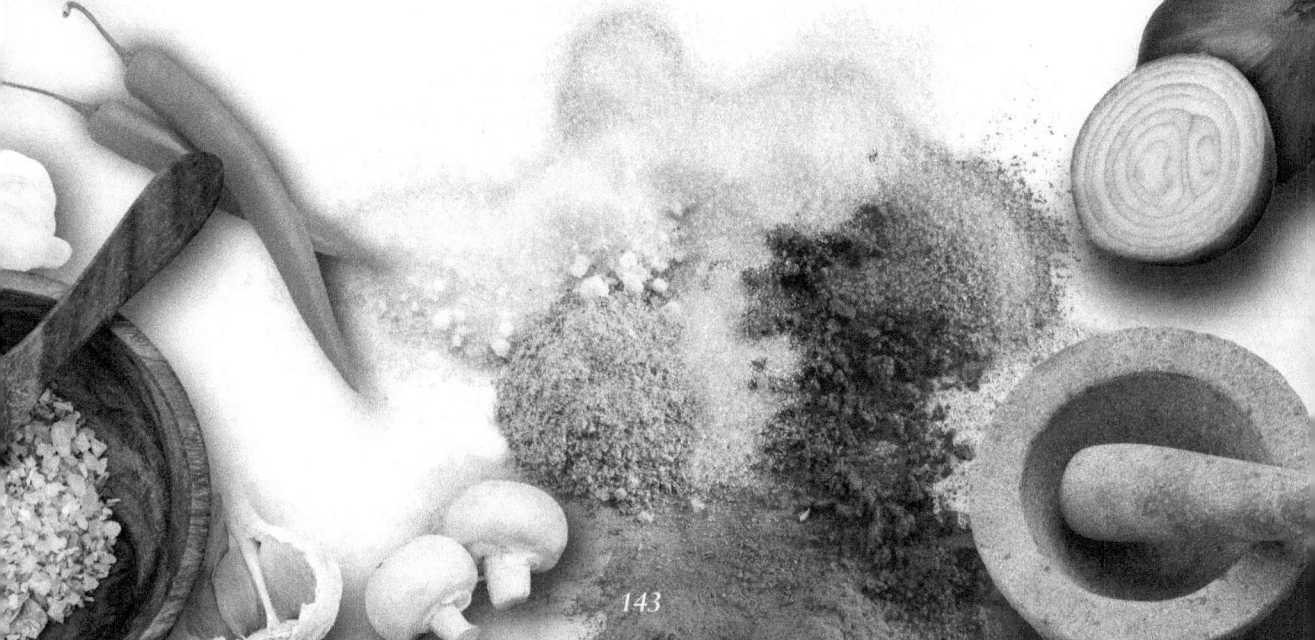

Curries

Chicken Curry Pie

Serves 4

INGREDIENTS
1 portion of Low carb Shortcrust Pastry (see page 97)

Filling
450 g Chickens Breasts
4 tablespoons (60 g) homemade Mayonnaise (see page 94)
3 medium Eggs (195 g)
1 small Egg yolk for glazing the pastry lid
175 g Green Pepper, finely chopped
1 tablespoon (15 g) curry powder
(we recommend Rajah or Fiddes Payne Madras curry powder)
½ teaspoon (2½ g) Paprika
½ teaspoon (2½ g) Onion powder
¼ teaspoon (1 ¼ g) ground Black Pepper
110 g half fat cream cheese
Pinch of salt
Small amount of Low fat (light) Spreadable Butter with rapeseed or olive oil (or both) for greasing the ovenproof pie dish

Nutrition in Grams
per Serving

Protein - 43.42
Fat - 39.6
Carbs - 4.79
Fibre - 8.86
Kcals - 577.24
Sat - 6.32
Mono - 9.02
Poly - 20.73
Trans - 0.18
Omega 3 - 14.09
Omega 6 - 6.53

Preheat the oven to 350°F (175°C). Once you have made the pastry, roll it out into a thin round shape (3-4 mm thick) and place into the base and sides of a 23 cm/10 inch - 5 cm/2 inch deep, slightly greased (with the spreadable butter) ovenproof pie dish. Bake the pastry in the centre of the oven for 15 minutes making sure that the inside of the pie crust is cooked before you put the contents in.

Crack 3 eggs into a large bowl and whisk together. Add the mayonnaise, half fat cream cheese, green pepper, curry powder, paprika, onion powder, black pepper and salt and mix thoroughly. Pour a little into the pie crust and place the chicken breasts on top. Pour the rest of the mixture over the top.

Mix the small egg yolk in a bowl and brush over the pie to glaze it, this gives a nice glisten to the pie and when cooked gives it a pleasant golden colour. Bake the pie for 35 - 40 minutes in the top half of the oven or until the pie has turned golden. Serve with a salad and salad dressing.

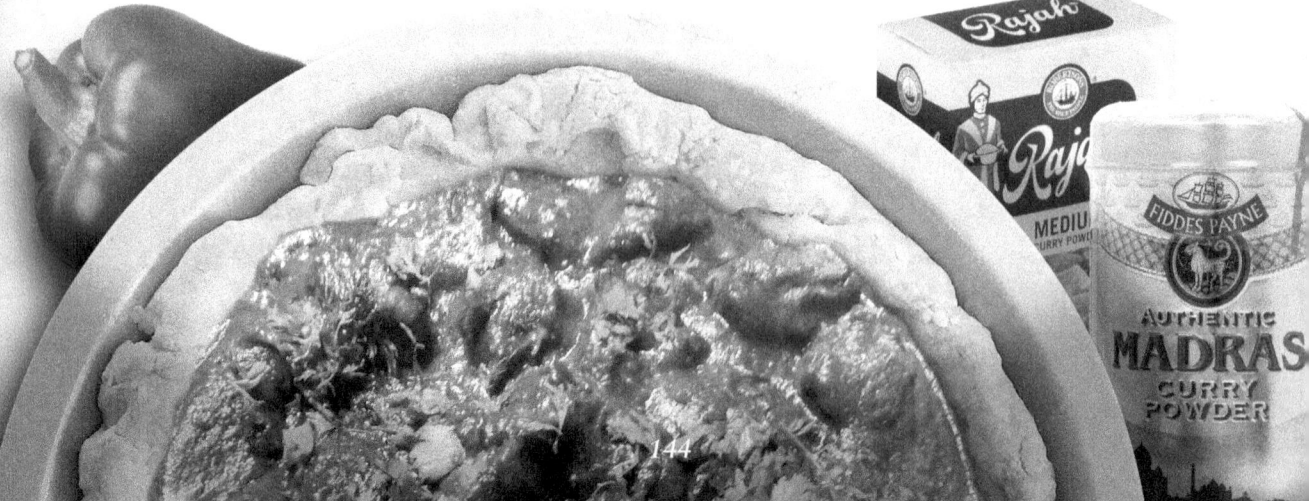

Curries

Chicken & Spinach Balti

This is an easy chicken curry best served in a small metal Balti dish for an authentic feel.

Serves 6

INGREDIENTS

Marinade

1 kg Chicken breasts, cut into bite-sized pieces
5 cm piece fresh Ginger (15 g), finely chopped
4 Garlic cloves (24 g), crushed
½ teaspoon Salt (2½ g)
The juice of 1 lime (30 ml)
1 teaspoon (5 g) ground Coriander
1 teaspoon (5 g) Chilli powder
1 teaspoon (5 g) ground Turmeric
1 teaspoon (5 g) ground Cumin
150 ml low fat Natural Yoghurt

For the curry

1 tablespoon (15 ml) Macadamia oil or Rapeseed Oil
2 small Red Onions (300 g), finely sliced
400 g Tomatoes, finely chopped
2 tablespoons (30 g) Tomato Purée
20 ml water
150 ml half fat Crème Fraiche
300 g Baby Spinach leaves

Garnish

Handful fresh Coriander leaves (40 g), chopped

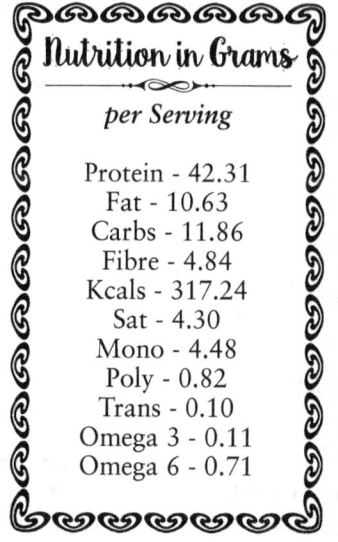

Nutrition in Grams

per Serving

Protein - 42.31
Fat - 10.63
Carbs - 11.86
Fibre - 4.84
Kcals - 317.24
Sat - 4.30
Mono - 4.48
Poly - 0.82
Trans - 0.10
Omega 3 - 0.11
Omega 6 - 0.71

First prepare the marinade for the chicken. Finely chop the ginger and garlic into a large bowl and add the salt. Add the lime juice, ground coriander, chilli powder, ground turmeric and ground cumin to the bowl and mix well. Add the chicken pieces and the yoghurt and stir the coating all the chicken. Cover the bowl with cling film and leave to marinate in the fridge for an hour.

5 minutes before the hour is up, heat the oil in a large frying pan over a low heat and add the onion. Fry for 1-2 minutes or until they are translucent, being careful not to burn them. Then add the tomatoes and the tomato purée and cook gently for about one minute. Now add the chicken to the pan along with the marinade and the water. Pour in the crème fraiche, turn up the heat until the mixture starts to boil, turn the heat down and simmer for 10-15 minutes, or until the chicken is cooked through. To check this, insert a knife into the chicken to see if the flesh is pink or not, if it is pink, carry on cooking until the chicken is white throughout. Add the spinach to the pan and stir for about 4 minutes. Sprinkle the fresh coriander over the top. Serve with low carb Naan bread (see page 36) or Spiced Cauliflower or Broccoli Rice (see page 160).

Curries

Lamb Curry

Lamb meat makes a great tasting curry. I prefer using diced lamb so that you get nice, big chunks of the succulent meat. Cooking this slowly enables the meat to become tender and delicate.

Serves 4

Nutrition in Grams
per Serving

Protein - 28.56
Fat - 13.07
Carbs - 19.47
Fibre - 6.52
Kcals - 316.75
Sat - 3.32
Mono - 7.21
Poly - 1.33
Trans - 0.33
Omega 3 - 0.26
Omega 6 - 1.06

INGREDIENTS

450 g minced or diced Lamb
1 medium sized (300 g) Aubergine, diced
1 x 400 g tin of Tomatoes or 400 g fresh Tomatoes
140 g Tomato puree
1 large Red Onion (265 g), finely chopped
4 cloves of Garlic (24 g), finely sliced
1 Courgette (175 g), sliced
1 teaspoon (5 g) ground Cumin
2 teaspoon (10 g) Coriander seeds, ground or ground Coriander
(grinding the seeds produces a fresher taste)
1 teaspoon (5 g) Turmeric, ground
1 teaspoon ground Ginger (5 g) or (7½ g) chopped fresh ginger
½- 1 teaspoon (2½ g - 5 g) chilli powder (dependent on taste)
1 tablespoon (15 ml) of Macadamia oil or Rapeseed Oil for frying
1 teaspoon ground Black Pepper (5 g)

In a large frying pan or saucepan, use a little Rapeseed Oil or Macadamia oil and fry the onions and garlic on a low heat until the onions are soft and translucent. Before the onions are done, add the diced aubergine, cumin, coriander, turmeric, black pepper and chilli powder and fry until the onions are done. Add the minced or diced lamb and mix thoroughly until slightly browned all over. Pour over the tinned tomatoes and add the tomato puree and stir together. Add the courgette and ginger and turn the heat up until the mixture is bubbling. Turn the heat down to simmer, place a lid on the frying pan or saucepan and cook for around 40 minutes, stirring regularly. Serve with cauliflower or broccoli rice.

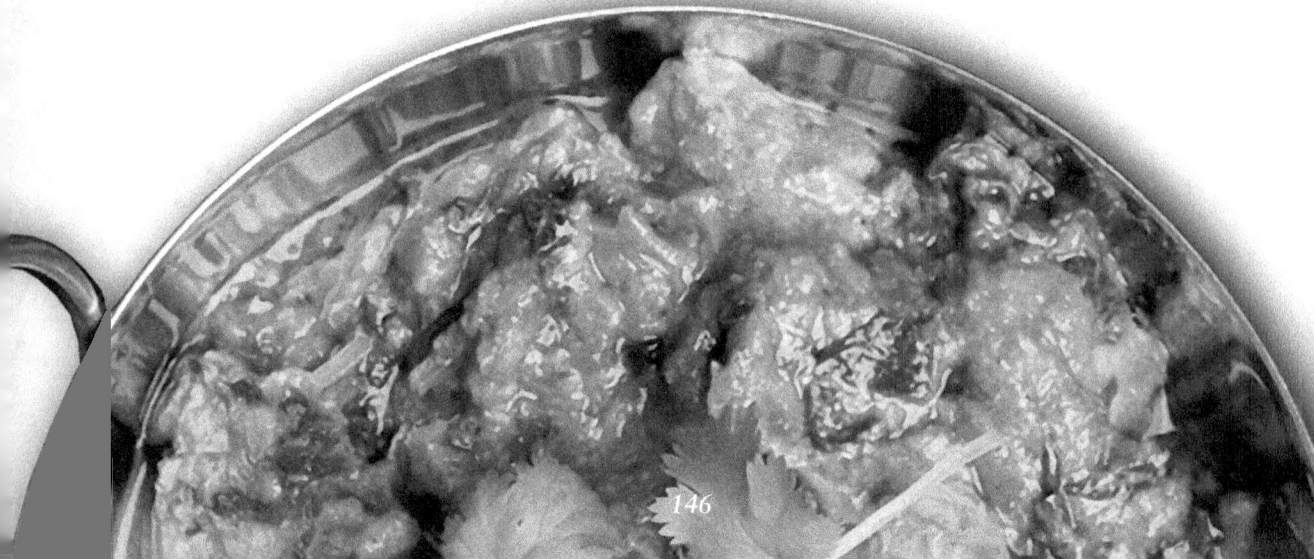

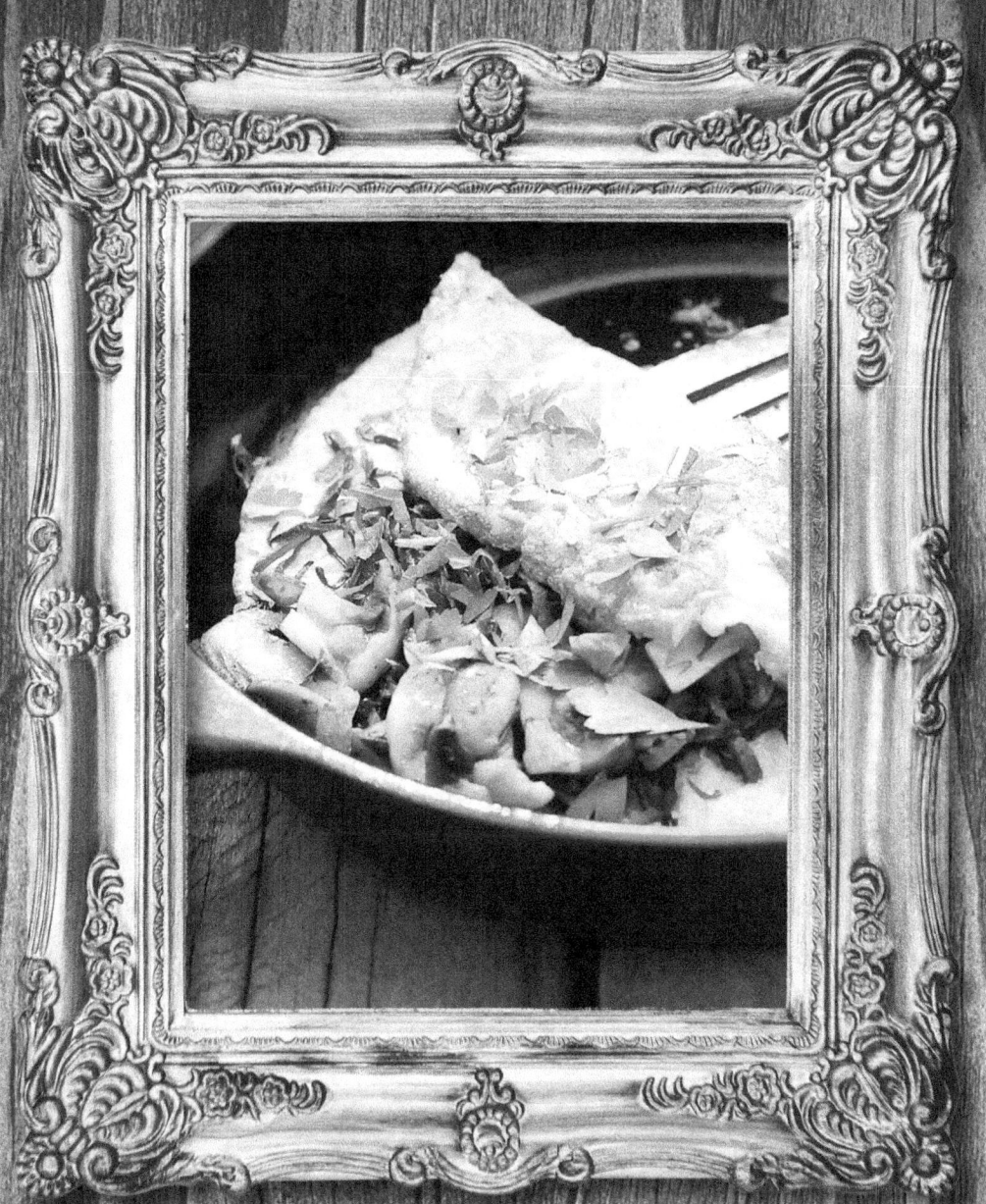

Eggs

Spanish Turnip Omelette

A Spanish Omelette is also known as a tortilla and is served flat and not folded in the pan. The various regions of Spain have different versions of this recipe with potatoes as one of the main ingredients. This recipe replaces the potato with turnips that are easier to use as they soften quicker and in my opinion are tastier than the traditional version.

Serves 2

Nutrition in Grams
per Serving

Protein - 23.80
Fat - 20.89
Carbs - 22.02
Fibre - 7.21
Kcals - 383.40
Sat - 4.59
Mono - 11.44
Poly - 2.11
Trans - 0.02
Omega 3 - 0.33
Omega 6 - 1.77

INGREDIENTS

4 large Eggs (300 g)

1 large Turnip (350 g), sliced

1 large Onion (265 g), peeled and finely chopped

25 g Chives, finely chopped

½ teaspoon (2½ g) Tarragon

2 large (200 g) Tomatoes, sliced

3 tablespoons (12 g) fresh Parsley, chopped

1 tablespoon (15 ml) Macadamia oil or Rapeseed oil for frying

Salt and freshly ground Black Pepper

Peel the turnip and chop them into 1 cm thick slices, then parboil them in water for about 10 minutes. Heat the oil and gently fry the onion and until they are soft and placed the boiled turnip slices evenly over the pan. Beat the eggs thoroughly in a small bowl and add the tarragon and chives. Pour the mixture over the turnip slices and onions and layer the sliced tomatoes all over the top. Allow the eggs to set on a low heat and the omelette to brown underneath, then either turn it over gently with a spatula or put the frying pan under the grill to cook the top. Slide the omelette on to a large plate and garnish with the parsley and serve immediately.

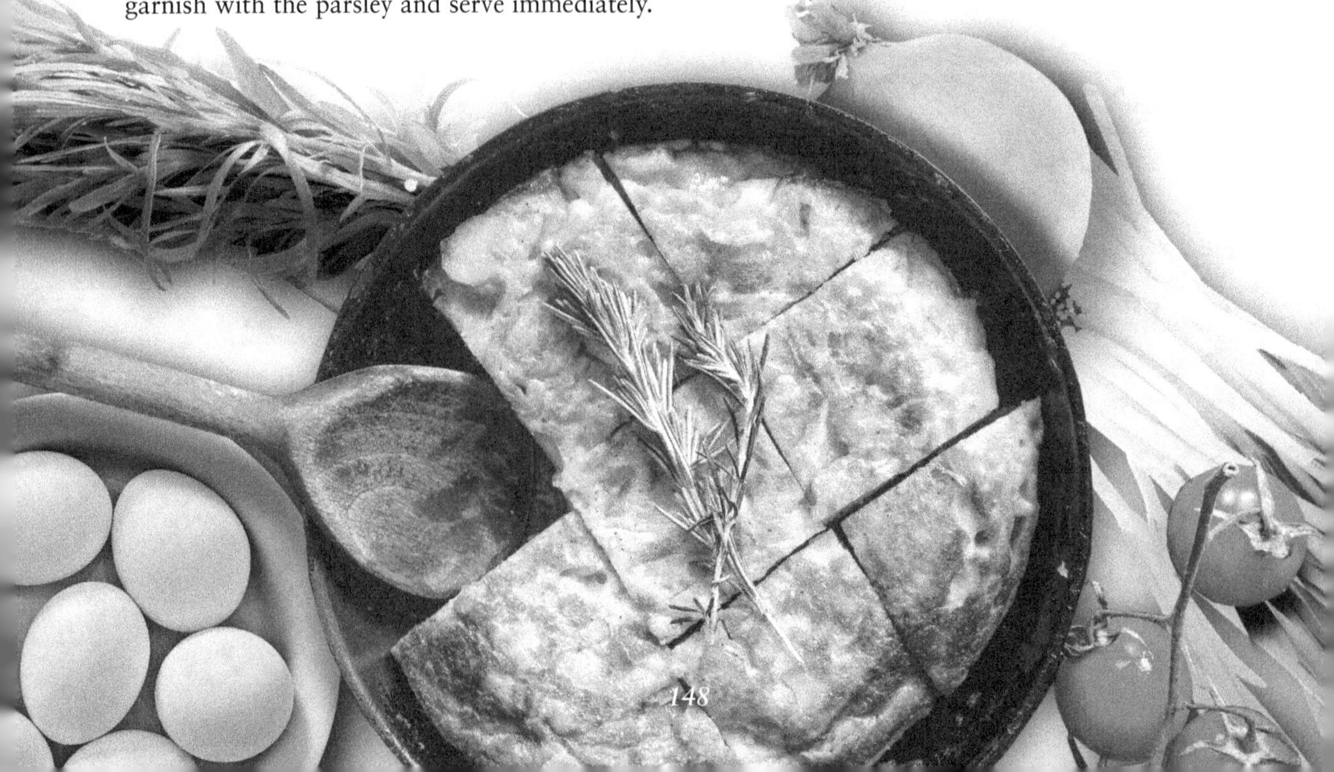

Mediterranean Eggs

Serves 3

INGREDIENTS

3 medium (195 g) Eggs
2 Garlic cloves (12 g), crushed
75 g Mushrooms, sliced
450 g Baby Spinach
1 x 400 g tin of chopped Tomatoes,
1 teaspoon (5 ml) Red hot sauce (such as Frank's Red Hot Original Cayenne Pepper Sauce)
1 teaspoon (5 g) ground Cumin
1 teaspoon (2 g) fresh Parsley, chopped
1 tablespoon (15 ml) Rapeseed oil or Macadamia oil for frying

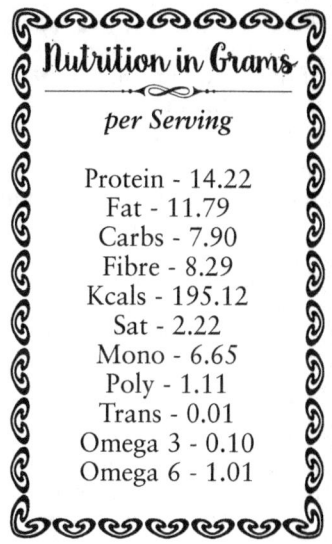

Nutrition in Grams
per Serving

Protein - 14.22
Fat - 11.79
Carbs - 7.90
Fibre - 8.29
Kcals - 195.12
Sat - 2.22
Mono - 6.65
Poly - 1.11
Trans - 0.01
Omega 3 - 0.10
Omega 6 - 1.01

Fry the onions and garlic in a little oil until soft. Add the mushrooms and cook for 3-5 minutes or until nicely browned. Then add the spinach, stir in the tomatoes, the hot sauce and cumin, simmer for 5 minutes. Make 3 holes in the mixture and crack the three eggs into the three holes. Add sea salt & pepper then cover and cook for 8 to 10 minutes or until the eggs reach your desired consistency. Top with fresh parsley.

Curried Eggs

These eggs are made with a curry powder you can mix yourself. As a rough guide, the strength and colour of curry comes from chilli powder, cayenne pepper, paprika and turmeric, and the flavour comes from ginger, cumin and coriander. Serve this dish with broccoli rice and a light green salad for a delicious meal.

Serves 3

INGREDIENTS

6 large Eggs (450 g)
4 small Onions (600 g), finely chopped
2 cloves Garlic (12 g), crushed
4 medium Tomatoes (360 g), skinned and chopped
2 teaspoons (10 g) ground Coriander
1 teaspoon (5 g) Turmeric
1 teaspoon (7½ g) fresh Ginger, grated
2 teaspoons (10 g) ground Cumin
½ teaspoons (2½ g) Cayenne Pepper
1 teaspoon Salt (5 g)
1 tablespoon (15 ml) Rapeseed oil or Macadamia oil

Nutrition in Grams
per Serving

Protein - 23.89
Fat - 19.92
Carbs - 22.85
Fibre - 7.38
Kcals - 372.33
Sat - 4.40
Mono - 10.57
Poly - 2.24
Trans - 0.02
Omega 3 - 0.23
Omega 6 - 1.99

Heat the oil gently in a frying pan and add the chopped onions and fry until soft and translucent. Bring a saucepan of water to the boil, turn off the heat and place the tomatoes into it and leave for a couple of minutes. This makes it easier to skin the tomatoes. Skin them and chop them into small pieces. Add them to the onions, followed by the garlic and spices and fry for a further 25-30 minutes over a low heat.

Meanwhile prepare the eggs. Put them in a pan of cold water, bring it to the boil and boil them for about 10 minutes. Then immediately crack the shell slightly and place them in cold water to prevent a dark ring forming around the yolk. Turn the heat down on the spicy onions and tomatoes. Shell the eggs, cut them in half, and place them on top of the sauce leave 5 minutes to warm the eggs through. Serve immediately.

Piperade

Piperade is a scrambled egg and vegetable dish that originated in the Basque region of France where the use of sweet red peppers is a culinary feature of their culture. This dish is delicious served with slices of toasted home-made low carb bread with garlic or herb butter, and a green salad.

Serves 4

INGREDIENTS

6 large Eggs (450 g)
1 large Onion (265 g), finely chopped
2 cloves Garlic (12 g), crushed
2 Green or Red Peppers (330 g), de-seeded and diced
4 large Tomatoes (400 g), roughly chopped
1 tablespoons (15 ml) Rapeseed oil or Macadamia oil
Salt and freshly ground black pepper
1 teaspoon (2 g) fresh Parsley, chopped

Nutrition in Grams

per Serving

Protein - 16.77
Fat - 13.75
Carbs - 11.05
Fibre - 4.06
Kcals - 239.50
Sat - 3.21
Mono - 7.02
Poly - 1.59
Trans - 0.01
Omega 3 - 0.16
Omega 6 - 1.34

Cook the onion and garlic for 5 minutes in the oil, then add the peppers and tomatoes and cook for a further 5 minutes. In a separate bowl beat the eggs, then pour these over the cooked vegetables and mix them in until they are lightly scrambled. Season to taste and serve garnished with parsley. Serve either hot or cold.

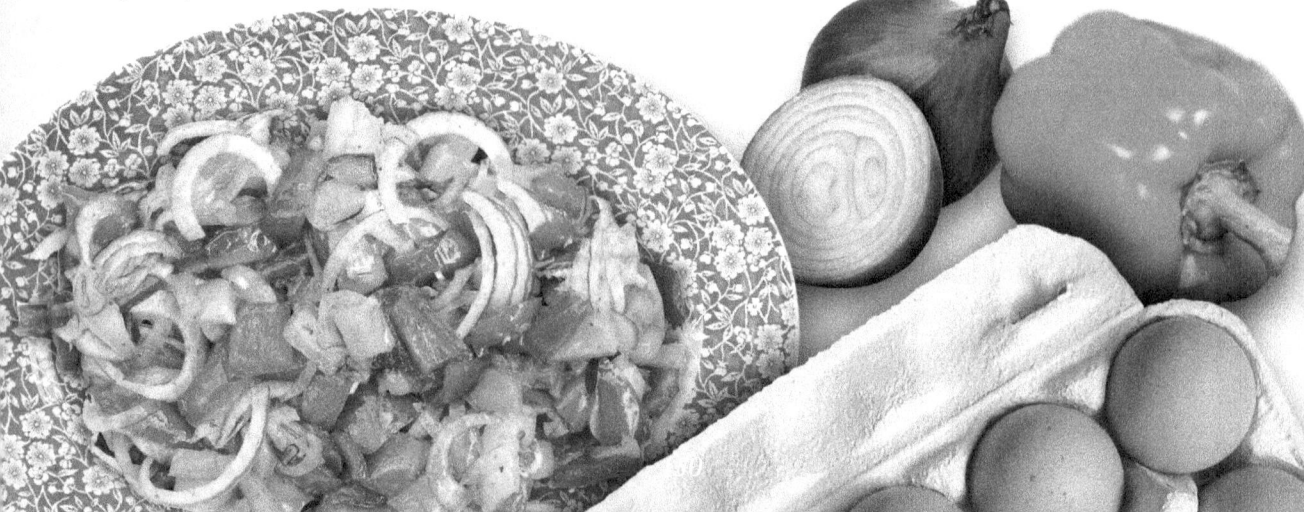

Eggs Primavera

In this recipe, sautéed mushrooms and crème fraiche add extra flavour to this baked egg dish. Serve it, with salads or a green vegetable for a light meal, or on its own as a starter.

Serves 4 ❶

Nutrition in Grams
per Serving

Protein - 10.82
Fat - 12.79
Carbs - 1.93
Fibre - 0.28
Kcals - 164.54
Sat - 5.06
Mono - 4.62
Poly - 1.49
Trans - 0.12
Omega 3 - 0.24
Omega 6 - 1.26

INGREDIENTS

4 large Eggs (300 g)

110 g Mushrooms, wiped and very finely chopped

25 g Low fat (light) Spreadable Butter with rapeseed or olive oil (or both)

70 ml half fat Crème Fraiche

Pre-heat the oven to gas mark 4, 350°F (180°C). Fry the mushrooms in the butter for 5 minutes. Divide the mixture between 4 individual ramekin dishes. Then break an egg into each dish and cover it with a tablespoon of half fat crème fraiche. Put the dishes on a tray in the oven and bake for 15-20 minutes, or until just set. Serve immediately.

Eggs Florentine

Spinach is a useful vegetable for combining with eggs or cheese in a variety of dishes. One of the best of these is Eggs Florentine where the eggs are served on a bed of spinach topped with cheese. The eggs can be poached first but I think it's easier to break them into nests formed from cooked spinach and finish off the dish in the oven. This is lovely when eaten with garlic bread (see page 60) and Classic Tomato Salad (see page 91)

Serves 4 ❷

INGREDIENTS

4 large Eggs (300 g)

900 g Spinach

100 ml half fat Crème Fraiche

Pinch of Nutmeg (1 g)

60 g Parmesan cheese, grated

Salt and freshly ground black pepper

Nutrition in Grams
per Serving

Protein - 19.82
Fat - 14.96
Carbs - 5.21
Fibre - 9.28
Kcals - 234.81
Sat - 6.55
Mono - 4.52
Poly - 1.20
Trans - 0.21
Omega 3 - 0.14
Omega 6 - 1.05

Pre-heat the oven to gas mark 6, 400°F (200°C). Wash the spinach several times, using fresh water each time. Then shake off all the excess water and put the spinach into a heavy bottomed pan. Cover and cook gently in its own liquid for 6-8 minutes until tender. Squeeze out as much moisture as you can and chop it finely. Return the spinach to the saucepan and add the half fat crème fraiche, salt, freshly ground black pepper and nutmeg. Stir this over a very gentle hear for 1 minute, then transfer to a lightly greased ovenproof dish and make 4 spaces for the eggs. Break the eggs into the spaces, then sprinkle the grated cheese on the top and bake the dish in the oven for 10-12 minutes until the eggs have set. Serve immediately.

Scotch Eggs

A Scotch egg consists of a hard-boiled egg wrapped in sausage meat, coated in bread crumbs and deep-fried. The London department store Fortnum & Mason claims to have invented Scotch eggs in 1738, but they may have been inspired by the Mughlai dish 'nargisi kofta' or Narcissus meatballs. The earliest printed recipe appears in the 1809 edition of Mrs. Rundell's 'A New System of Domestic Cookery' in which she served them hot, with gravy. This recipe uses minced pork (as sausage meat is cured) and is baked in the oven as opposed to deep frying them to keep the fats down.

Makes 4 eggs

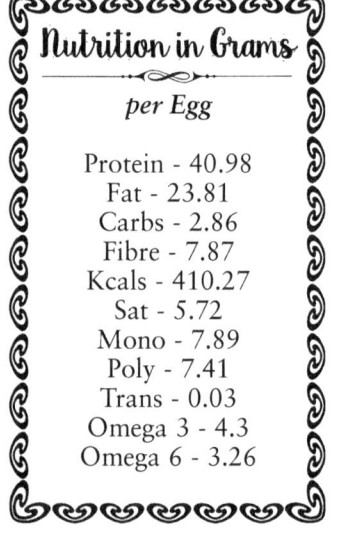

Nutrition in Grams

per Egg

Protein - 40.98
Fat - 23.81
Carbs - 2.86
Fibre - 7.87
Kcals - 410.27
Sat - 5.72
Mono - 7.89
Poly - 7.41
Trans - 0.03
Omega 3 - 4.3
Omega 6 - 3.26

INGREDIENTS

6 large Eggs (450 g)

400 g minced Pork

1 teaspoon Worcestershire Sauce (5 g) (see page 94)

1 teaspoon (5 g) Mustard Powder

1 teaspoon Mace, ground (5 g)

1 tablespoons fresh Parsley, finely chopped (15 g)

42 g Flaxseed, finely ground

100 g dried low carb Breadcrumbs (see page 58)

Have a large bowl of cold water ready. Put 4 of the eggs into a large saucepan of water and bring to the boil. Once boiling, simmer for 5 minutes. After 5 minutes, remove the eggs with a spoon and plunge them into the bowl of cold water. Prepare a baking tray with a sheet of baking paper over the surface.

In another bowl, put the minced pork, parsley, Worcestershire sauce, mustard powder and mace into a bowl with plenty of seasoning. Break one of the remaining eggs into the mixture and mix together thoroughly. Split the mixture into roughly 4 equal amounts and flatten each one into the size of your hand. Crack open the remaining egg into a bowl, beat with a fork, then sieve into a small bowl. Tip the flaxseed flour into another bowl and season well. Finally, tip the breadcrumbs into another bowl.

Preheat the oven to gas mark 5 - 190°C (275°F). When the eggs are cool, tap lightly on a hard surface to crack the shell and peel them. Place the egg onto the flattened meat and wrap the mince so that it covers the egg, smoothing out the joins and keeping the thickness over the egg consistent. Roll the eggs in the chia flour, shaking off any excess, then roll in the breadcrumbs and coat completely. Place the egg onto the baking tray and stick a cocktail stick through the egg at an angle pointing downwards to prevent it from rolling around.

Place the baking tray of eggs into the top half of the oven and cook for 25 minutes or until they are lightly browned.

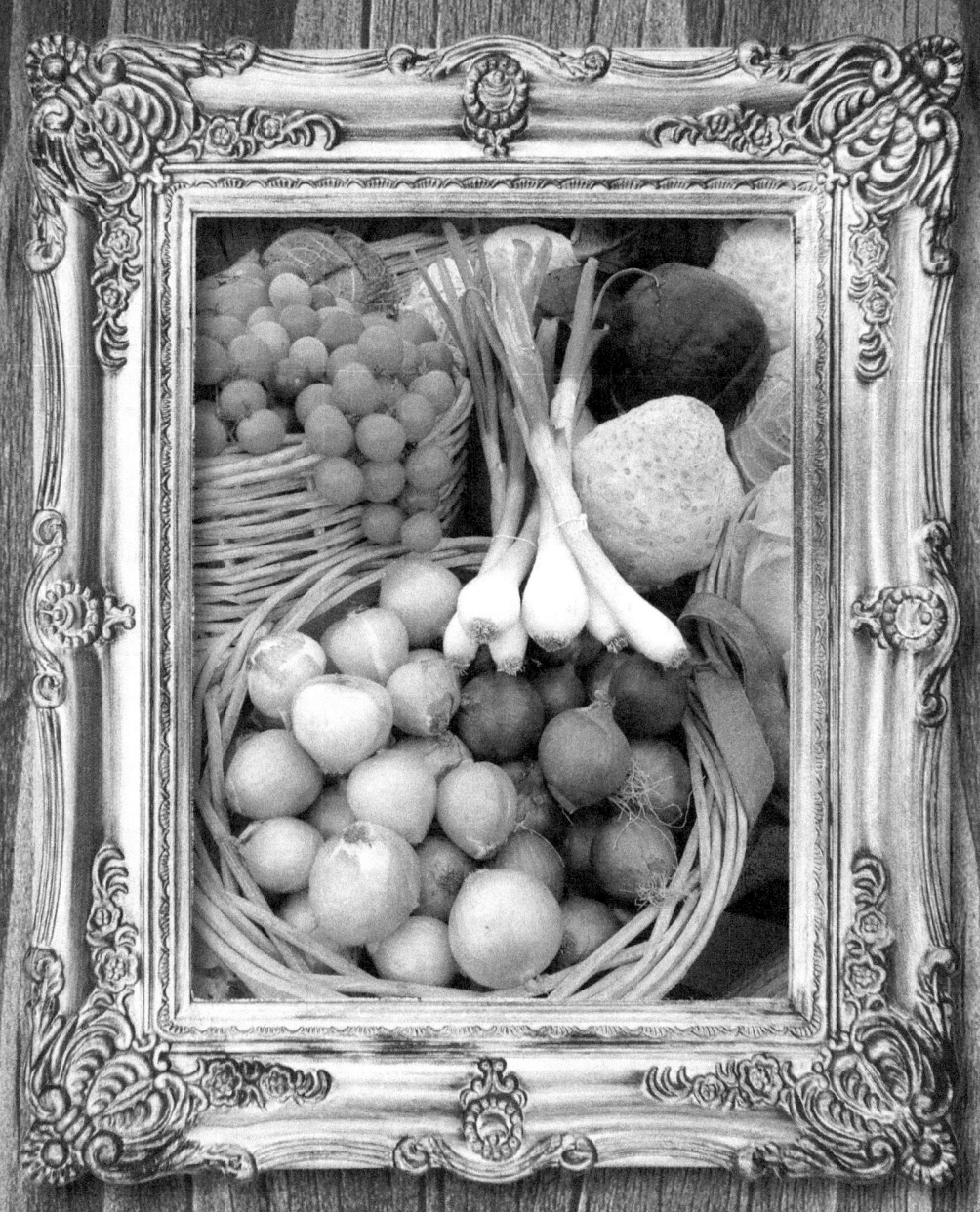

Accompanying Vegetables

Vegetable Preparation

Vegetable	Pre-Cook Preparation
Artichoke	Cut off the stalk and remove the hard outside leaves. Cut off about 2.5 cm from the outside leaves to make an opening in the centre top. Wash well and drain heads down.
Asparagus	Wash the sticks carefully, cutting off a little of the white base of the stalk.
Aubergine or Egg Plant	Wipe or wash. Peel if to be fried or sautéed.
Beans (French or Runner)	Wash and string the beans. French beans can be cooked whole. Runner beans are best cut into thin slices.
Beetroot	Wash carefully, taking care not to break the skin.
Broccoli	Cut off stalks and coarse outer leaves. Wash in cold water.
Brussel Sprouts	Wash and peel. Cut into pieces or finely dice.
Cabbage	Remove any discoloured outer leaves. Cut off the end of thick stalks. Wash in cold water.
Cabbage (Savoy or Red)	Remove discoloured outer leaves. Cut into quarters. Cut out the centre stalk. Wash or soak in cold water. Shred finely with a sharp knife.
Carrots	Scrape and slice length wise or chop into circles.
Cauliflower	Cut off the thick stalk and outer leaves. Soak for 15 minutes in cold salted water, then drain. Leave whole, in florets, or slice cutting across the stump.
Celery	Wash and scrub. Scrape outside leaves if necessary. Cut into short lengths as required.
Chicory	Cut off a thin slice from the base of each head, and remove the core. Wash in salt water.
Courgettes	Wash and cut lengthwise. Saute: Wash and remove top and bottom, then cut into slices.
Endive	Wash thoroughly, discarding the coarse outer leaves. Separate leaves from the root.
Leeks	Remove coarse outside leaves. Cut off tops and root. Wash thoroughly and split down the centre.
Marrow	Peel, cut in half and remove the seeds. Cut into even sized pieces.
Mushrooms	Cultivated mushrooms: Wipe with a damp cloth. Field mushrooms: Skin and washed thoroughly.
Onions	Peel. (can be done under cold water, to stop eyes watering)
Peas (Garden)	Shell and rinse in cold water.
Peppers (Green or Red)	Wash and wipe. Cut off stalk. Take out the hard stalk. To stuff, cut a hole in the middle.
Pumpkins	Cut in quarters, peel off skin and discard seeds. Slice thickly.
Sea Kale	Trim off the thick ends of the stalks and wash thoroughly.
Shallots	Peel as onions.
Spinach	Wash well, and remove coarse stalks.
Swede	Remove discoloured outer leaves and trim stalks. Cut a cross in bottom of each.
Tomatoes	Usually eaten with skin on, but to remove skin, dip in very hot water.
Turnips	Wash and peel. Cut into pieces or finely dice.

and Cooking Times

Cooking Method	Approx Cooking Time
Place heads downwards in enough boiling water to cover them. When cooked, the leaves can easily be removed.	30 to 45 minutes
Lie flat in a steamer or stand in a tall pan. Boil gently in water.	15 to 20 minutes
Bake: Parboil first if they are to be stuffed. Fry in slices dipped in flour or batter.	Parboil: 20 mins Bake: 30 mins Fry: 10 to 12 mins
Cook in boiling water.	10 to 15 minutes
Cook in boiling water until soft.	1 to 2 hours
Cook in boiling water.	10 to 15 minutes
Cook in boiling water.	10 to 15 minutes
Cook in a little fast boiling water.	10 to 12 minutes
Cook in a little fast boiling water.	10 to 15 minutes
Cook in boiling water.	15 to 20 minutes
Cook (stem down if whole) in boiling water.	Whole: 15 to 20 minutes Florets: 10 to 15 minutes
Cook in boiling water.	20 to 30 minutes
Cook in boiling water. Optionally, add the juice of half a lemon to the water.	30 minutes
Cook in boiling water. Saute: In garlic flavoured butter. Add a little black pepper.	10 to 15 mins Saute until golden
Although usually served shredded in a salad, it may be braised or stewed.	20 to 30 minutes
Cook in boiling water. Braise: Use in soups or stews.	Boil: 15 to 25 minutes Braise: 45 to 60 minutes
Cook in boiling water.	10 to 20 minutes
Fry: lightly in a little oil, turning to cook both sides. Grill: brush with oil and grill on each side.	2 to 3 minutes each side
Fry: slice and fry until golden brown. Boil: in water. Bake: in casserole in oven.	Fry: 5 to 8 mins Boil: 20 to 30 mins Bake: 40 mins
Cook in a little boiling water. A sprig of mint and a little sugar can be added.	10 to 15 minutes
Bake: boil first in water. Then stuff and bake. Salad: shred and serve.	Boil: 5 minutes, remove skins, stuff and bake for 30 minutes
Cook in boiling water.	30 minutes or until tender
Cook in boiling water.	30 minutes to 1 hour
Bake in casserole in oven. Cook in boiling water.	Bake: 30 mins Boil: 35 to 45 mins
Place in a pan with no water. Cook gently at first, stirring, then boil rapidly.	15 minutes
Cook in boiling water.	Young: 15 mins Old: 50 mins
Grill: cut in half, brush with a little oil and season. Bake: whole or in half.	Grill: 5 to 10 mins Bake: 15 to 20 mins
Cook in boiling water.	Young: 15 to 20 mins Old: 30 mins

Accompanying Vegetables

Ratatouille

The name Ratatouille comes from the French term 'touiller', which means 'to stir up'. Ratatouille originated in the area around Nice in southern France. It was originally a peasant dish, and was made in the summer season with fresh summer vegetables. The original recipe uses courgettes (zucchini), tomatoes, green and red peppers (bell peppers), onions, and garlic. The best Ratatouille is made when the vegetable flavours are well blended, and the vegetables are soft but not mushy. This can be served as a side vegetable with Mushroom flan (page 126) I also like to serve it cold, strongly flavoured with herbs, as a salad dish.

Serves 4

Nutrition in Grams
per Serving

Protein - 4.46
Fat - 4.46
Carbs - 15.12
Fibre - 7.23
Kcals - 130.46
Sat - 0.67
Mono - 3.04
Poly - 0.30
Trans - 0.00
Omega 3 - 0.05
Omega 6 - 0.16

INGREDIENTS

2 small Onions (300 g), peeled and finely chopped

2 cloves Garlic (12 g), crushed

2 small Aubergines (500 g), unpeeled and chopped into cubes

225 g Courgettes, washed and sliced

2 large Green or Red Peppers (330 g), de-seeded and diced

225 g Tomatoes, roughly chopped

1 tablespoon (15 g) Tomato Puree

1 tablespoon (15 ml) Macadamia oil or Rapeseed oil

Salt and freshly ground black pepper to taste

Heat the oil in a large saucepan and gently fry the onions and garlic for 5-7 minutes so they become translucent. Meanwhile prepare all the other vegetables and add them to the pan with the tomato puree. Cover and cook the whole mixture over a gentle heat for 30-35 minutes until the vegetables are soft but not mushy. Season to taste.

Serve immediately, or leave to cool and serve cold as a salad.

Spiced Cider Carrots

Carrots have the advantage of being both cheap and available most of the year round. In this dish their natural sweetness is complemented by the cider and an extra tang is given with the mustard and rosemary. Serve with Macadamia and Mushroom Roast (see page 106) or any meat roast and a side dish of Lemon Broccoli (see page 134) to spice up your side vegetables.

Serves 4

INGREDIENTS

450 g Carrots, scrubbed

15 g Spreadable butter cut with rapeseed or olive oil or both

75 ml Apple Cider

Accompanying Vegetables

Nutrition in Grams
per Serving

Protein - 1.20
Fat - 2.76
Carbs - 8.83
Fibre - 3.73
Kcals - 79.96
Sat - 1.10
Mono - 0.92
Poly - 0.46
Trans - 0.04
Omega 3 - 0.09
Omega 6 - 0.37

75 ml water
2 teaspoons (7 g) fresh chopped Rosemary or
1 teaspoon (5 g) dried Rosemary
1 teaspoon (5 g) Mustard powder

First chop the carrots into dice. Then melt the butter in a small saucepan, add the carrots and cook over a gentle heat, for 5 minutes. Pour in the cider and water. Add the rosemary &nd mustard, bring the liquid to the boil and then simmer in a covered par. for 10 minutes. Check half-way through the cooking time that there is enough liquid.

When the carrots are tender, put them in a warm serving dish and boil the remaining liquid until it is thick and syrupy. Pour this as a glaze over the top. Serve straight away.

Stuffed Courgettes

Courgette is the French word for a small marrow. Sometimes sold under their Italian name, Zucchini, they are good value during the summer months. A rich celery and tomato sauce is the basis of the filling for this dish and I like to serve it with Tomato Sauce (see page 67) and Cauliflower Rice (see page 136 without the spices).

Serves 4

INGREDIENTS

4 large (700 g) Courgettes
225 g Onions, peeled and finely chopped
1 clove Garlic (6 g), crushed
2 sticks Celery (80 g), washed and finely chopped
1 x 400 g tin of Tomatoes, drained
2 tablespoons (8 g) fresh parsley, finely chopped
100 g Extra Mature Cheddar Cheese, grated
3-4 tablespoons Vegetable stock or water
1 tablespoon (15 ml) Macadamia oil or Rapeseed oil
Salt and freshly ground black pepper

Nutrition in Grams
per Serving

Protein - 9.90
Fat - 13.07
Carbs - 12.86
Fibre - 4.32
Kcals - 214.96
Sat - 5.44
Mono - 5.41
Poly - 0.71
Trans - 0.23
Omega 3 - 0.16
Omega 6 - 0.53

Pre-heat the oven to gas mark 4, 350°F (180°C). First, prepare the courgettes. Wipe and blanch them for 5 minutes in boiling water. Then cut them in half lengthways, scoop out the flesh and chop it finely. Now prepare the onions and lightly fry them in the oil for 2 or 3 minutes. Add the garlic and fry for a further 2-3 minutes. Next add the celery and continue cooking the vegetables for about 5 minutes. Then add the tomatoes, parsley and chopped courgette flesh. Cook this mixture uncovered, stirring occasionally, until it has reduced to a thick rich sauce. (This takes about 20 minutes.) Season well. Let the mixture cool slightly and then pile it into the prepared courgette shells. Place the filled shells in a lightly greased ovenproof dish and sprinkle them with grated cheese. Pour in a Little stock or water, then bake for 20 minutes or until the shells are tender and the cheese on top is golden brown and bubbling. Serve straight away.

== *Accompanying Vegetables* ==

Turnip Paprika Goulash

This dish is warming to eat and to look at. Paprika comes from grinding sweet red peppers of which the Hungarian type is one of the most well known. Paprika is a powder made from grinding sweet red peppers and unlike other red pepper powders, such as cayenne and chilli, can be used liberally as it isn't hot. Paprika is the spice used in traditional Hungarian goulash, usually garnished with soured cream. This is great served with a green salad or you could use it without the yoghurt for a side dish.

Serves 4

INGREDIENTS

450 g Turnips, peeled and thinly sliced

450 g Leeks, cleaned and sliced thinly

350 g Mushrooms, wiped and quartered

½ teaspoon (2½ g) Paprika

Salt and freshly ground black pepper

1 tablespoon (15 ml) Rapeseed oil or Macadamia oil

Garnish

150 ml Thick Low fat Greek Yoghurt

Nutrition in Grams
per Serving

Protein - 6.17
Fat - 4.69
Carbs - 11.47
Fibre - 6.60
Kcals - 116.02
Sat - 0.58
Mono - 3.04
Poly - 0.30
Trans - 0
Omega 3 - 0.06
Omega 6 - 0.25

First prepare all the vegetables. Parboil the Turnips for 10 minutes, then drain, reserving the cooking liquid. Heat the oil in a frying pan and gently fry the leeks, mushrooms and paprika for 8-10 minutes in a covered pan over a low heat. Then add the parboiled Turnips and mix well very gently so as not to break up the vegetables too much. Continue cooking for 5 minutes, adding a little of the Turnip stock if necessary. Season to taste and serve the dish immediately, garnished with Greek Yoghurt.

Lemon Broccoli

Broccoli is a member of the cabbage family and is a close relation of the cauliflower. There is the purple-headed or 'purple sprouting' type and also the green-headed variety which is known as Calabrese. You can use either in this dish. The sauce has a subtle lemon tang and can be made just before the broccoli is cooked and kept warm over a pan of hot water.

Serves 4 as a side dish

INGREDIENTS

450 g Broccoli

40 g Low fat (light) Spreadable Butter with rapeseed or olive oil (or both)

1 teaspoon (5 g) flour

225 ml Milk

Accompanying Vegetables

2 large Egg yolks (100 g)

2 tablespoons (30 ml) Lemon juice

Salt and freshly ground black pepper

Garnish

Crushed Coriander seeds or coarsely ground Black Pepper

Prepare the broccoli by dividing it into even-sized heads or spears and trimming the base of each stalk. Split the thicker stalks to ensure even cooking. Melt 10 g of the butter cut with rapeseed in a pan, add the flour and cook this roux for 1-2 minutes. Add the milk gradually and bring the sauce to the boil, stirring continually. Then remove the pan from the heat. Beat the egg yolks in a small bowl and mix in a little of the sauce. Add this to the rest of the sauce, stirring well. Transfer the mixture to a double-boiler Return to the Heat and stir in the remaining butter and lemon juice. Heat the sauce gently until it begins to thicken. Season to taste.

Meanwhile steam or cook the broccoli in a very small amount of boiling salted water for about 5-7 minutes. When it is cooked, put it into a warm serving dish, pour the sauce over the top and garnish with a few crushed coriander seeds or coarsely ground black pepper. Serve straight away.

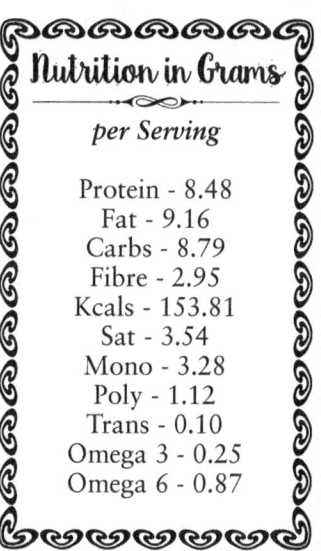

Nutrition in Grams

per Serving

Protein - 8.48
Fat - 9.16
Carbs - 8.79
Fibre - 2.95
Kcals - 153.81
Sat - 3.54
Mono - 3.28
Poly - 1.12
Trans - 0.10
Omega 3 - 0.25
Omega 6 - 0.87

White Turnip Rydan Celtic Mash

If you mash swede and vegetables together to serve as a side dish, you are making Stwnsh Rydan, a popular dish in North Wales. This is a delicious alternative to mashed potatoes as a tasty side dish for roasts and pies or as a topping for a shepherd's pie. It actually has more flavour than mashed potatoes and if mashed well has a creamy texture just like mashed potatoes, with less of the carbs.

Serves 1

INGREDIENTS

125 g Swede, chopped into small chunks

125 g Turnips, chopped into small chunks

15 g Low fat (light) Spreadable Butter with rapeseed or olive oil (or both)

40 ml semi-skimmed Milk

Salt and Pepper to taste

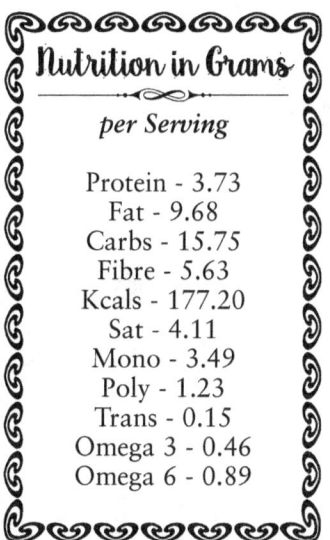

Nutrition in Grams

per Serving

Protein - 3.73
Fat - 9.68
Carbs - 15.75
Fibre - 5.63
Kcals - 177.20
Sat - 4.11
Mono - 3.49
Poly - 1.23
Trans - 0.15
Omega 3 - 0.46
Omega 6 - 0.89

Chop the swede into small chunks so that when you boil them they soften easier. Put them in a saucepan with plenty of water and boil them for 25 minutes, or until really soft. Meanwhile put the chopped turnip in a pan of water and boil them for 15 minutes, or until soft. Drain both vegetables thoroughly and put them both into a saucepan. Add the milk and butter and thoroughly mash until soft and creamy. Serve immediately.

Accompanying Vegetables

Spiced Shredded Green Cabbage

Green cabbage is a great low carb alternative to potatoes, pasta and rice and when fried in butter it tastes great as a side dish for your main meal. You can have it just plain for a roast or as in this recipe spice it up a little for a Curry or a Chilli.

Serves 4

INGREDIENTS

700 g Green Cabbage, shredded

40 g Low fat (light) Spreadable Butter with rapeseed or olive oil

1 teaspoon (5 g) medium Curry Powder (strength is dependent on your personal choice, so keep tasting until it suits your needs)

1 teaspoon (5 g) Cumin

A pinch of Saffron (½ g) - optional

Salt and pepper to taste

Nutrition in Grams per Serving

Protein - 3.6
Fat - 7.57
Carbs - 6.55
Fibre - 8.5
Kcals - 128.68
Sat - 2.77
Mono - 3.19
Poly - 1.1
Trans - 0.1
Omega 3 - 0.22
Omega 6 - 0.88

Shred the cabbage into thin 1 inch long pieces. Melt the Sunflower spread in a frying pan. Place the Cabbage in the pan and sprinkle over the spices. Cook the shredded cabbage on medium heat, stirring continuously, for 15 minutes or until the cabbage softens and is good to taste. Add Salt and pepper to taste.

If using with a chilli add ½ tsp of Chilli powder at the beginning and after a few minutes taste to see if it is hot enough for your taste. Add more if needed. If using as an accompanying vegetable for a roast, add ½ teaspoon of Thyme at the beginning.

Spiced Cauliflower or Broccoli Rice

This is a great alternative to rice in curry or chilli dishes. The Cauliflower works best for look or taste but Broccoli has lower carbs. Although it is fiddly to make (unless you have a food processor), your effort will be rewarded. You can omit the spices for other rice dishes.

Serves 4

INGREDIENTS

450 g Cauliflower or Broccoli cut into individual florets

1 small Onion (150 g), very finely chopped

1 Garlic clove (6 g), crushed

1 teaspoon (5 g) ground Turmeric

1 teaspoon (5 g) ground Coriander

1 tablespoon (15 ml) Macadamia oil or Rapeseed oil

First, the fiddly bit, unless you're using a food processor. Holding the stalk end of the Cauliflower or Broccoli floret (I advise wearing some gloves to protect from grating your fingers) grate the heads of the florets on the smallest setting on your grater. If you have no protection stop grating when you reach the top of the stalk, you really only want the flowery heads of the florets anyway. If you use a food processor, use the grating blade if you have one or if you only have the standard blade, only process for about 20 seconds or until the cauliflower or broccoli becomes rice-like otherwise you are in danger of producing a vegetable pulp.

Pour a little Sunflower Oil into a large frying pan and add the finely chopped Onions and crushed Garlic and fry on a gentle heat, stirring continually, until the Onions are translucent. Add the spices and fry gently for about 5 minutes, mixing thoroughly.

Add the grated Cauliflower or Broccoli and mix well. Fry on a low heat for around 10 minutes, continually stirring the mixture so that it doesn't burn. The best thing is to keep tasting the rice until the vegetable has slightly softened and becomes palatable. Delicious, served with a Curry or a Chilli.

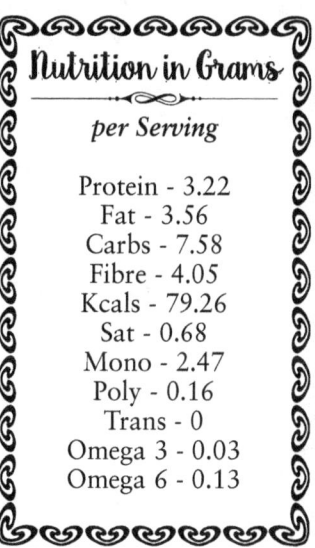

Nutrition in Grams
per Serving

Protein - 3.22
Fat - 3.56
Carbs - 7.58
Fibre - 4.05
Kcals - 79.26
Sat - 0.68
Mono - 2.47
Poly - 0.16
Trans - 0
Omega 3 - 0.03
Omega 6 - 0.13

Swede or Turnip Paprika Chips

The great low carb alternative to chips or French fries with the zing of smoked Paprika.

Serves 1

INGREDIENTS
175 g Swede or Turnips, chopped into chips
1 teaspoon (5 g) smoked Paprika
1 tablespoon (15 ml) Rapeseed oil or Macadamia oil

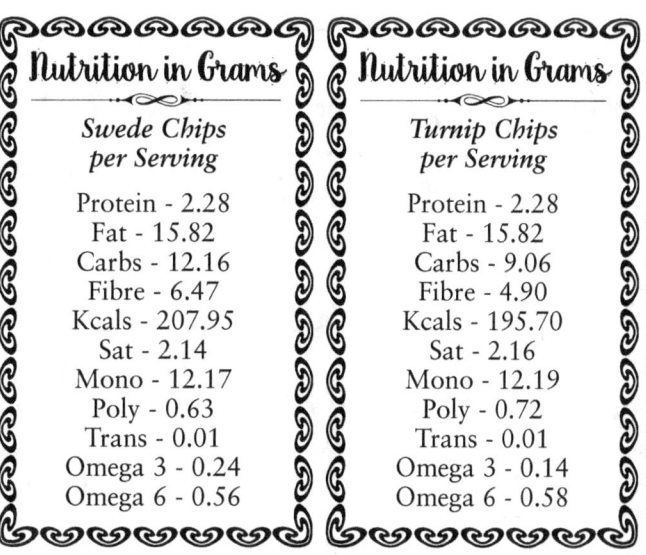

Nutrition in Grams
Swede Chips per Serving

Protein - 2.28
Fat - 15.82
Carbs - 12.16
Fibre - 6.47
Kcals - 207.95
Sat - 2.14
Mono - 12.17
Poly - 0.63
Trans - 0.01
Omega 3 - 0.24
Omega 6 - 0.56

Nutrition in Grams
Turnip Chips per Serving

Protein - 2.28
Fat - 15.82
Carbs - 9.06
Fibre - 4.90
Kcals - 195.70
Sat - 2.16
Mono - 12.19
Poly - 0.72
Trans - 0.01
Omega 3 - 0.14
Omega 6 - 0.58

Swede - Put the chipped swede into a saucepan of boiling water and boil for 10 minutes. Drain and add the oil to the pan and shake so that the oil covers the chips completely. Sprinkle the paprika over the chips and again shake so that the paprika covers the chips. Pour on to a frying pan and using a fork, separate all the chips and fry on a medium heat. Keep turning the chips until they are browned all over. Serve hot.

Turnip - The turnip is a softer and more fragile vegetable to the swede, so there is no need to boil them before you fry them. Just cut them into chips and place them in a saucepan and add the oil and shake the pan until the chips are covered in the oil, add the paprika and likewise shake the pan until the chips are covered in the spice. Pour on to a frying pan and using a fork, separate all the chips and fry on a medium heat. Keep turning the chips until they are browned all over. Serve hot.

Accompanying Vegetables

Salt & Vinegar Courgette Crisps

A delicious alternative to potato crisps as a snack or even as a side dish with a Tomato Sauce (see page 91),

Serves 1

INGREDIENTS

1 Courgettes, thinly sliced (175 g)

1 tablespoon (15 ml) Rapeseed oil or Macadamia oil

Salt

Sprinkle of Malt Vinegar (10 ml)

Nutrition in Grams
per Serving

Protein - 2.13
Fat - 15.56
Carbs - 3.69
Fibre - 1.75
Kcals - 164.75
Sat - 2.18
Mono - 12.11
Poly - 0.40
Trans - 0.01
Omega 3 - 0.15
Omega 6 - 0.25

Preheat the oven to 250°F (120°C). Slice the courgettes into crisp thick slices (about 2-3 mm). Place the slices on a large board and carefully salt each one. Leave to stand for about 10 minutes. Brush or spray the oil onto the courgette slices. Place the slices on a slightly oiled baking tray.

Put the baking tray in the centre of the oven and cook until they have dried out and crisped up. Check them after half an hour and lower the heat to 150°F (75°C) or lower and continue to dry. Keep checking every 10 minutes to make sure they don't burn, as they will taste bitter. They may take up to an hour to fully dry out and become crispy. Remove the crisps from the oven when they are dry drizzle a little malt vinegar on each. Let them cool, ideally on a rack. You can eat them as they are, or serve with a salsa dip, mayonnaise or tomato sauce.

Creamed Green Cabbage

A rich and creamy side dish with a fresh flavour of lemon zest, garlic and parsley.

Serves 4

Nutrition in Grams
per Serving

Protein - 5.54
Fat - 7.06
Carbs - 10.23
Fibre - 5.63
Kcals - 138.75
Sat - 3.13
Mono - 2.55
Poly - 0.85
Trans - 0.12
Omega 3 - 0.20
Omega 6 - 0.65

INGREDIENTS

700 g Green Cabbage, shredded into bite-size chunks

40 g Low fat (light) Spreadable Butter with rapeseed or olive oil (or both)

150 g Thick Low fat Greek Yoghurt

30 g fresh parsley, finely chopped

The zest of a half a Lemon (7½ g)

2 cloves Garlic, crushed (12 g)

Salt and pepper to taste

Melt the butter in a frying pan on medium heat and add the shredded green cabbage, sprinkle a clove of the crushed garlic over the cabbage and sauté for a few minutes until golden brown. Add the yoghurt and cook on a low heat. Do not bowl. Lower the heat towards the end. Season to taste. Mix together the remaining garlic, the parsley and the lemon zest in a small bowl and add to the cabbage just before serving.

Accompanying Vegetables

Mushroom Pâté

Once made, this pâté will keep for several days in the fridge.

Serves 6

INGREDIENTS

1.4 kg Mushrooms, very finely chopped
2 large Onions (530 g), finely chopped
4 Garlic cloves (24 g), finely chopped
125 ml White Wine
2 tablespoons dried Parsley (8 g)
A pinch of dried Thyme (1 g)
A pinch of Nutmeg (1 g)
1 tablespoon (15 ml) of Macadamia oil or Rapeseed oil
Salt and black pepper
6 slices of Toasted Low carb Bread (see page 58)

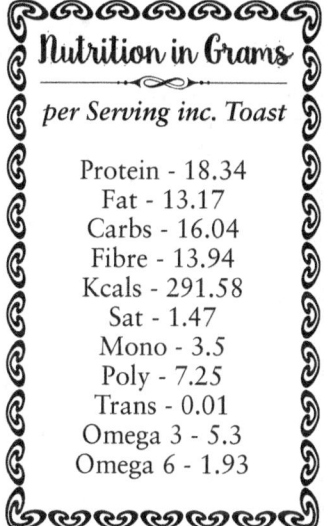

Nutrition in Grams
per Serving inc. Toast

Protein - 18.34
Fat - 13.17
Carbs - 16.04
Fibre - 13.94
Kcals - 291.58
Sat - 1.47
Mono - 3.5
Poly - 7.25
Trans - 0.01
Omega 3 - 5.3
Omega 6 - 1.93

Put the oil in a frying pan and fry the onions and garlic until soft. Add the mushrooms, stir, add the wine, season, and cook until very soft. Drain the liquor from the mushrooms, reserving the mushrooms and onions, into another pan, and then reduce this liquid to a thick syrupy texture.

Pass the mushrooms through a food mill or chop finely, then add back to the thick liquor. Add the herbs and nutmeg. The consistency should be firm. Taste and adjust seasoning if necessary. Serve on low carb toast.

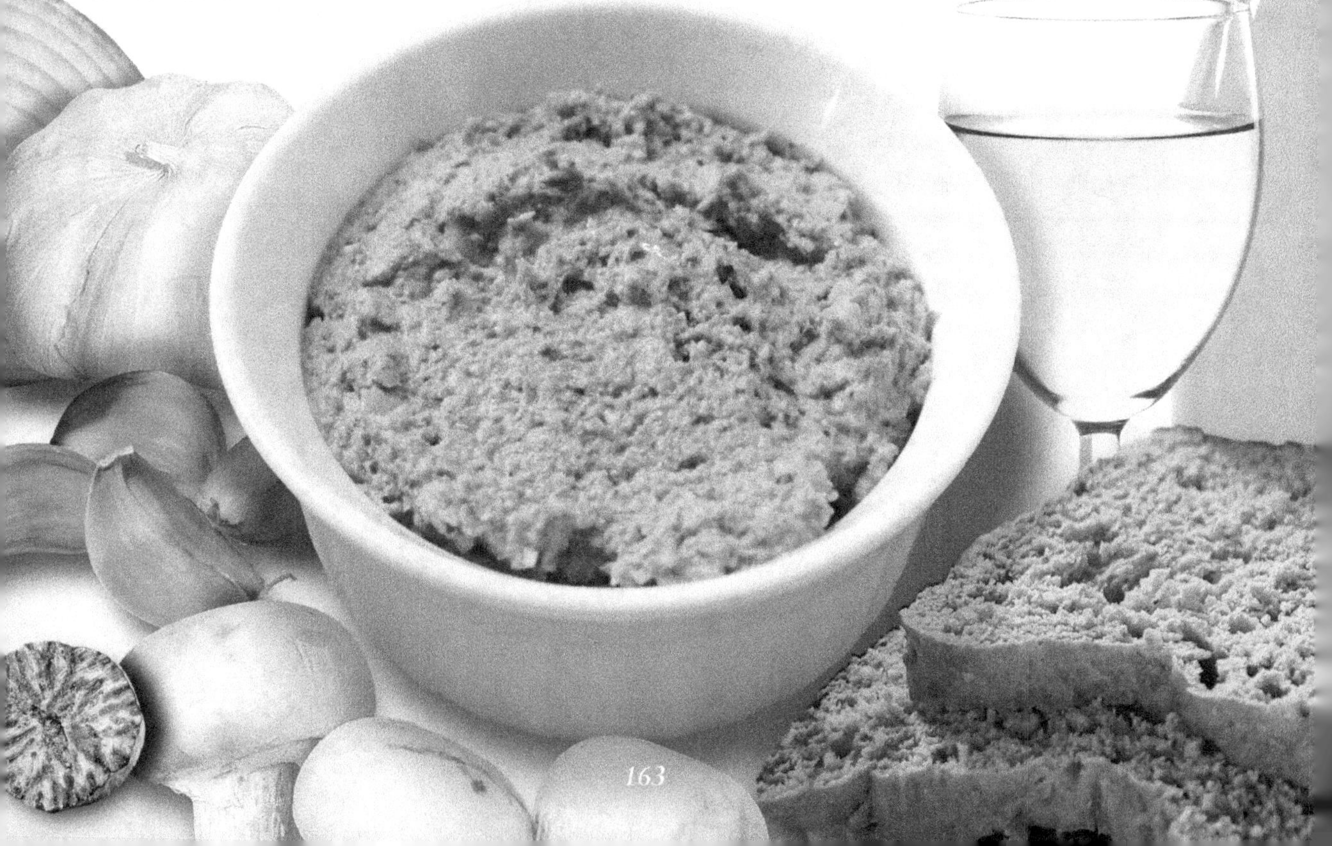

Accompanying Vegetables

Stuffed Artichoke Tomatoes

This stuffed tomato dish with its light filling makes a delicious starter, or side salad. The combination of eggs, artichoke hearts and mushrooms mixed with fresh herbs and a little wine vinegar is delicious, and a dab of cream cheese on the top of the tomatoes not only secures the lid, but also adds a rich finish.

Serves 4

INGREDIENTS

1 large Egg (75 g), hard boiled

50 g Mushrooms, wiped and sliced

10 g Low fat (light) Spreadable Butter with rapeseed or olive oil (or both)

2 Artichoke Hearts (100 g), tinned

½ tablespoon fresh Parsley (2 g), finely chopped

1 tablespoon (5 ml) White Wine Vinegar

8 medium Tomatoes (720 g)

25 g half fat Cream Cheese

Salt and freshly ground Black Pepper

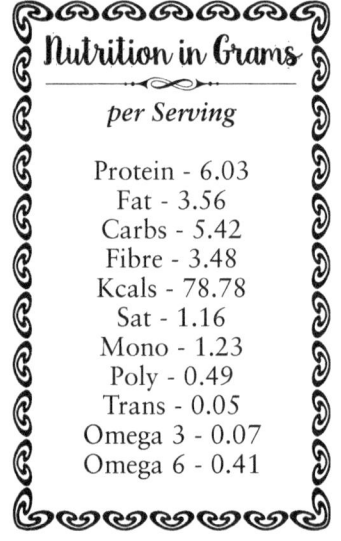

Nutrition in Grams

per Serving

Protein - 6.03
Fat - 3.56
Carbs - 5.42
Fibre - 3.48
Kcals - 78.78
Sat - 1.16
Mono - 1.23
Poly - 0.49
Trans - 0.05
Omega 3 - 0.07
Omega 6 - 0.41

First boil the egg. Remember that when eggs are hard-boiled, they must be cracked and put straight away into cold water after they are cooked to prevent a dark ring forming between the yolk and the white. Next fry the mushrooms in the melted butter until they are just soft. Finely chop the artichoke hearts, parsley, egg and sautéed mushrooms, and put all the ingredients into a bowl. Season thoroughly and mix in up to 1 tablespoon of white wine vinegar. Slice the bottoms off the tomatoes.

Reserve the bottoms for lids. Scoop out the centres of the tomatoes, keeping the flesh and seeds for a sauce or stock. Then season the insides of the tomatoes with the salt and pepper and fill them with the vegetable and egg mixture. Dab a little cream cheese on the top of each one and replace the lids. Serve chilled.

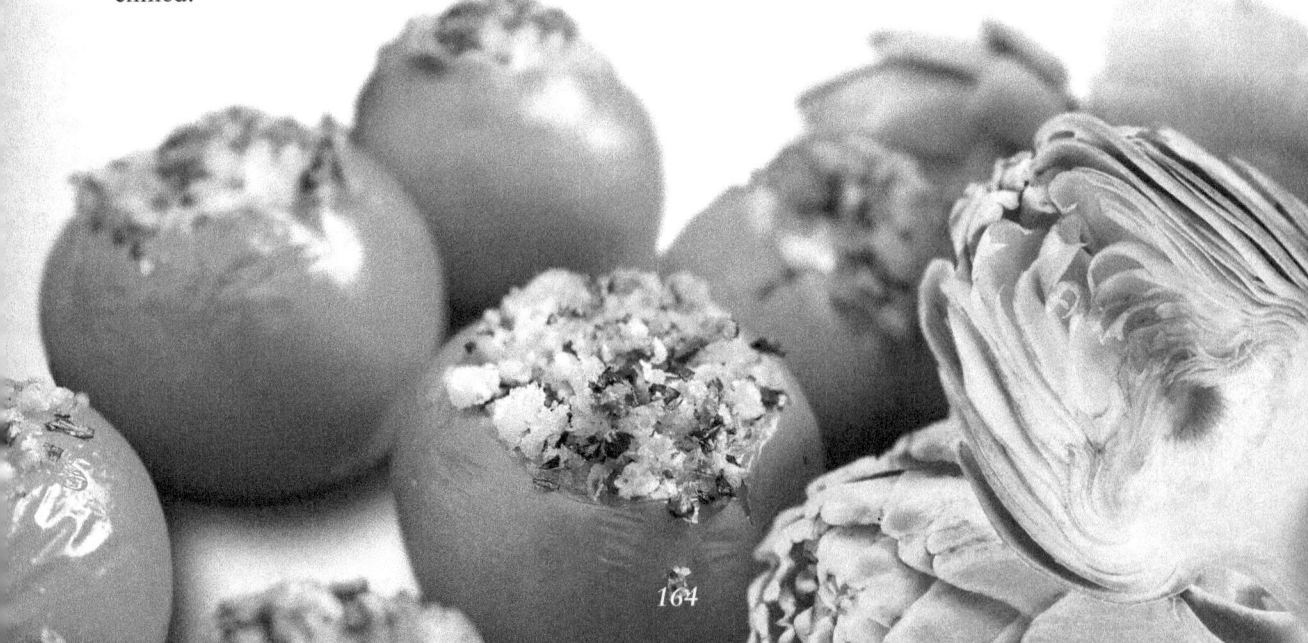

Accompanying Vegetables

Onion Rings

Make your own low carb onion rings in the oven. They go great with a burger or as a side dish.

Serves 4

INGREDIENTS

1 large Onion, (265 g)

1 medium Egg (65 g)

60 g Flaxseeds, ground

60 g white Chia seeds, ground

60 g grated Parmesan cheese

1 teaspoon (5 g) Garlic powder

½ tablespoon (2½ g) Chilli powder or Paprika

1 pinch Salt

1 tablespoon (15 ml) Macadamia oil or Rapeseed oil

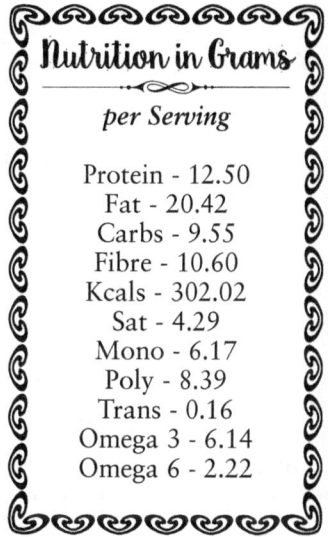

Nutrition in Grams

per Serving

Protein - 12.50
Fat - 20.42
Carbs - 9.55
Fibre - 10.60
Kcals - 302.02
Sat - 4.29
Mono - 6.17
Poly - 8.39
Trans - 0.16
Omega 3 - 6.14
Omega 6 - 2.22

Preheat the oven to gas mark 6 - 400°F (200°C). Peel the onion and slice into rings, about 5 mm thick. To make the flour, mix the ground flax seeds, ground white chia seeds, garlic powder, chilli powder or paprika, salt and parmesan cheese in a bowl. Crack the egg into another bowl and whisk thoroughly. Lightly oil a baking tray. One by one, immerse the onion rings into the egg mix and then into the flour mix, making sure they are completely covered by the flour. Place the rings on the baking tray and either drip or spray a little onto them and bake in the oven for 15–20 minutes, using the oven's grill setting. They're done when they are golden brown and crisp.

Stuffed Peppers

Peppers seem to have been specifically designed to hold a savoury stuffing and they are very easy to prepare. This recipe with its cauliflower rice, mushroom filling and rich tomato sauce is a complete meal on its own.

Serves 4

INGREDIENTS

170 g Cauliflower

275 ml pint water

For the sauce

4 Green Peppers (660 g)

2 medium Onions (400 g), peeled and finely chopped

2 cloves Garlic (12 g), crushed

2 x 400 g tins of Tomatoes

4 tablespoons (60 g) Tomato Puree

Nutrition in Grams

per Serving

Protein - 7.42
Fat - 8.91
Carbs - 29.27
Fibre - 10.18
Kcals - 243.36
Sat - 1.36
Mono - 6.08
Poly - 0.77
Trans - 0
Omega 3 - 0.04
Omega 6 - 0.55

Accompanying Vegetables

Salt and freshly ground black pepper to taste
1 tablespoon (15 ml) Macadamia oil or Rapeseed oil

For the stuffing
1 tablespoon (15 ml) Macadamia oil or Rapeseed oil
1 large Onion (265 g), peeled and finely chopped
110 g button Mushrooms, wiped and sliced
2 teaspoons (8 g) fresh chopped Thyme or 1 teaspoon (5 g) dried Thyme
1 teaspoon (6 ml) Soy Sauce

Pre-heat the oven to gas mark 4 - 160°C (320°F). For the cauliflower, we are basically doing the same that we did for the Cauliflower rice (see page 136, without the spices), except we won't be frying it. Holding the stalk end of the cauliflower, grate the heads of the florets on the smallest setting on your grater. To protect from grating your fingers, stop grating when you reach the top of the stalk, you really only want the flowery heads of the florets anyway. Grate 170 g of the cauliflower, rather than weighing it before you grate it as you will have some left over, unless of course you have grated your fingers. Pour the rice into a saucepan and cover with water, bring to the boil and simmer for about 5 minutes.

Now prepare the sauce. Fry the finely chopped onion and crushed garlic in the Rapeseed oil or Macadamia oil for about 5 minutes. Add the tomatoes and tomato puree and simmer this for about 30 minutes in a covered pan while the cauliflower rice is cooking. Season well.

Meanwhile prepare the peppers. Slice off the tops (reserving them for lids) and de-seed them carefully, then blanch in boiling water for 5 minutes. Heat 1 tablespoon of oil in a frying-pan and gently fry the onion for a few minutes. Add the sliced mushrooms and thyme and cook on a low heat for a few minutes. When the Cauliflower is cooked, drain away any excess water and mix with the fried onions and mushrooms. Season well with salt, freshly ground black pepper and a little soy sauce. Then fill each pepper with some of the mixture, and replace the lids.

Stand the filled peppers in a lightly oiled, deep ovenproof dish and pour the tomato sauce round the peppers. Cover the dish with foil or a matching lid and bake the peppers for 30 minutes until they are tender but not limp. Serve immediately.

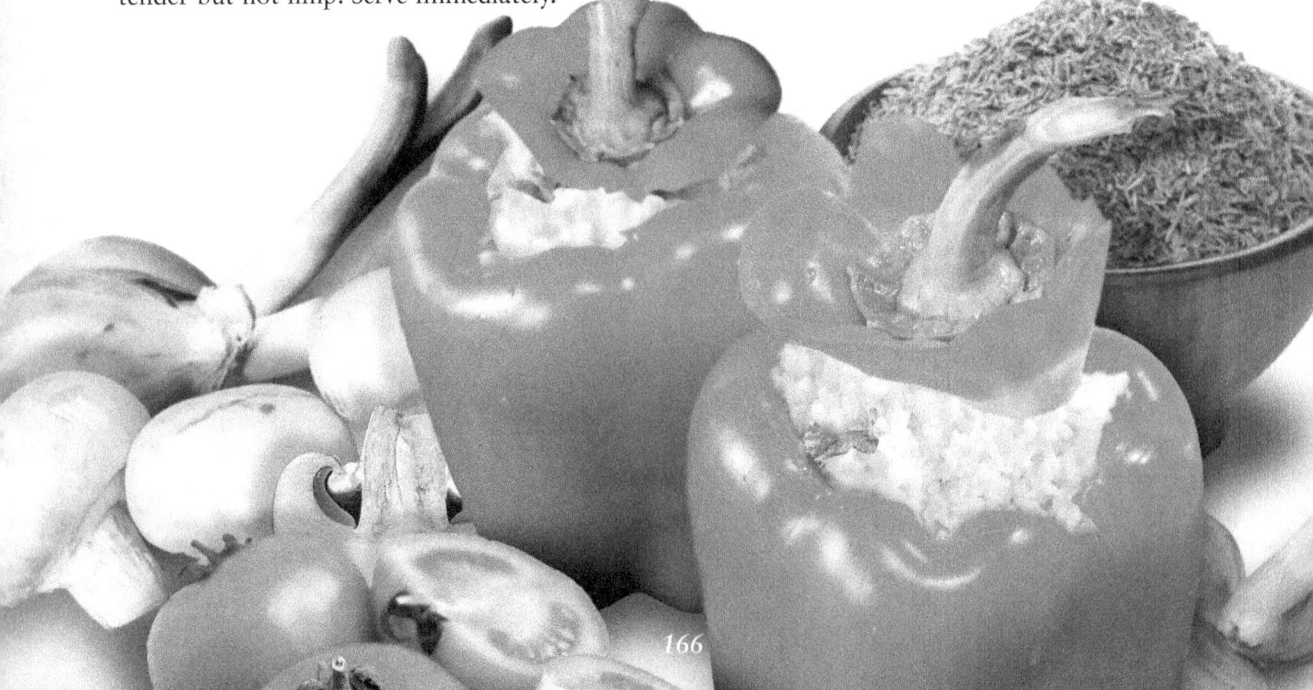

Accompanying Vegetables

Leek & Mushroom Gratin

The flavours of leeks and wine blend together especially well in this supper dish which could be served as a side dish or as a main course if accompanied by steamed vegetables.

Serves 4

INGREDIENTS

460 g Leeks, cleaned, trimmed and sliced
110 g Mushrooms, wiped and sliced
1 tablespoon (15 ml) Macadamia oil or Rapeseed oil
275 ml Vegetable stock or water
1 Bay leaf (0.3 g)
1 tablespoon (4 g) fresh Parsley
Juice of 1 Lemon (50 ml)
80 g Extra Mature Cheddar cheese, grated
150 ml Semi-skimmed Milk
3 tablespoons (35 ml) White Wine
55 g fresh low carb Breadcrumbs
1 teaspoon (5 ml) Macadamia oil or Rapeseed oil
Salt and freshly ground black pepper

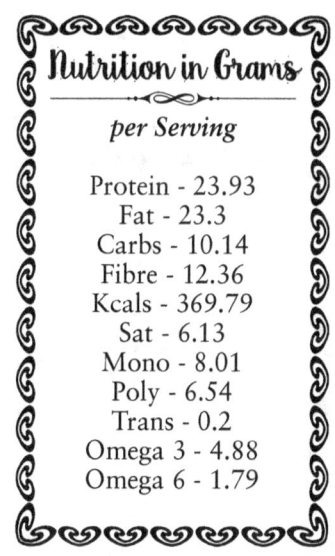

Nutrition in Grams

per Serving

Protein - 23.93
Fat - 23.3
Carbs - 10.14
Fibre - 12.36
Kcals - 369.79
Sat - 6.13
Mono - 8.01
Poly - 6.54
Trans - 0.2
Omega 3 - 4.88
Omega 6 - 1.79

Pre-heat the oven to gas mark 6 - 200°C (400°F). First prepare the vegetables. Then heat the oil in a small saucepan and fry the vegetables very lightly to seal in the flavour. Pour in the stock or water, bay leaf and lemon juice and cook this uncovered for about 10 minutes. Then lift the vegetables from the pan with a slotted spoon and transfer to a lightly greased ovenproof dish. Boil up the remaining liquid and reduce it until you are left with ¼ pint (150 ml). Next, sprinkle half the cheese over the leeks and mushrooms in the ovenproof dish. Mix together the reduced stock with the cream and wine and season to taste. Pour this mixture over the vegetables. Mix the remaining cheese and breadcrumbs with a teaspoon of oil and sprinkle this over the top of the vegetables to form a crunchy topping. Bake this dish for 15-20 minutes until the top is brown and crispy.

Cauliflower Mash

Serves 4

INGREDIENTS

450 g Cauliflower
100 g grated Parmesan cheese
½ lemon juice and zest (30 ml)
Salt and freshly ground pepper to taste

Cut the cauliflower into florets. Boil the cauliflower in plenty of lightly salted water for about 5 minutes, just enough to retain a fairly firm texture. Pour into a colander and leave until all the water has drained off. Put the cauliflower back in the saucepan and add the Parmesan cheese. Grate the zest of the lemon onto a saucer (just the yellow skin, not the white pulp underneath). Add this and the lemon juice to the Cauliflower and mash thoroughly. Season to taste.

The Ultimate Mash

Serves 1

INGREDIENTS

50 g Swede, chopped into small chunks

50 g Turnips, chopped into small chunks

1 Carrot (40 g), sliced

40 g Brussel Sprouts, halved

10 g Low fat (light) Spreadable Butter with rapeseed or olive oil (or both)

20 ml semi-skimmed Milk

Salt and Pepper to taste

Nutrition in Grams per Serving

Protein - 3.63
Fat - 7.14
Carbs - 10.92
Fibre - 5.59
Kcals - 134.40
Sat - 3.10
Mono - 2.45
Poly - 0.96
Trans - 0.12
Omega 3 - 0.32
Omega 6 - 0.69

Nutrition in Grams per Serving

Protein - 9.34
Fat - 7.29
Carbs - 7.00
Fibre - 2.46
Kcals - 134.85
Sat - 4.00
Mono - 1.82
Poly - 0.39
Trans - 0.22
Omega 3 - 0.04
Omega 6 - 0.33

This mash, with its combination of colours and flavours produces a beautiful, rich mash that can be used as a side dish or an alternative topping to a shepherd's pie. In plenty of water boil the small chunks of swede on their own as they take longer to soften. Boil the turnips and carrot together. The swedes will take about 25 minutes to be soft enough to mash, while the turnip and carrot will take about 15 minutes. I like to boil and mash the sprouts separately as their colour looks great when stirred with the other mashed vegetables at the end. The sprouts will also take about 15 minutes to soften. For the spinach, just put it into a colander and pour boiling water over it, this enough for it to shrink so you can add it to the mash. When soft drain the vegetables thoroughly (ideally using a colander) and put the spinach, swede, turnip and carrot back in a saucepan, add the milk and 10 g of the butter and mash together, making sure you get all the lumps. Drain the sprouts and put them in another saucepan, add the remaining butter and mash thoroughly. Finally season both to taste and stir the sprouts into the other vegetables and serve.

Pickled Onions

Makes 2 x 500 ml jars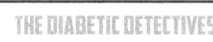

INGREDIENTS

300 ml Malt Vinegar

200 ml Apple Cider Vinegar

500 g small pickling Onions (approximately 24 onions)

25 g table Salt

1 teaspoon (5 g) Stevia

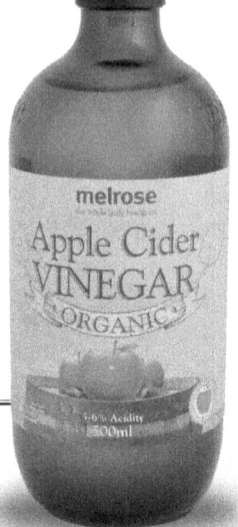

Accompanying Vegetables

10 Peppercorns (2 g)
2 teaspoons (10 g) Mustard seeds
1 teaspoon (5 g) Coriander seeds
1 teaspoon (5 g) Fennel seeds
2 Bay leaves (0.6 g)
2 teaspoons (5 ml) Lemon juice

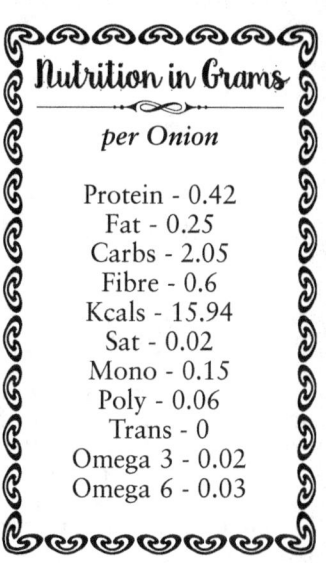

Nutrition in Grams

per Onion

Protein - 0.42
Fat - 0.25
Carbs - 2.05
Fibre - 0.6
Kcals - 15.94
Sat - 0.02
Mono - 0.15
Poly - 0.06
Trans - 0
Omega 3 - 0.02
Omega 6 - 0.03

Boil a kettle full of water. Place the onions in a large bowl. Pour the kettle of boiling water over the onions and leave for 20 seconds. Then pour them into a colander and when they have fully drained, return them to the bowl and pour over lots of very cold water. The skins should now peel off easily. Put back on the bowl and sprinkle salt over every onion. Cover the bowl and leave overnight for 24 hours. Meanwhile pour the malt vinegar and apple cider vinegar into a large saucepan and add the Stevia, peppercorns, mustard seeds and bay leaves. Cover the saucepan and place on a medium heat and bring to the boil. When boiling, remove from the heat and set aside for 24 hours.

When the 25 hours are up, put the onions in a colander and rinse them thoroughly under a cold water running tap and then dry them with a tea towel. Put them into clean jars. Pour the vinegar mixture into a jug and pour the jug all over the onions, making sure you cover them completely. Seal the jars and leave for 6 weeks, when the will be ready to eat.

Dill Pickled Gherkins

Fresh gherkins (or pickling Cucumbers) are in season from June to October. When buying fresh gherkins, look for small, firm, unblemished specimens. There's something special pickling your own and the flavour is better than shop bought one. However, note that these need to be prepared at least 2 weeks in advance of using, but they are easy to prepare and last for up to 2 years.

Makes 2 x 500 ml jars

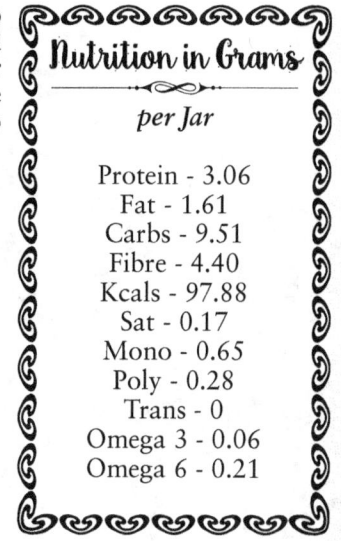

Nutrition in Grams

per Jar

Protein - 3.06
Fat - 1.61
Carbs - 9.51
Fibre - 4.40
Kcals - 97.88
Sat - 0.17
Mono - 0.65
Poly - 0.28
Trans - 0
Omega 3 - 0.06
Omega 6 - 0.21

INGREDIENTS

500 g small pickling or ridged Cucumber
40 g coarse Sea Salt

For the Pickling Vinegar

½ tablespoon (2½ g) black Peppercorns
½ tablespoon (2½ g) Coriander seeds
½ tablespoon (2½ g) yellow Mustard seeds
¼ teaspoon (1¼ g) Chilli Powder
5 cloves (2 g)
A few pieces of Mace blades (1 g) Mace is the outer shell of the nutmeg fruit. It has a lighter, sweeter flavour

Accompanying Vegetables

4 Shallots (100 g)
1 Bay leaf
350 ml white Wine Vinegar
A handful of Dill sprigs (25 g), stalks removed

Cut the pickling or ridged cucumbers into sticks or slices. Peel and slice the shallots in half through the root, then into three. Next, place a layer of the cucumbers into a large bowl and evenly cover with the sea salt and then add a layer of the shallots and again coat with the salt, repeat until all the cucumbers and shallots are used. Place a plate over them and leave them overnight so the salt can draw out the excess moisture. The following day, pour away the drawn water, then rinse.

To make the pickling vinegar, put all the spices into a medium saucepan. Toast them over a low heat until they begin to smell aromatic. Add the bay leaf, pour in all of the vinegar and stir thoroughly, then bring to a simmer. Add the dill sprigs. Pack the cucumber and shallots into jars with airtight seals (thoroughly clean the jars and dry then pop them in a medium oven gas mark 5 - 180°C (375°F) for 5 minutes to sterilise them), pour over the hot vinegar and seal. They will be ready to use in 2 weeks but are best after around three months and can last tightly sealed in a jar, either in the fridge or a cool place for up to 2 years.

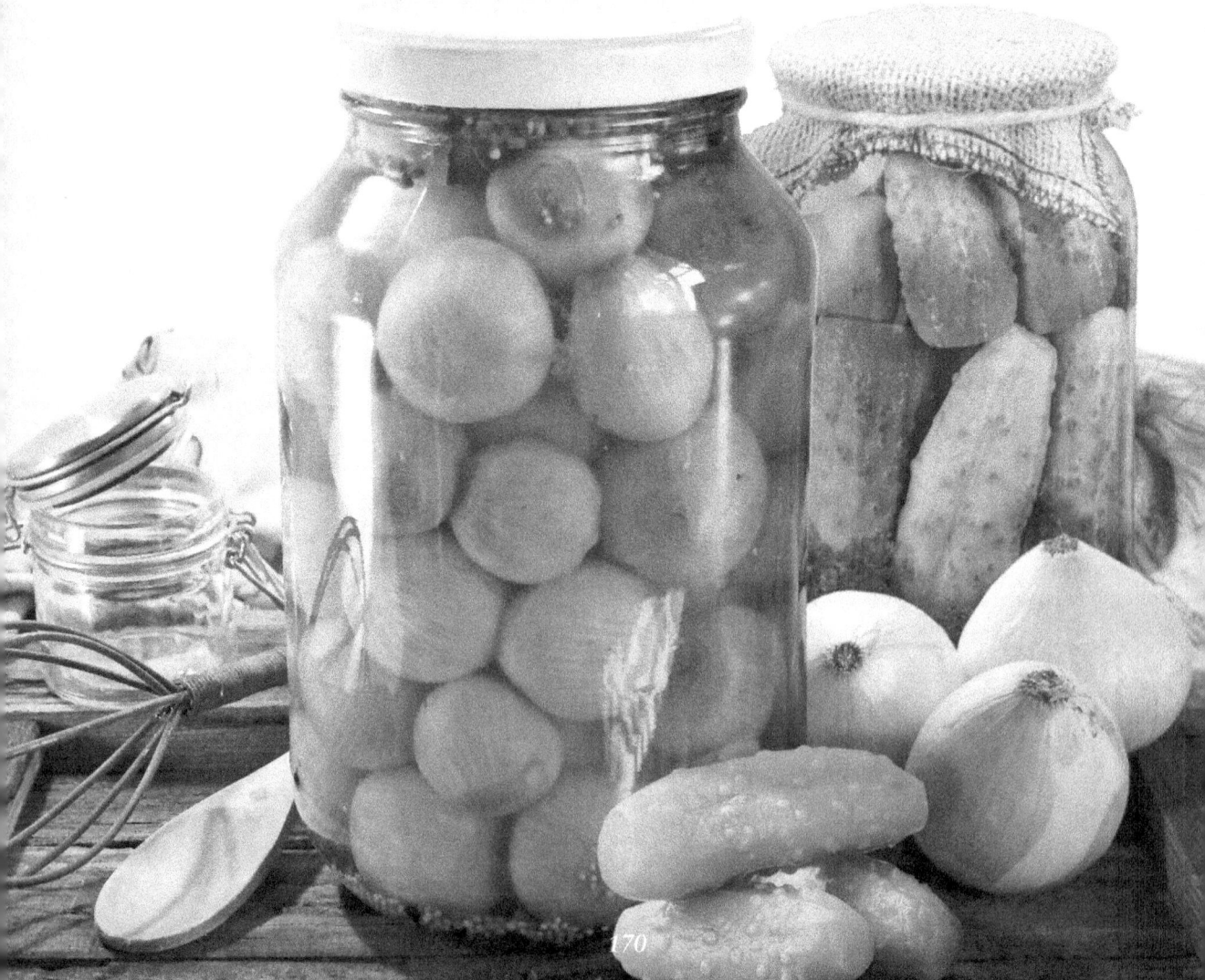

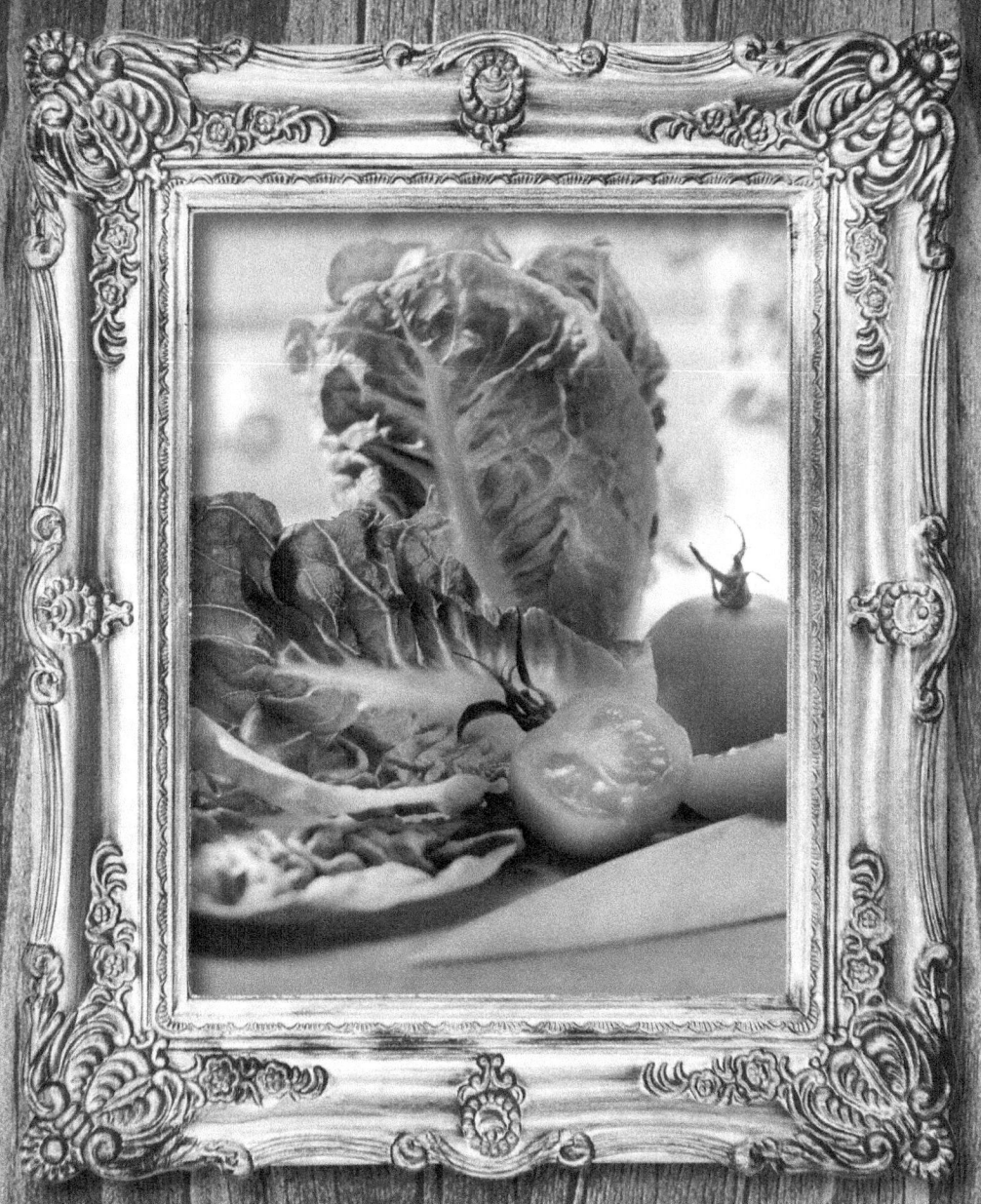

Salads & Dressings

═══════ Salad & Dressings ═══════

Mixed Green Salad

Green salads can be a meal in themselves once you think beyond the lettuce leaf. The range of greenery available is enormous from the dark shades of watercress to the pale hue of spring onions. It's worth making salads a feature of a meal rather than an afterthought.

Serves 4

INGREDIENTS

1 small Lettuce (700 g)

1 bunch Spring Onions (90 g), finely chopped

4 sticks Celery (160 g), trimmed and chopped

½ Cucumber (155 g), sliced into rings

240 g Radishes

1 bunch Watercress (60 g), cleaned

1 quantity of Vinaigrette Dressing (see page 177)

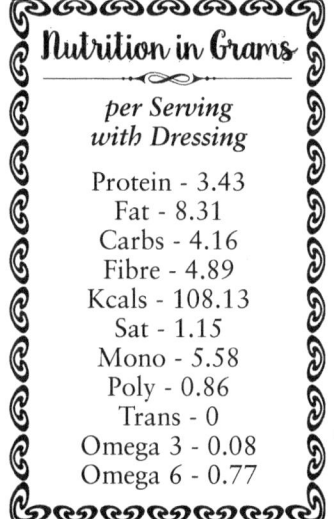

Nutrition in Grams

per Serving with Dressing

Protein - 3.43
Fat - 8.31
Carbs - 4.16
Fibre - 4.89
Kcals - 108.13
Sat - 1.15
Mono - 5.58
Poly - 0.86
Trans - 0
Omega 3 - 0.08
Omega 6 - 0.77

First prepare the lettuce by separating out the leaves and wiping them with a damp cloth. Then prepare all the other vegetables, put all the ingredients into a large salad bowl and sprinkle over the Vinaigrette dressing. It is best to toss green salads with your hands as this prevents the fragile leaves from becoming bruised.

Summer Salad

Raw food plays an important part in a diet for everyone interested in healthy eating. Salads are an excellent way of providing essential vitamins and minerals which might otherwise be lost in the cooking process.

Serves 4

INGREDIENTS

1 small Lettuce (700 g)

A handful of Baby Spinach leaves (50 g)

1 medium Carrot (70 g), scrubbed and grated

4 sticks Celery (160 g), trimmed and sliced

A third of a Cucumber (100 g), diced

2 large Eggs (150 g), hard boiled (see page 68)

1 small Onion (150 g), peeled and finely chopped

450 g Tomatoes, washed and sliced

1 teaspoon (5 g) Mustard, preferably Dijon

A handful of Watercress (30 g)

1 quantity of Vinaigrette Dressing (see page 177)

Nutrition in Grams

per Serving with Dressing

Protein - 9.96
Fat - 12.12
Carbs - 11.11
Fibre - 7.32
Kcals - 200.68
Sat - 2.12
Mono - 6.9
Poly - 1.43
Trans - 0
Omega 3 - 0.13
Omega 6 - 1.29

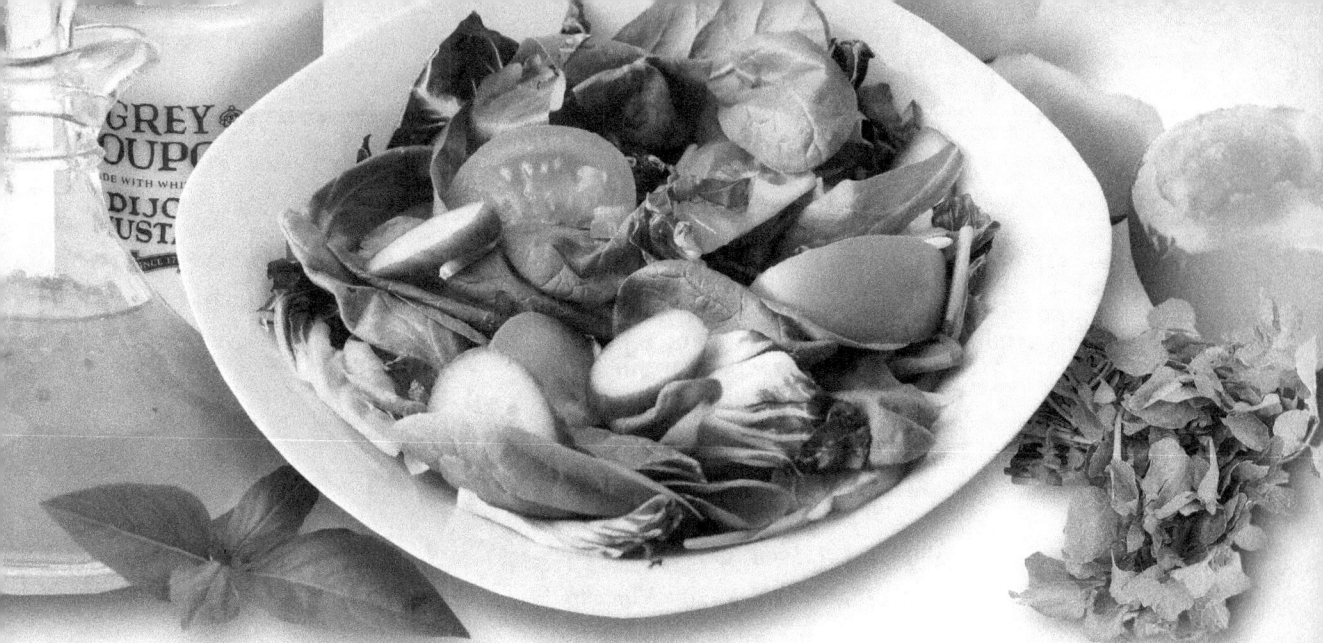

Put up a saucepan of water to boil, big enough for the water to flow freely around the eggs while they're boiling. Once the water is boiling, use a large spoon to gently lower the eggs into the water. Lower the heat to a simmer and set a timer for 12 minutes. After 12 minutes, turn the heat off, drain the water and run cold water over the eggs until the shells are cold to the touch. Peel the shell off and put aside to fully cool down.

Prepare all the other ingredients and put them into a large salad bowl. Mix them straight away with the dressing as this coating of oil and vinegar prevents some of the vitamins and minerals from being destroyed by contact with the air. Now slice the cooled eggs and place evenly over the salad. Serve chilled.

Classic Tomato Salad

This is a really simple way of serving tomatoes, as the Salt, Pepper and Stevia mixture draws out juices from them so that they create their own dressing. Serve this as a side salad, garnished with watercress.

Serves 4 ❶

Nutrition in Grams
per Serving

Protein - 1.19
Fat - 0.13
Carbs - 3.26
Fibre - 1.51
Kcals - 18.85
Sat - 0.01
Mono - 0
Poly - 0.01
Trans - 0
Omega 3 - 0
Omega 6 - 0

INGREDIENTS
450 g Tomatoes, sliced
1½ teaspoons (7½ g) Salt
½ teaspoon (2½ g) freshly ground Black Pepper
¼ teaspoon (1¼ g) Stevia
A little Cider Vinegar (5 ml)

Garnish
1 bunch Watercress (50 g)

Slice the tomatoes and lay them on a plate. Mix together the Salt, Pepper and Stevia and sprinkle this mixture over the tomatoes. Leave them to stand, preferably in the fridge, for 15 minutes. Put them into a serving dish lined with watercress, and sprinkle on a little extra Vinegar if you like a sharper flavour.

Greek Salad with Feta Cheese

This recipe can become a full meal when served with low carb French bread (see page 36, without the garlic butter) you can simply use it as a side salad piled on top of a bed of Lettuce or Endive (Endive is a member of the chicory family. It has a crisp texture and a sweet, nutty flavour with a mild bitterness - great served raw or cooked).

Serves 6

INGREDIENTS

100 g Feta Cheese

1 tablespoon (15 ml) Olive Oil

1 tablespoon (15 ml) White Wine Vinegar

2 sticks of Celery (80 g), sliced

1 quantity of Classic Tomato Salad (see page 91)

50 g Green Pepper, chopped into 8 cm/3 inch strips

1 bunch Spring Onions (90 g), finely chopped

1 teaspoon (5 g) Fennel Seed

Freshly ground Black Pepper

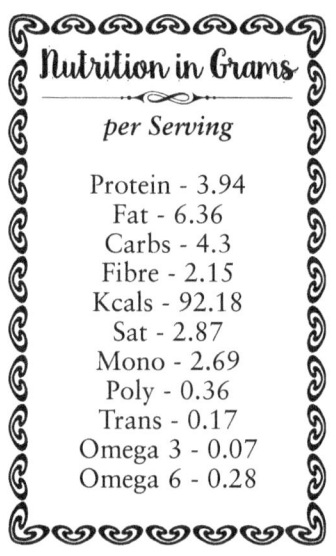

Nutrition in Grams

per Serving

Protein - 3.94
Fat - 6.36
Carbs - 4.3
Fibre - 2.15
Kcals - 92.18
Sat - 2.87
Mono - 2.69
Poly - 0.36
Trans - 0.17
Omega 3 - 0.07
Omega 6 - 0.28

Cut the cheese into cubes, put them into a bowl and grind some Black Pepper over the top. Mix together the Oil and Vinegar and pour this over the cheese. Chill for at least 30 minutes in the fridge to marinate. Arrange the Tomato salad in a serving dish and pile the marinated Feta Cheese over the top. Sprinkle with the Green Pepper, finely chopped Spring Onions and Fennel Seed.

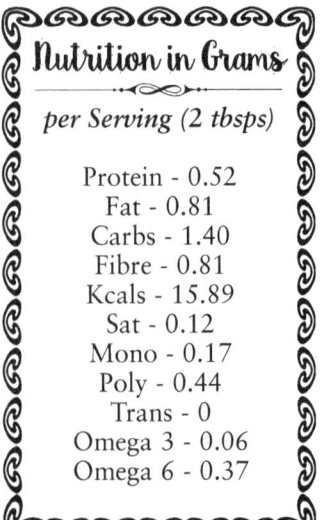

Nutrition in Grams

per Serving (2 tbsps)

Protein - 0.52
Fat - 0.81
Carbs - 1.40
Fibre - 0.81
Kcals - 15.89
Sat - 0.12
Mono - 0.17
Poly - 0.44
Trans - 0
Omega 3 - 0.06
Omega 6 - 0.37

Classic Coleslaw

Makes about 540 g - 2 tablespoons (30 g) per portion

INGREDIENTS

2 tablespoons (30 g) homemade Mayonnaise (see page 94)

1 tablespoons (15 g) Lemon Juice

½ teaspoon (2½ g) Mustard, preferably Dijon

¼ Red Cabbage (250 g), trimmed and shredded

½ small Onion (75 g), peeled and finely chopped

2 large Carrots (160 g), peeled and coarsely grated

Salt and freshly ground Black Pepper

Place the mayonnaise, lemon juice and mustard in a large serving bowl. Season well with salt and freshly ground black pepper and mix. Once you've peeled and sliced all your vegetables add the red cabbage, onion and carrots and stir well to coat in the dressing. Cover and chill for an hour before serving.

Salad & Dressings

Tuna & Tomato Salad

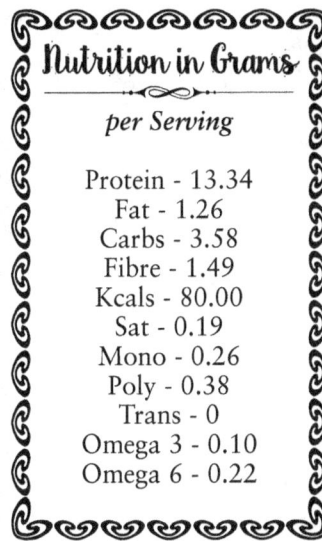

Nutrition in Grams
per Serving

Protein - 13.34
Fat - 1.26
Carbs - 3.58
Fibre - 1.49
Kcals - 80.00
Sat - 0.19
Mono - 0.26
Poly - 0.38
Trans - 0
Omega 3 - 0.10
Omega 6 - 0.22

This healthy tomato salad recipe is great as a meal in itself or as a side dish replacing cooked vegetables. This recipe contains Radicchio, which is a leaf chicory, also known as Italian chicory. It has a bitter and spicy taste and has crisp white veined red leaves, which gives this salad a fresh.

Serves 4

INGREDIENTS
200 g tinned Tuna in brine, drained
40 g Radicchio, diced
180 g fresh Tomatoes, diced
300 g red Radishes, thinly sliced
2 tablespoons (30 ml) Apple Cider Vinegar
2 tablespoons (30 ml) Lime juice
1 teaspoon (5 g) Green Pesto (see page 93)

Drain the tinned tuna thoroughly and using a fork, empty into a salad bowl. Add the pesto and mix with the tuna with a fork. Add half the sliced radishes, cider vinegar and the lime juice. Mix the ingredients together and leave for 10 minutes. Then add the remainder of the radishes and the sliced tomatoes. Best served immediately.

Chicken Caesar Salad

A Caesar salad is a salad of Romaine Lettuce, chicken and croutons dressed with parmesan cheese, lemon juice, olive oil, egg, Worcestershire sauce, garlic, and black pepper. The creation of the salad is thought to be by Italian immigrant and restaurant owner Caesar Cardini, who ran restaurants in both Mexico and the United States.

Serves 4

INGREDIENTS
2 boneless (500 g), skinless Chicken breasts
1 Romaine Lettuce (800 g)
10 cherry tomatoes (150 g), halved
4 slices of low carb bread, each about 1.5 cm thick
Sea salt and freshly ground black pepper
1 tablespoon (15 ml) Macadamia oil or Rapeseed oil for frying

Nutrition in Grams
per Serving

Protein - 40.55
Fat - 15.81
Carbsv5.74
Fibre - 13.62
Kcals - 359.27
Sat - 2.04
Mono - 5.31
Poly - 7.4
Trans - 0.02
Omega 3 - 5.52
Omega 6 - 1.88

Lay some cling film on a board and place the chicken breasts upon it and cover with cling film. Using a rolling pin, bang the chicken until it is about 1 cm thick, then season the breasts on both sides with a little salt and plenty of freshly ground black pepper. Fry some Rapeseed oil in a large frying pan, place on a medium heat and add the chicken and cook for 2 minutes. Turn the breasts over and repeat on the other side until nicely browned and cooked through. Remove from the heat put aside to cool down.

For the salad, break up the lettuce leaves into small pieces and put into a large serving dish and scatter over the tomatoes. Toast the slices of low carb bread and cut them into pieces about 1½ cm square. Cut the cooked chicken breasts into thick strips and add to the salad and toss together lightly. Serve with Caesar salad dressing.

Caesar Salad Dressing

Makes approximately 250 ml (50 ml per serving)
Serves 5

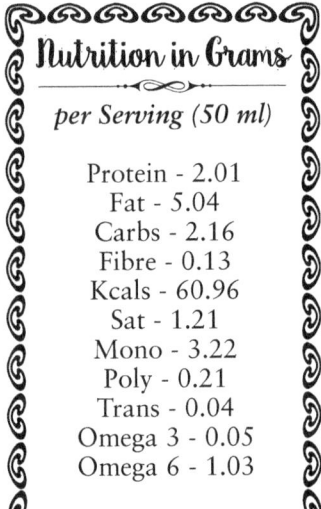

Nutrition in Grams
per Serving (50 ml)

Protein - 2.01
Fat - 5.04
Carbs - 2.16
Fibre - 0.13
Kcals - 60.96
Sat - 1.21
Mono - 3.22
Poly - 0.21
Trans - 0.04
Omega 3 - 0.05
Omega 6 - 1.03

INGREDIENTS

2 Garlic cloves (12 g), crushed
1 teaspoon (5 g) Anchovy paste
2 tablespoons (30 ml) lemon juice
1 teaspoon (5 g) Dijon mustard
1 teaspoon (5 g) Worcestershire sauce (see page 94)
225 ml Mayonnaise (see page 94)
20 g freshly grated Parmesan Cheese
¼ teaspoon (1¼ g) Salt
¼ teaspoon (1¼ g) freshly ground Black Pepper

In a bowl, whisk together the garlic, anchovy paste, lemon juice, Dijon mustard and Worcestershire sauce. Add the mayonnaise, Parmesan cheese, salt and pepper and whisk until well combined. This dressing will keep in the fridge for about a week.

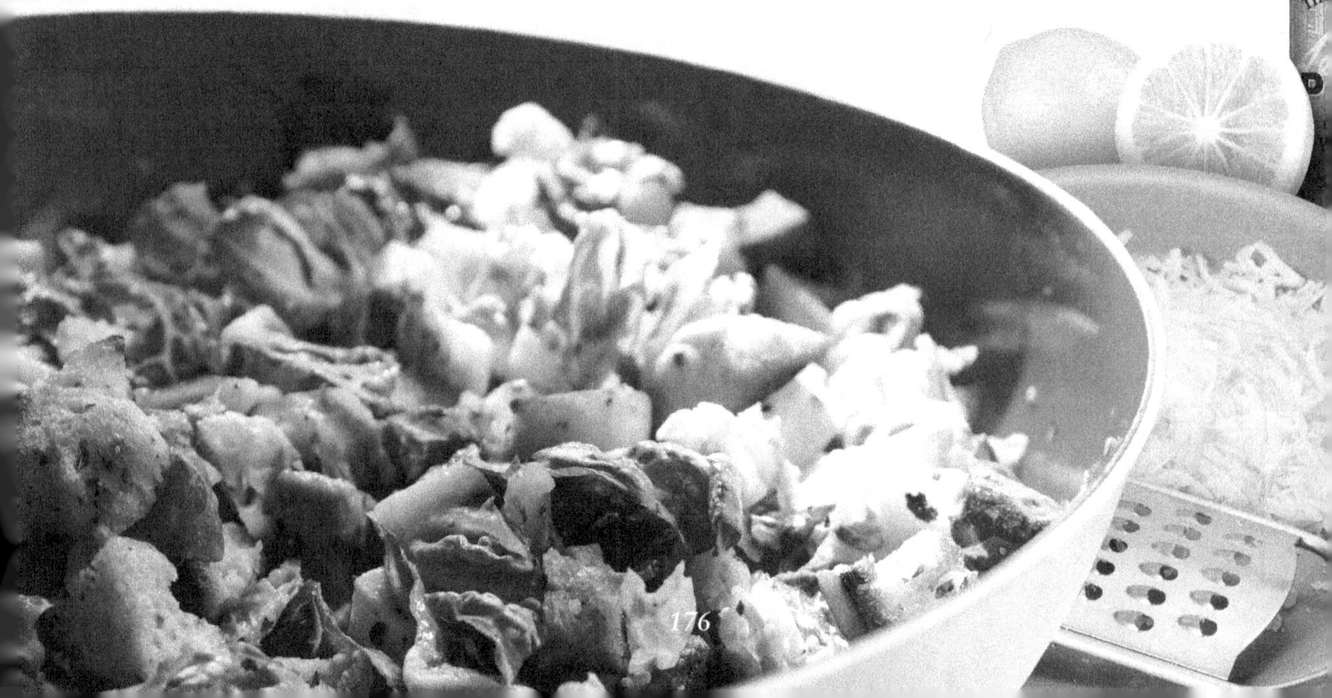

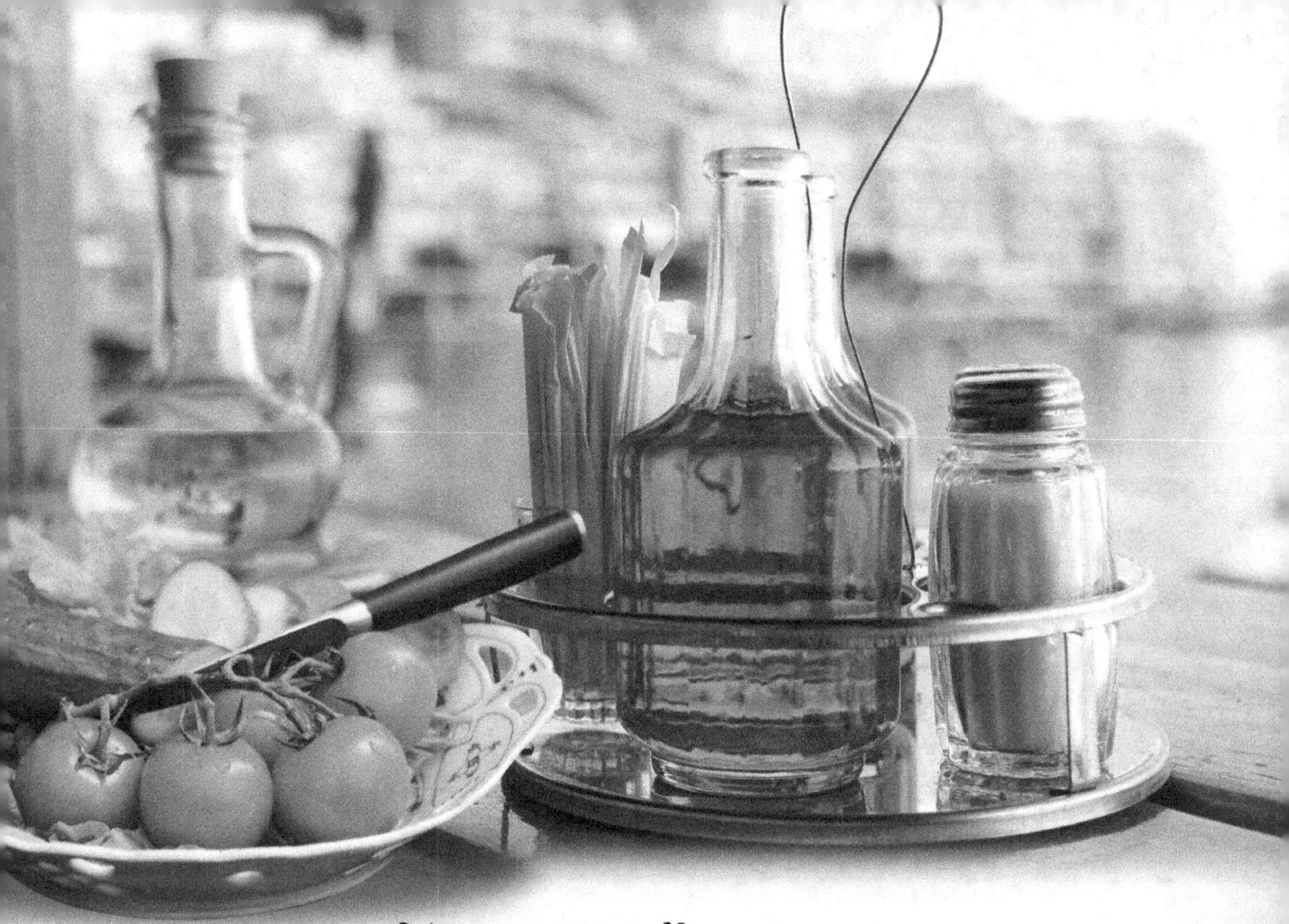

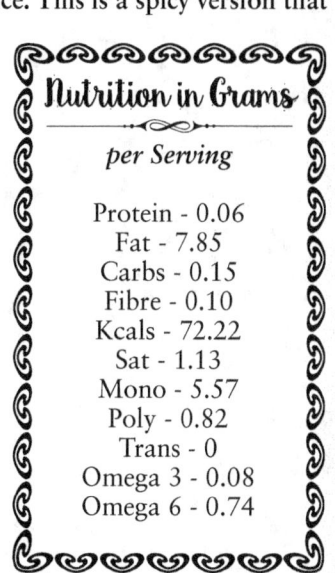

Vinaigrette Dressing

There are no hard and fast rules about vinaigrette dressing but the most common ratio is three parts olive oil to one of vinegar, this dressing however cuts down the oil. The oil can be either olive oil or rapeseed and the vinegar can be wine, herb or cider vinegar or lemon juice. This is a spicy version that ideally complements any green salad.

Serves 4

INGREDIENTS

1 tablespoon (15 ml) Apple Cider Vinegar
A pinch (1 g) of Mustard powder
A pinch (1 g) of Paprika
½ teaspoon (2½ g) Horseradish sauce (see page 95)
2 tablespoons (30 ml) Olive Oil

Put the vinegar in a bowl or preferable a screw-top jar and add the mustard powder, horseradish and paprika. Mix thoroughly or if you are using a jar, screw the lid on tightly and shake. When the spices are blended add the olive oil and mix or shake again until all the ingredients have combined. This dressing can then be used straight away or kept for a couple of days in the fridge. Always shake thoroughly before using.

Nutrition in Grams
per Serving

- Protein - 0.06
- Fat - 7.85
- Carbs - 0.15
- Fibre - 0.10
- Kcals - 72.22
- Sat - 1.13
- Mono - 5.57
- Poly - 0.82
- Trans - 0
- Omega 3 - 0.08
- Omega 6 - 0.74

THE DIABETIC DETECTIVES

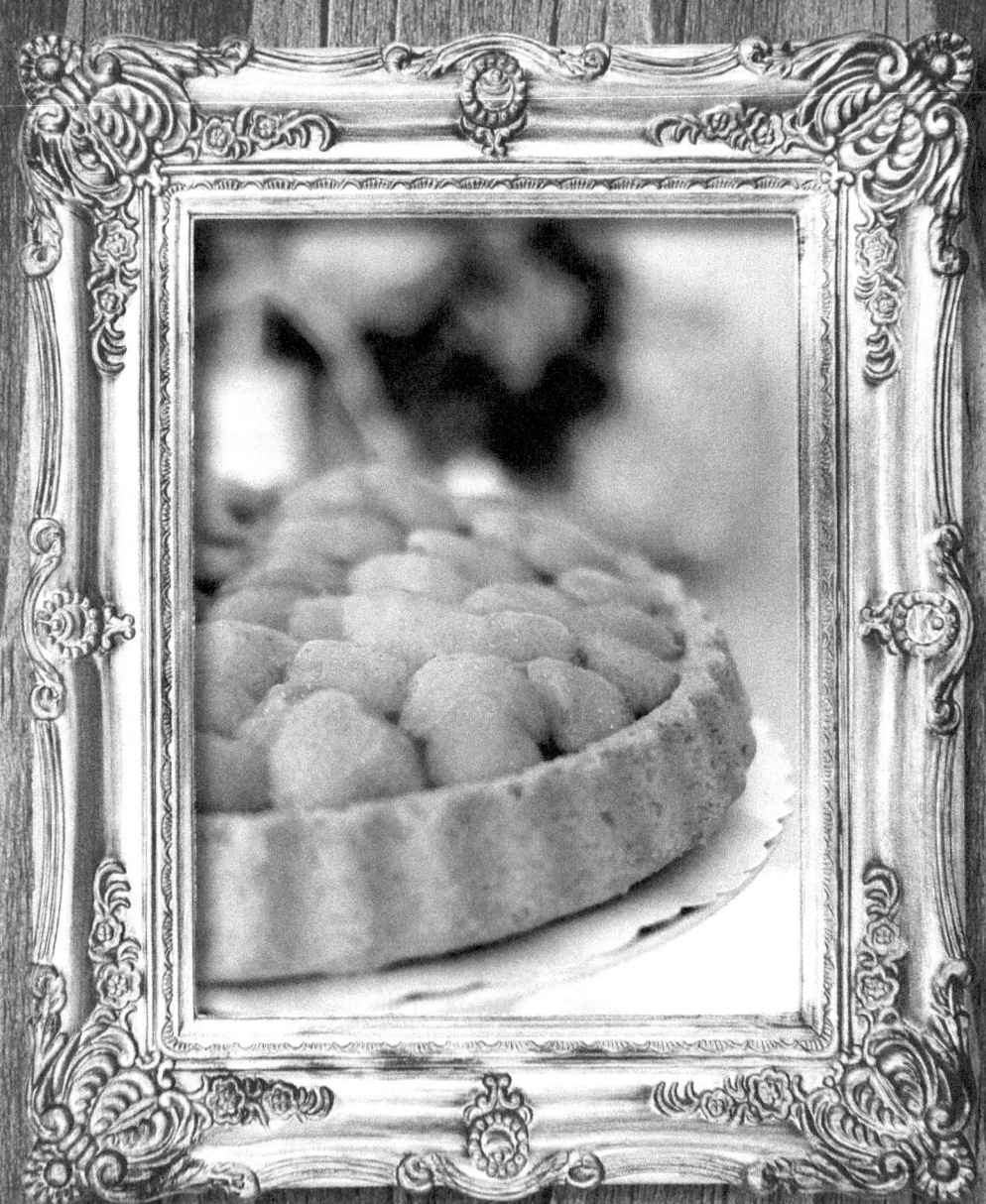

Desserts

Desserts

Strawberry Egg Custard

Serves 6

INGREDIENTS

720 ml unsweetened Almond Milk
4 large Eggs (300 g)
20 g Vanilla flavoured low fat Natural Yoghurt
2 teaspoons (10 g) pure Vanilla Extract
¼ teaspoon Salt
1 teaspoon (5 ml) liquid Vanilla Stevia
1 teaspoon (5 g) Cinnamon or ½ teaspoon (2½ g) ground Nutmeg
3 Strawberries (36 g)
A little Spreadable Butter (cut with rapeseed oil or olive oil or both) for greasing the ramekins

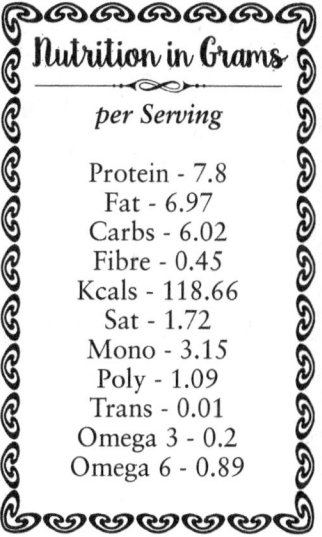

Nutrition in Grams

per Serving

Protein - 7.8
Fat - 6.97
Carbs - 6.02
Fibre - 0.45
Kcals - 118.66
Sat - 1.72
Mono - 3.15
Poly - 1.09
Trans - 0.01
Omega 3 - 0.2
Omega 6 - 0.89

Pre-heat the oven to gas mark 4 - 180°C (350°F). In a mixing bowl, crack in the eggs and whisk thoroughly. Add the vanilla flavoured natural yoghurt, vanilla extract, Stevia and salt. Blend well together. In a large saucepan, pour in the almond milk or semi-skimmed Milk and heat up until just below boiling point (if you accidentally boil it, just leave it to stand for a minute). Slowly add a little of the hot milk into the egg mixture and stir well. Then pour in the rest of the milk gradually. Grease 6 ramekins with a little spreadable butter and pour the egg custard mixture evenly into each dish (a ramekin is small dish for baking and serving an individual portion of food). Sprinkle a little cinnamon or nutmeg over each custard and place the 6 ramekins into an ovenproof dish or roasting tin that is big enough to accommodate all of them. Pour hot water into the dish so that it reaches half way up the sides of the ramekins. Put the ovenproof dish in the centre of the oven. Cook for 25-30 minutes and then remove from the oven and take out the ramekins and leave to cool down. Cut the strawberries in half and place a half on top of the custard cut side down. These can be eaten immediately or you can put them in the fridge and eat chilled.

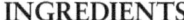

Brandy Pancakes

Serves 1

INGREDIENTS

1 medium Egg (65 g)
20 g white Chia seeds, ground
20 g Flaxseed, ground
75 ml semi-skimmed Milk
75 ml Water
¼ teaspoon (1.25 g) Baking Powder (optional)
1 teaspoon (5 g) Macadamia oil or Rapeseed oil for frying

Desserts

Grind the white chia seeds and flaxseed in a nut mill or blender until they become a fine flour. Place them in a mixing bowl and crack the egg into the bowl and mix thoroughly. Gradually add the milk and water, stirring continuously until you have a smooth texture. Pour a little Rapeseed oil or Macadamia oil in a frying pan and heat it on a low heat for about 3 minutes. Pour in the pancake mix and spread over the surface of the pan (by tilting the pan). Wait 90 seconds to 2 minutes or until the underside starts to brown nicely, then flip and cook for another 90 seconds on the other side. Put on a plate and douse liberally with Brandy. Alternatively you can put a little lemon juice on the pancake.

Nutrition in Grams
per Serving including 25 ml Brandy

Protein - 17.77
Fat - 25.86
Carbs - 5.58
Fibre - 12.34
Kcals - 415.00
Sat - 4.02
Mono - 8.46
Poly - 11.33
Trans - 0.04
Omega 3 - 8.22
Omega 6 - 3.10

Chocolate Brownies

Makes 9 x 5 cm square Brownies

INGREDIENTS ❷

80 g Flaxseed, ground
6 g Psyllium Husk
16 g Low fat (light) Spreadable Butter with rapeseed or olive oil (or both)
40 g Cocoa Powder or 50 g of melted 85% Cocoa chocolate bar
1 g Stevia - only necessary if using cocoa powder which is very bitter
1 g Baking Powder
1 zest of one Orange (28 g) or 8 ml of Cointreau
2 medium Eggs (130 g)
100 ml semi-skimmed Milk
120 ml Water

Nutrition in Grams
per Brownie (Cocoa)

Protein - 4.89
Fat - 7.21
Carbs - 1.76
Fibre - 4.28
Kcals - 100.94
Sat - 1.78
Mono - 1.91
Poly - 2.93
Trans - 0.02
Omega 3 - 2.08
Omega 6 - 0.86

Nutrition in Grams
per Brownie (Chocolate)

Protein - 4.33
Fat - 8.6
Carbs - 3.1
Fibre - 3.81
Kcals - 117.3
Sat - 2.57
Mono - 2.3
Poly - 2.97
Trans - 0.02
Omega 3 - 2.08
Omega 6 - 0.89

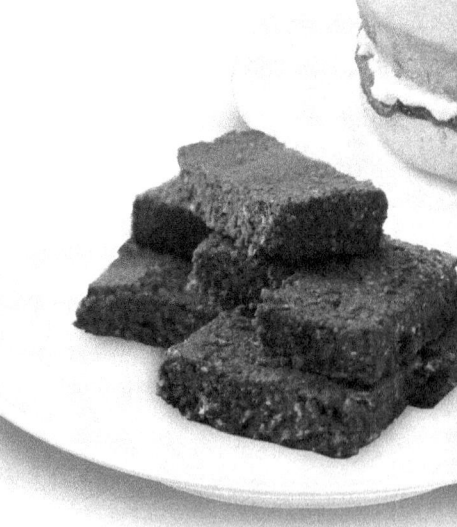

Get a 15 cm x 15 cm non stick baking tin with a removable bottom (makes it so much easier to remove the brownies).

Grind the flaxseed in a nut mill or blender until they become a fine flour. Pre heat the oven to gas mark 4 - 180°C (350°F). In a mixing bowl, whisk the eggs together into a smooth consistency. In another bowl mix together the flaxseed flour, cocoa powder, baking powder and orange zest (if using). Add the dry ingredients to the eggs and stir in well. (If you are using the chocolate, you need to bring a medium sized saucepan of water to the boil, and then turn the heat down to low. Snap the chocolate bar into small chunks and place in a heatproof bowl small enough to fit into the saucepan, the chocolate will now melt. When it is runny enough to pour out, you can add it to the egg mixture). Add the spreadable butter and melted chocolate/Cocoa powder. If you are using the zest of an orange, grate the orange with the lowest setting on your grater (just the orange part not the white pith just underneath) and add this or add the lid full of Cointreau and beat it all together into a smooth, just pourable mix. (Add more water if necessary to make it just pourable).

Pour the mix into the brownie tin. Spread the mix out using a plastic spatula, so that evenly fills the bottom of the tin. It will only be around 1 cm/½ inch deep at this point. But don't worry, it will rise. Bake in the lower part of the oven for around 40 minutes, or until firm to the touch. Try not to chop the Brownies up until you are ready to eat them. They will last longer that way. The idea behind this is to create a satisfying size of chocolate fix from the chocolate bar, whilst preserving its taste.

Sponge Cakes
Serves 4 ❷

INGREDIENTS

120 g Flaxseed, ground

8 g Psyllium Husk

24 g Low fat (light) Spreadable Butter with rapeseed or olive oil (or both) and a little more for greasing the cake tins

120 ml semi-skimmed milk

150 g Water

3 medium (195 g) Eggs

3 g Baking Powder

2 teaspoons (10 ml) Vanilla Essence

Grind the flaxseed in a nut mill or blender until it becomes a fine flour. Pre heat the oven to gas mark 4 - 180°C (350°F). In a mixing bowl, whisk the eggs together into a smooth consistency. In another bowl mix together the chia seed and flaxseed flour and baking powder. Add the dry ingredients to the eggs. Add the vanilla essence and stir in well. Use 2 (one for each half of the cake) 15 cm/6 inch diameter cake tins) and grease them with a little spreadable butter and pour in the mix and spread evenly over the 2 tins. Bake on the middle shelf of the oven for around 45 minutes or until slightly golden in colour and firm to the touch. Store in a cake tin or in the fridge.

Strawberry Vanilla Cake Filling ❷

INGREDIENTS

40 g Strawberries, sliced

60 g thick Low fat Greek Yoghurt or half fat Crème Fraiche

2 teaspoons (10 ml) Vanilla Extract

In a mixing bowl, mix the yoghurt or crème fraiche with the vanilla essence. Spread this evenly on the top of one of the sponge halves. Then lay out the sliced strawberries evenly over the vanilla spread. Place the top half of the cake on top of the strawberries and position correctly.

Nutrition in Grams
per Serving including Sponge

Protein - 13.94
Fat - 21.07
Carbs - 4.78
Fibre - 10.03
Kcals - 299.68
Sat - 4.14
Mono - 5.5
Poly - 9.68
Trans - 0.08
Omega 3 - 7.03
Omega 6 - 2.66

Macadamia Vanilla Cake Filling

 INGREDIENTS

40 g Macadamia nut butter

60 g thick Low fat Greek Yoghurt or half fat Crème Fraiche

2 teaspoons (10 ml) Vanilla Extract

In a mixing bowl, mix the yoghurt or crème fraiche with the vanilla essence. Spread the macadamia nut butter evenly on the top of one of the sponge halves. Then spread vanilla mixture evenly over the nut butter. Place the top half of the cake on top of the nut butter and position correctly.

Nutrition in Grams
per Serving including Sponge

Protein - 14.67
Fat - 28.62
Carbs - 4.73
Fibre - 10.69
Kcals - 368.28
Sat - 5.35
Mono - 11.39
Poly - 9.82
Trans - 0.08
Omega 3 - 7.04
Omega 6 - 2.78

Nutrition in Grams
per Serving including Sponge

Protein - 14.89
Fat - 28.66
Carbs - 5.52
Fibre - 12.23
Kcals - 375.1
Sat - 5.36
Mono - 11.39
Poly - 9.83
Trans - 0.08
Omega 3 - 7.05
Omega 6 - 2.79

Lemon Cake Filling

INGREDIENTS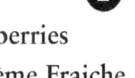

40 g Macadamia nut butter or sliced Strawberries

60 g thick Low fat Greek Yoghurt or half fat Crème Fraiche

1 Lemon Zest and Juice (58 g)

2 teaspoons (10 ml) Vanilla Extract

Follow the instructions for the Macadamia Vanilla Cake filling, but add the zest and juice of the lemon to the yoghurt or crème fraiche mixture.

Chocolate Cake Filling

 **INGREDIENTS**

40 g Macadamia nut butter

60 g Low fat Greek Yoghurt or half fat Crème Fraiche

1 Lemon Zest (15 g)

30 g Cocoa Powder

1 g of Stevia

2 teaspoons (10 ml) Vanilla Extract

Follow the instructions for the Macadamia Vanilla Cake filling, but add the cocoa and Stevia to the yoghurt or crème fraiche mixture.

Nutrition in Grams
per Serving including Sponge

Protein - 16.41
Fat - 30.27
Carbs - 6.02
Fibre - 12.89
Kcals - 398.47
Sat - 6.31
Mono - 11.93
Poly - 9.86
Trans - 0.08
Omega 3 - 7.04
Omega 6 - 2.84

Desserts

French Custard Strawberry Tart

A beautiful strawberry tart recipe made with low carb shortcrust pastry case with thick custard and glazed strawberries. Serve with a tablespoon of half fat crème fraiche for a delicious dessert.

Serves 8

Nutrition in Grams
per Serving

Protein - 7.41
Fat - 6.2
Carbs - 14.64
Fibre - 1.46
Kcals - 139.94
Sat - 2.69
Mono - 1.87
Poly - 0.69
Trans - 0.05
Omega 3 - 0.11
Omega 6 - 0.59

INGREDIENTS
1 portion of low carb short crust Pastry (see page 97)
A little ground White Chia Seeds for rolling out the pastry
500 g small Strawberries, cut in half
60 g Strawberry Jelly

For the thick Custard
350 ml semi-skimmed Milk
1 Vanilla Pod, split lengthways (45 g)
4 large Egg yolks (300 g)
40 g Stevia
10 g cornflour
Finely grated zest of 1 Lemon (15 g)

Garnish
1 tablespoon (15 g) of crème fraiche per serving

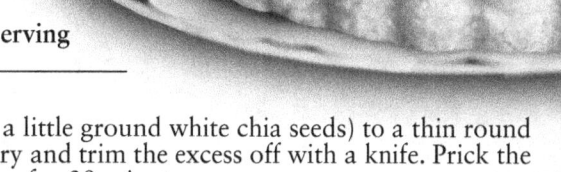

Roll the pastry out on a lightly floured surface (using a little ground white chia seeds) to a thin round shape. Line a deep, 23 cm/9 inch tart tin with the pastry and trim the excess off with a knife. Prick the base gently all over with a fork. Then, put in the fridge for 30 minutes.

Meanwhile, make the thick custard. Put the milk and vanilla pod in a large sauce pan and bring to the boil, then turn off the heat. In a large mixing bowl, whisk the egg yolks and Stevia thoroughly. Then beat in the lemon zest. Put the cornflour in a cup and add a tablespoon of water and mix thoroughly into a paste and add to the egg yolk mixture. Gradually add the warm milk to the egg mixture, whisking continuously. Pour the mixture back into the saucepan and gently bring to the boil, stirring constantly until it has thickened. Take the saucepan off the heat, put aside and leave to cool.

Preheat the oven to gas mark 4 - 160°C (320°F). Put the cooled pastry case into the centre of the oven and blind bake for 15 minutes, then transfer to a wire rack to cool completely. When cooled, spoon the thick custard into the tart, then spread evenly with the back of a spoon. Place a strawberry half in the centre of the tart, and then arrange concentric rings of strawberries around it until the whole tart is covered. Bring a medium sized saucepan of water to the boil, and then turn the heat down to low. Put the strawberry jelly in a heatproof bowl small enough to fit into the saucepan, add 2 tablespoons of hot water from the saucepan and pour it onto the jelly. Mix it up until all the jelly has melted (turn the heat on to very low if it is not melting). Now, brush the melted jelly over the strawberries and leave for a few minutes to set. Garnish each serving with a tablespoon of crème fraiche and serve.

Vanilla Cheesecake

Serves 8

INGREDIENTS

Pastry Base

Half portion of Low Carb Flax and Chia Pastry

(see page 97 for the recipe)

Filling

680 g half fat Cream Cheese

3 medium Eggs (195 g)

1 tablespoon (15 ml) Vanilla Extract

1 teaspoon (5 ml) almond extract

Nutrition in Grams
per Serving

Protein - 18.09
Fat - 9.95
Carbs - 7.01
Fibre - 1.92
Kcals - 200.91
Sat - 2.07
Mono - 2.23
Poly - 4.88
Trans - 0.29
Omega 3 - 3.49
Omega 6 - 1.38

Preheat the oven to gas mark 5 - 190°C (375°F). Prepare the pastry as per the recipe on page? Roll out the pastry to be a 23 cm/ 9 inch circle and line the base only of a 23 cm / 9 inch flan dish and bake blind in the centre of the oven for 15 minutes. Remove the flan dish from the oven and turn the oven down to gas mark 4 - 180°C (350°F). In a mixing bowl mix together the half fat cream cheese and the Vanilla and Almond extracts. Then crack the eggs into the mixture and beat thoroughly until creamy. Pour over the pastry and cook in the centre of the oven for 35 minutes at or until golden brown.

Remove from the oven. When you tap with your fingers on the side of the flan dish the centre of the cheesecake should wobble very slightly while being firm at the edges. If it's wobbly throughout, return to the oven and check every 5 minutes. Cover until the cheesecake has cooled down and then chill it in the fridge for several hours, preferably overnight to let the cake completely set. Serve straight from the fridge.

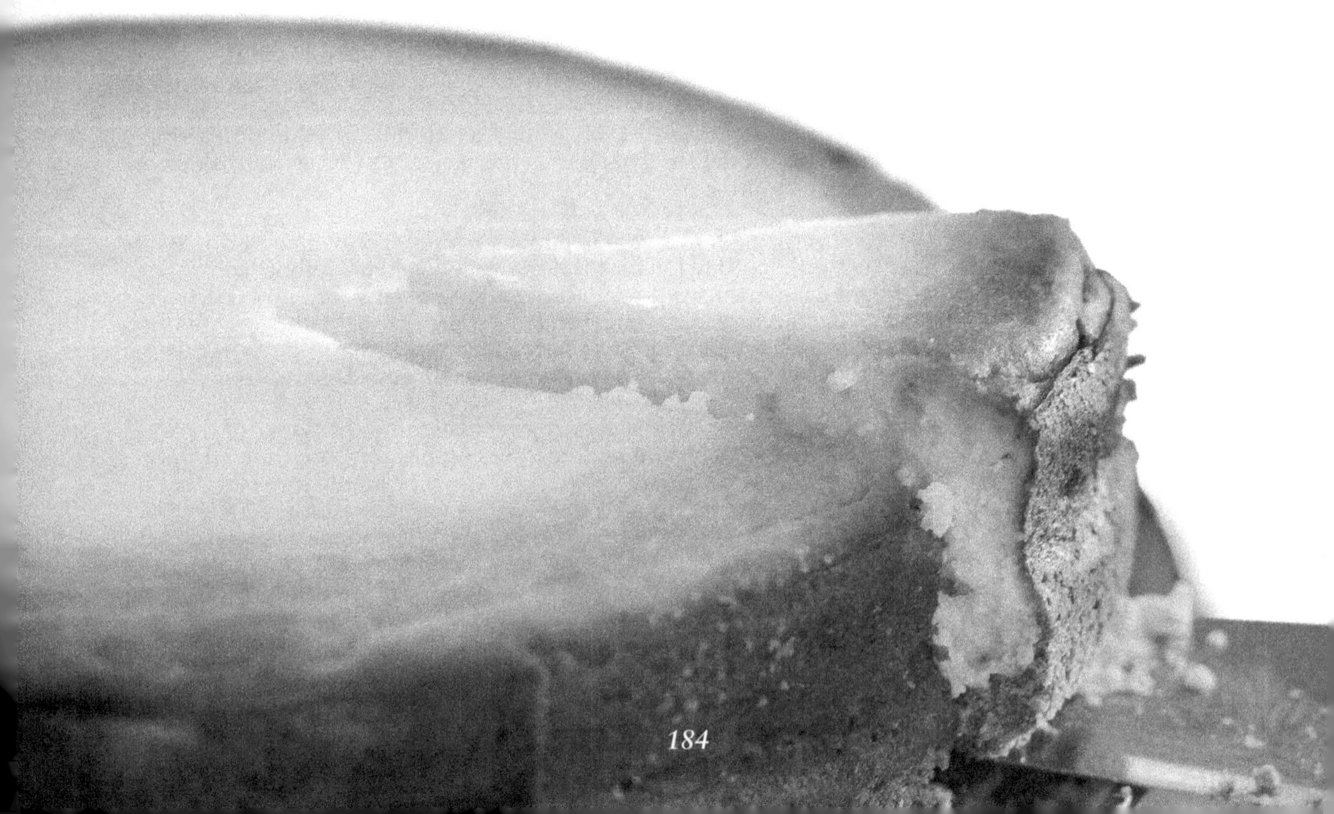

Desserts

Marbled Strawberry Cheesecake

This strawberry cheesecake has a pleasing swirl of pureed strawberries with a hint of lemon.

Serves 8

INGREDIENTS

Pastry Base

Half portion of Low Carb Flax and Chia Pastry
(see page 97 for the recipe)

Filling

480 g half fat Cream Cheese

2 medium Eggs (130 g)

1 tablespoon of lemon juice (15 ml)

200 g Strawberries, pureed

1 tablespoon (15 ml) Vanilla Extract

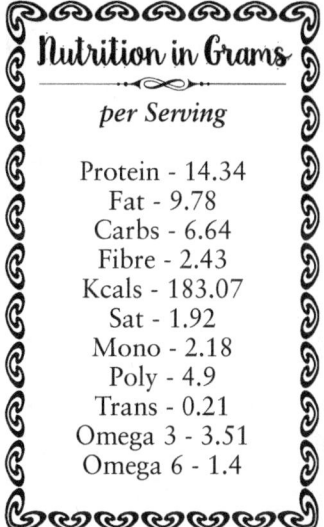

Nutrition in Grams

per Serving

Protein - 14.34
Fat - 9.78
Carbs - 6.64
Fibre - 2.43
Kcals - 183.07
Sat - 1.92
Mono - 2.18
Poly - 4.9
Trans - 0.21
Omega 3 - 3.51
Omega 6 - 1.4

As with the previous cheese cake recipe, preheat the oven to gas mark 5 - 190°C (375°F). Prepare the pastry as per the recipe in the Pastry chapter. Roll out the pastry to be a 23 cm/9 inch circle and line the base only of a 23 cm/9 inch, 5 cm/2 inch deep flan dish and bake blind in the centre of the oven for 15 minutes. Remove the flan dish from the oven and turn the oven down to gas mark 4 - 180°C (350°F). In a mixing bowl mix together the half fat cream cheese and the lemon juice. Then crack the eggs into the mixture and beat thoroughly until creamy. Pour the mixture over the pastry base.

Liquidise the strawberries until they are a smooth paste and add the Stevia to the mix. Using a spoon, drop the strawberry mix over the surface of the cake and then using a fork gently swirl the pureed strawberries very gently into the mixture to create a marbled effect. Don't mix fully into the mixture.

Cook in the centre of the oven for 35 minutes or until golden brown. Remove from the oven. When you tap with your fingers on the side of the flan dish the centre of the cheesecake should wobble very slightly while being firm at the edges. If it's wobbly throughout, return to the oven and check every 5 minutes. Cover until the cheesecake has cooled down and then chill it in the fridge for several hours, preferably overnight to let the cake completely set. Serve straight from the fridge.

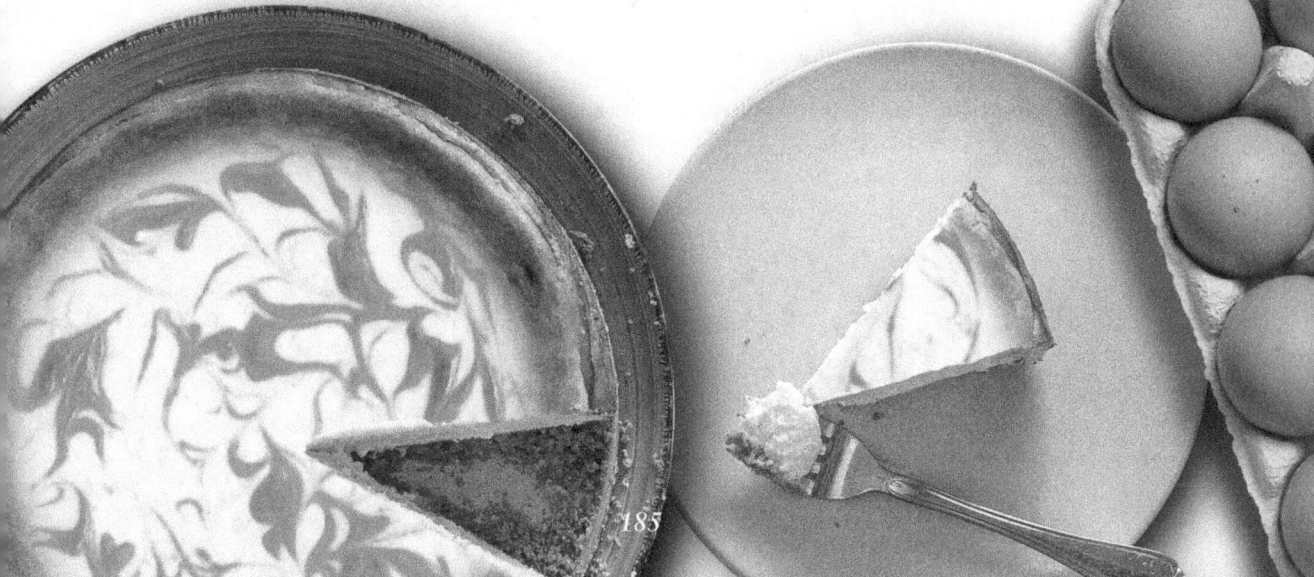

New York Cheesecake

Serves 8

INGREDIENTS

Pastry Base

Half portion of Low Carb Flax and Chia Pastry
(see page 97 for the recipe)

Filling

550 g half fat Cream Cheese

100 g half fat Crème Fraiche

2 medium Eggs (130 g)

Zest of 1 Lemon, finely grated (about 2 teaspoons) 10 g

1 tablespoon (15 ml) Vanilla Extract

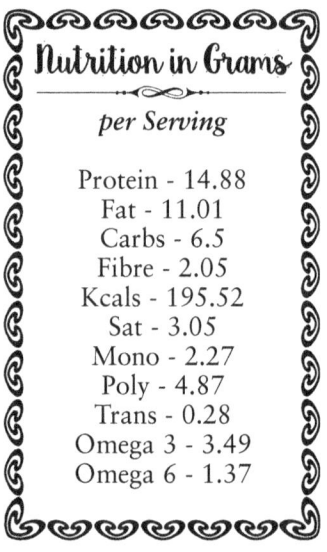

Nutrition in Grams per Serving

Protein - 14.88
Fat - 11.01
Carbs - 6.5
Fibre - 2.05
Kcals - 195.52
Sat - 3.05
Mono - 2.27
Poly - 4.87
Trans - 0.28
Omega 3 - 3.49
Omega 6 - 1.37

Preheat the oven to gas mark 5 - 190°C (375°F). Prepare the pastry as per the recipe in the Pastry chapter. Roll out the pastry to be a 23 cm/ 9 inch circle and line the base only of a 23 cm/ 9 inch flan dish and bake blind in the centre of the oven for 15 minutes. Remove the flan dish from the oven and turn the oven down to gas mark 4 - 180°C (350°F). In a mixing bowl mix together the half fat cream cheese and the lemon zest. Then crack the eggs into the mixture and beat thoroughly until creamy. Add the crème fraiche and vanilla extract and mix thoroughly. Pour the mixture over the pastry base.

Cook in the centre of the oven for 45 minutes at or until golden brown. Remove from the oven. When you tap with your fingers on the side of the flan dish the centre of the cheesecake should wobble very slightly while being firm at the edges. If it's wobbly throughout, return to the oven and check every 5 minutes. Cover until the cheesecake has cooled down and then chill it in the fridge for several hours, preferably overnight to let the cake completely set. Serve straight from the fridge.

Carrot & Cinnamon Cake

There are recipes dating from the Roman times in which carrots were used for their sweetness and colour. This carrot cake has a rich colour and close texture, and it is heavily spiced with cinnamon and nutmeg. It will freeze or keep well for several days in an air tight tin.

Makes a 450 g cake - Serves 8

INGREDIENTS

150 g Flaxseed, ground

75 g White Chia Seeds, ground

1 tablespoon cinnamon (15 g)

1 teaspoon nutmeg (5 g)

Desserts

2 tablespoon baking powder (30 g)
110 g Low fat (light) Spreadable Butter with rapeseed or olive oil (or both)
40 g Stevia
225 g Carrots, peeled and finely grated

Nutrition in Grams
per Serving

Protein - 5.62
Fat - 19.39
Carbs - 10.14
Fibre - 10.25
Kcals - 246.37
Sat - 4.75
Mono - 4.78
Poly - 8.71
Trans - 0.15
Omega 3 - 6.21
Omega 6 - 2.49

Pre-heat the oven to gas mark 3 - 170°C (325°F). Mix together the flaxseed and chia seed flour, spices and baking powder in a large bowl. Then melt the butter and Stevia together in a saucepan, and stir this mixture into the flour, combining all the ingredients thoroughly. Next stir in the grated carrots. Put the mixture into a well greased 1 lb (450 g) loaf tin and bake for 60-80 minutes, or until it feels firm to the touch and a skewer inserted into the centre comes out clean. Leave the cake in the tin for 10 minutes, then turn it out onto a cooling rack.

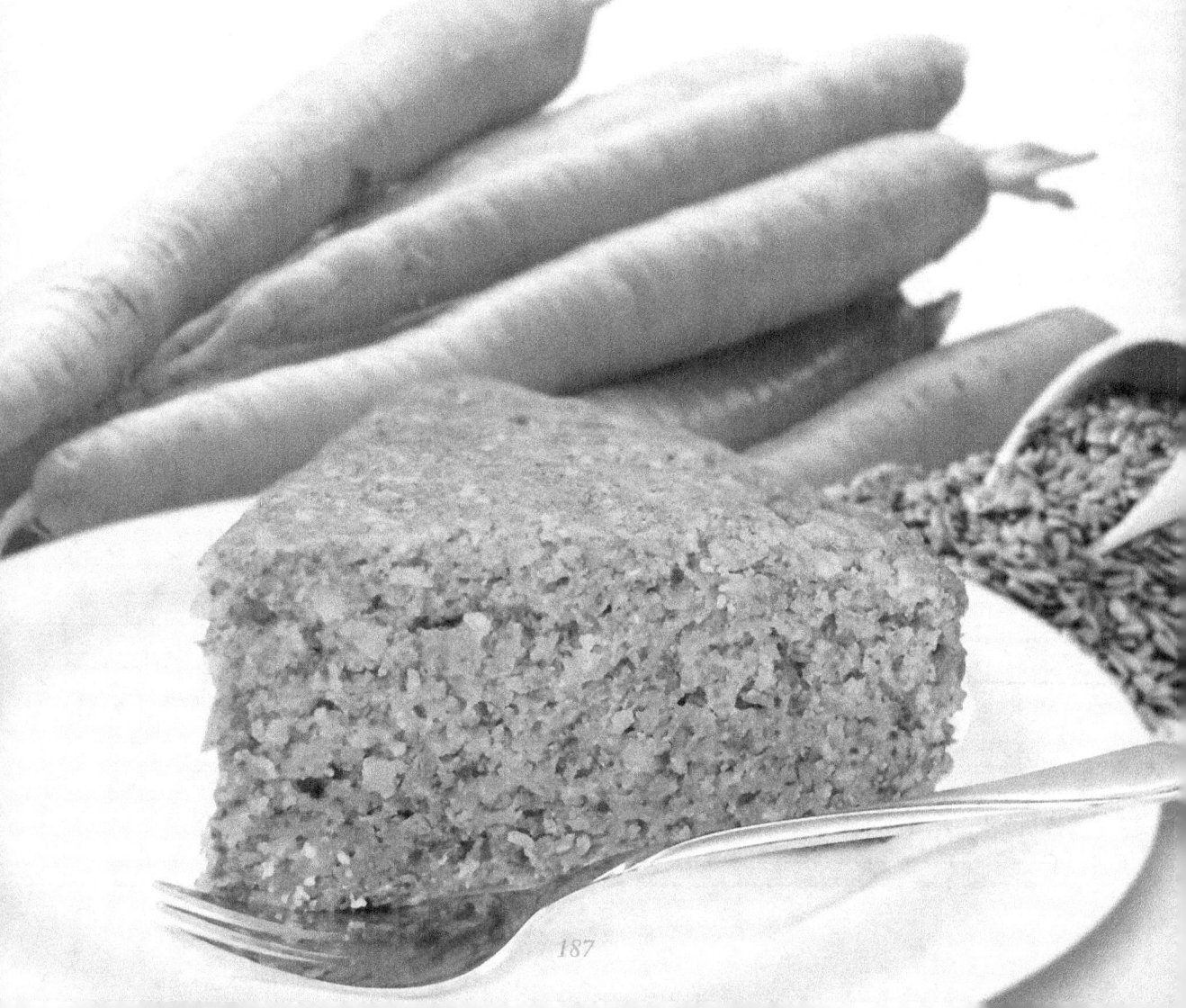

Food Names
Trans Atlantic Food Name Differences

English	American English	Notes
Aubergine	Eggplant	
Biscuit	Cookie	
Chicory	Endive	*This is for Belgian endive, not all chicory*
Chips	French Fries	
Cider	Hard Cider	
Clingfilm	Saran wrap	
Coriander	Cilantro	
Cornflour	Cornstarch	
Cos lettuce	Romaine lettuce	
Courgette	Zucchini or Summer Squash	
Crisps	Chips	
Cutlet	Chop	
French Beans	String Beans	
Frying Pan	Skillet	
Gammon	Ham	
Greaseproof Paper	Wax Paper/Parchment paper	
Green / Red Peppers	Bell Peppers	
Grill	Broiler	
Hull	Shuck	
Jam	Jelly	
Jelly	Jello	
Liquidiser	Blender	
Main Course	Entrée	
Mince	Ground	
Pastry case	Pie case	
Pie	Pot Pie	
Pint	Pint	*Though the names are the same, a pint in the UK is equivalent to 568 ml whereas in the US it is 473 ml.*
Plain flour	All purpose flour	
Porridge	Oatmeal, Cooked	
Pudding	Dessert	
Rocket	Arugula	
Self-raising flour	Self-rising flour	
Spirit	Liquor	
Spring Onions	Green Onions	
Swede	Rutabaga	*Also known as a yellow turnip and in Scotland these are called Neeps*
Sweet	Dessert	*Dessert is used in the UK too*
Tart	Pie	*In the UK pies have lids and are savoury,*
Tin Foil	Aluminum Foil	
Tinned	Canned	

Oven Temperatures

All oven temperatures are for fan assisted ovens. For non fan assisted ovens, we suggest you increase the temperature by 20 degrees or check the manufacturer's handbook, although cannot guarantee the results in the same way we can for fan assisted ovens. We also strongly recommend you use an oven thermometer at all times.

Conversions (UK/US)

Weights

Imperial	Metric
½ oz	10 g
¾ oz	20 g
1 oz	25 g
1½ oz	40 g
2 oz	50 g
2½ oz	60 g
3 oz	75 g
4 oz	110 g
4½ oz	125 g
5 oz	150 g
6 oz	175 g
7 oz	200 g
8 oz	225 g
9 oz	250 g
10 oz	275 g
12 oz	350 g
1 lb	450 g
1 lb 8 oz	700 g
2 lb	900 g
3 lb	1.35 kg

Volume

Imperial	Metric
2 fl oz	55 ml
3 fl oz	75 ml
5 fl oz (¼ pint)	150 ml
10 fl oz (½ pint)	275 ml
1 pint	570 ml
1¼ pint	725 ml
1¾ pint	1 litre
2 pint	1.2 litre
2½ pint	1.5 litre
4 pint	2.25 litres

Liquid Measurements

1 tsp	5 ml
1 tbsp	15 ml
⅛ cup	30 ml
¼ cup	60 ml
½ cup	120 ml
1 cup	240 ml

Oven Temperatures

Gas Mark	°F	°C
1	275°F	140°C
2	300°F	150°C
3	325°F	170°C
4	350°F	180°C
5	375°F	190°C
6	400°F	200°C
7	425°F	220°C
8	450°F	230°C
9	475°F	240°C

US Cup Conversions

US	Imperial	Metric
1 cup flour	5 oz	150 g
1 cup butter	8 oz	225 g
1 cup grated cheese	4 oz	110 g
1 stick butter	4 oz	110 g

General Guide

US	Imperial	Metric
¼ Cup	1½ oz	38 g
½ Cup	3 oz	75 g
⅔ Cup	4 oz	100 g
¾ Cup	4½ oz	113 g
1 Cup	6 oz	150 g

Glossary of Cooking Terms

This is a generalised list of the most common cooking terms (not necessarily used in this book).

Al Dente
Italian term used to describe pasta that is cooked until it offers a slight resistance to the bite. Can also apply to vegetables.

Bake
To cook by dry heat, usually in the oven.

Barbecue
Usually used generally to refer to grilling done outdoors or over an open charcoal or wood fire. More specifically, barbecue refers to long, slow direct- heat cooking, including liberal basting with a barbecue sauce.

Baste
To moisten foods during cooking with meat juices or a special sauce to add flavour and prevent drying.

Batter
A mixture containing flour and liquid, thin enough to pour.

Beat
To mix rapidly in order to make a mixture smooth and light by incorporating as much air as possible.

Blanch
To immerse in rapidly boiling water and allowing to cook slightly.

Blend
To incorporate two or more ingredients thoroughly.

Boil
To heat a liquid until bubbles break continually on the surface.

Broil
To cook on a grill under strong, direct heat.

Caramelise
To heat sugar in order to turn it brown and give it a special taste.

Chop
To cut solids into pieces with a sharp knife or other chopping device.

Clarify
To separate and remove solids from a liquid, thus making it clear.

Cream
To soften a fat, especially butter, by beating it at room temperature. Butter and sugar are often creamed together, making a smooth, soft paste.

Cure
To preserve meats by drying and salting and/or smoking.

Deglaze
To dissolve the thin glaze of juices and brown bits on the surface of a pan in which food has been fried, sautéed or roasted. To do this, add liquid and stir and scrape over high heat, thereby adding flavour to the liquid for use as a sauce.

Degrease
To remove fat from the surface of stews, soups, or stock. Usually cooled in the refrigerator so that fat hardens and is easily removed.

Dice
To cut food in small cubes of uniform size and shape.

Dissolve
To cause a dry substance to pass into solution in a liquid.

Dredge
To sprinkle or coat with flour or other fine substance.

Drizzle
To sprinkle drops of liquid lightly over food in a casual manner.

Dust
To sprinkle food with dry ingredients. Use a strainer or a jar with a perforated cover.

Fillet
As a verb, to remove the bones from meat or fish. A fillet (or filet) is the piece of flesh after it has been boned.

Glossary

Flake
To break lightly into small pieces.

Flambé
To flame foods by dousing in some form of potable alcohol and setting alight.

Fold
To incorporate a delicate substance, such as whipped cream or beaten egg whites, into another substance without releasing air bubbles. Cut through the mixture with a spoon, whisk, or fork; go across bottom of bowl, up and over, close to surface. The process is repeated, while slowing rotating the bowl, until the ingredients are thoroughly blended.

Fricassee
To cook by braising; usually applied to fowl or rabbit.

Fry
To cook in hot fat. To cook in a fat is called pan-frying or sautéing; to cook in a thin layer of hot fat is called shallow-fat frying; to cook in a deep layer of hot fat is called deep-fat frying.

Garnish
To decorate a dish both to enhance its appearance and to provide a flavoursome addition. Parsley, lemon slices, raw vegetables, chopped chives, and other herbs are all forms of garnishes.

Glaze
To cook with a thin sugar syrup cooked to crack stage; mixture may be thickened slightly. Also, to cover with a thin, glossy icing.

Grate
To rub on a grater that separates the food in various sizes of bits or shreds.

Gratin
From the French word for "crust." Term used to describe any oven-baked dish (usually cooked in a shallow oval gratin dish) on which a golden brown crust of bread crumbs, cheese or creamy sauce is formed.

Grill
To cook on a grill over intense heat.

Grind
To process solids by hand or mechanically to reduce them to tiny particles.

Julienne
To cut vegetables, fruits, or cheeses into thin strips.

Knead
To work and press dough with the palms of the hands or mechanically, to develop the gluten in the flour.

Liquidise
To puree in a blender or food processor.

Marinate
To flavour and moisturize pieces of meat, poultry, seafood or vegetable by soaking them in or brushing them with a liquid mixture of seasonings known as a marinade. Dry marinade mixtures composed of salt, pepper, herbs or spices may also be rubbed into meat, poultry or seafood.

Meuniere
Dredged with flour and sautéed in butter.

Mince
To cut or chop food into extremely small pieces.

Mix
To combine ingredients usually by stirring.

Pan-Broil
To cook uncovered in a hot frying pan, pouring off fat as it accumulates.

Pan-Fry
To cook in small amounts of fat.

Parboil
To boil until partially cooked; to blanch.

Pare
To remove the outermost skin of a fruit or vegetable.

Peel
To remove the peels from vegetables or fruits.

Pickle
To preserve meats, vegetables, and fruits in brine.

Pinch
A pinch is the very small amount you can hold between your thumb and forefinger.

Glossary

Pit
To remove pits from fruits.

Plump
To soak dried fruits in liquid until they swell.

Poach
To cook very gently in hot liquid kept just below the boiling point.

Puree
To mash foods until perfectly smooth by hand, by rubbing through a sieve or food mill, or by whirling in a blender or food processor.

Reduce
To boil down to reduce the volume by evaporation.

Refresh
To run cold water over food that has been parboiled, to stop the cooking process quickly.

Render
To make solid fat into liquid by melting it slowly.

Roast
To cook by dry heat in an oven.

Sauté
To cook and/or brown food in a small amount of hot fat.

Scald
To bring to a temperature just below the boiling point.

Scallop
To bake a food, usually in a casserole, with sauce or other liquid. **Crumbs often are sprinkled over.**

Score
To cut narrow grooves or gashes partway through the outer surface of food.

Sear
To brown very quickly by intense heat. This method increases shrinkage but develops flavour and improves appearance.

Shred
To cut or tear in small, long, narrow pieces.

Sift
To put one or more dry ingredients through a sieve or sifter.

Simmer
To cook slowly in liquid over low heat at a temperature of about 100°C (180°F). The surface of the liquid should be barely moving, broken from time to time by slowly rising bubbles.

Skim
To remove impurities, whether scum or fat, from the surface of a liquid during cooking, thereby resulting in a clear, cleaner-tasting final result.

Steam
To cook in steam in a pressure cooker, deep well cooker or a double boiler. A small amount of boiling water is used, more water being added during steaming process, if necessary.

Steep
To extract colour, flavour, or other qualities from a substance by leaving it in water just below the boiling point.

Sterilise
To destroy micro organisms by boiling with a dry heat, or with steam.

Stew
To simmer slowly in a small amount of liquid for a long time.

Stir
To mix ingredients with a circular motion until they are well blended or of uniform consistency.

Toss
To combine ingredients with a lifting motion, usually associated with salads.

Truss
To secure poultry with string or with skewers, so that it holds its shape while cooking.

Whip
To beat rapidly to incorporate air and produce expansion, as in heavy cream or egg whites.

Appendix I

THE DEMONIC ORIGIN OF COVID19

Please allow me to prove the demonic origin of COVID19 from the bible...

Simply put. The Crown of thorns put on Jesus' head, is a Corona of Spike proteins. It is COViD19. The soldiers braided/platted/double helixed/Gene spliced that crown. Then the soldiers spat upon Jesus. That is how COVID is transferred.

27 Then the soldiers of the governor [Demon possessed members of the US military, since the 1NC churches, the Watchtower and Laodicea, have their Head Quarters in the US] took Jesus into the governor's palace and gathered the whole body/coil together to him [all of the first new covenant saints finished being gather to him by baptism into the reappointed Laodicea, the 7th congregation of Revelation3].

28 And disrobing him [destroyed his priesthood], they draped him with a scarlet cloak [General's/Military cloak: Hiding his body - lockdown hiding?],

29 and they braided/plaited/double helixed [US military personnel gene spliced the COVID19 RNA from synthetic DNA, which is twisted, braided, plaited RNA in a double Helix, a molecular plait. Plaits/Braids are helical!] a crown out of thorns [2x. corona is a Latin feminine noun meaning crown. So a crown of spike proteins] and put it on his head [Jesus' head is the first new covenant (1NC) saints of the 3rd Holy Spirit. 1NC reserves on earth, are protected from COVID by Psalm91 and Genesis15. But they are not protected from the vaccines] and a reed in his right [hand] [a satanic reed, demon possessed people became the rulers of Laodicea and 1NC Zoar]. And, kneeling before him [They kneel before the Laodicean or 1NC Zoarite priest who represents Jesus], they made fun of him, saying: Good day, you King of the Jews! [Literally he was not. But in the end times fulfilment he is the secular King of the Jews. He is Caesar when the fulfilment occurs]

30 And they spit upon him [that is how Coronavirus (COVID19) is transferred. Demon possessed soldiers released it into the world targeting Jesus, the 1NCs] and took the reed and began hitting him upon his head [forcing the Coronavirus spike proteins into his head, the 1NC reserves - through the vaccine - using the demon possessed reed of the administration of 1NC Zoar. So there are demon possessed fake 1NCs in 1NC Zoar along with sealed married true 1NCs who have not yet been inducted into the 3rd Holy Spirit, but are still on the substitute bench. There is a Judas class that is known to Jesus but not removed from the congregation].

31 Finally, when they had made fun of him, they took the cloak off and put his outer garments upon him and led him off for impaling/crucifixion *(Matthew 27 NWT)*

For those who are interested, our latest decoded bible interpretations are on www.truebiblecode.com. Our chronology although very detailed has been wrong over 700 times. But as of 2021May8, we believe it is now good enough, whereas our doctrine is and always has been wonderful and is a major advance in love over standard Christianity.

Regrettably the light of our church, the Lords Witnesses, has always been hidden under the measuring basket of our historically inaccurate chronology. But the light is still shining in the darkness and the darkness has not overpowered it.

So this was the project that deflected me from building the Quadrocopter drone. I did not want to give my drone to mankind. I thought it would be used for genocide. And that is one prophecy I made in 1990 that looks like being correct. Today in 2021, Drone swarms are the latest military technology. They are widely used for extra judicial killings.

www.ingramcontent.com/pod-product-compliance
Lightning Source LLC
Chambersburg PA
CBHW081428220526
45466CB00008B/2303